Building Trust in Veterinary Practice

Building Trust in Veterinary Practice

Ryan Barba, MBA

WILEY

Published by John Wiley & Sons, Inc., Hoboken, New Jersey.

For general information on our other products and services or for technical support, please contact our Customer Care Department within the United States at (800) 762-2974, outside the United States at (317) 572-3993 or fax (317) 572-4002.

Wiley also publishes its books in a variety of electronic formats. Some content that appears in print may not be available in electronic formats. For more information about Wiley products, visit our web site at www.wiley.com.

Library of Congress Cataloging-in-Publication Data:

Names: Barba, Ryan author
Title: Building trust in veterinary practice / Ryan Barba.
Description: Hoboken, New Jersey : Wiley, [2026] | Includes index.
Identifiers: LCCN 2026009765 | ISBN 9781394424238 paperback | ISBN
  9781394424252 adobe pdf | ISBN 9781394424245 epub | ISBN 9781394424269
Subjects: LCSH: Veterinary care teams | Leadership
Classification: LCC SF604.5 .B37 2026
LC record available at https://lccn.loc.gov/2026009765

Cover Design: Wiley
Cover Images: © Prasert Krainukul/Getty Images, Grace Maina/Getty Images, OLIVEIA/stock.adobe.com, anuwat/stock.adobe.com
Printed and bound by CPI Group (UK) Ltd, Croydon, CR0 4YY

C9781394424238_150526

For the leaders and mentors who believed in me when I needed it most: Robert Blaney, Robert Best, Brendan Lynch, Steven Theroux, Kimberly and Christian Petrucci, Louis Ventura, and Nicholas Uva.

And for Buddy.

Table of Contents

Foreword

A Blueprint for the Next Era of Veterinary Medicine

The history of companion animal veterinary medicine is one of relentless scientific progress and profound compassion. In the span of a single human generation, we have moved from a profession primarily focused on farm animals and infectious disease control to one defined by advanced specialty care, sophisticated diagnostics, and—most importantly—the emotional depth of the human–animal bond. Our pets are no longer property; they are family. They are our confidants, our comfort, and often, the silent anchors in our increasingly turbulent lives.

Yet, for a profession built on such a beautiful, vital foundation, the present moment is marked by a deep and pervasive tension. We are living through an unprecedented golden age of clinical capability, yet the system designed to deliver this care is buckling under its own weight.

This tension—between the impeccable standard of care we are trained to provide and the unsustainable operational and emotional environment we must work within—is the critical gap this book courageously seeks to bridge.

The Unspoken Crisis of the Golden Age

To understand the immense importance of the concepts contained within these pages, we must first clearly define the crisis. It is not merely a staffing shortage or a cyclical downturn; it is a fundamental Crisis of Trust, as Chapter 1 so accurately names it, that threatens the very sustainability of the profession we cherish.

The challenges are multifaceted and interlocking. Inside the clinic, teams struggle with soaring rates of burnout and moral injury. These compassionate professionals—driven by an innate desire to heal—are systematically fractured by the gap between the care they know is possible and the care they are forced to deliver due to financial constraints, time limits, and the sheer volume of demand. This pressure cooker environment erodes mental health, drives high turnover, and ultimately diminishes the quality of interaction with the client. It is a slow, silent attrition of the soul, and its consequences ripple outward into every consultation room.

Simultaneously, the client landscape has changed dramatically. The pet owner of today is more informed, more invested, and more financially committed than ever before. But this deeper bond also comes with deeper vulnerability and higher expectations. When clients arrive at the hospital, they are often terrified, stressed, and emotionally drained. When faced with the Money Problem—the unavoidable truth of rising healthcare costs—they often interpret the necessary financial conversation not as an objective discussion of advanced medical options, but as a moral judgment or a betrayal of trust.

The heartbreaking reality is that clinical excellence alone can no longer guarantee practice success or professional well-being. A complex surgery performed flawlessly can still be overshadowed by a rushed check-in, an indifferent tone, or a confusing invoice. The moment the client feels unheard, unseen, or judged, the entire relationship—and the ability to deliver care—is compromised. The veterinary world has focused intensely on advancing the science of medicine, but it has critically underestimated the necessity of perfecting the delivery of that medicine. This book is the indispensable guide to perfecting that delivery.

Redefining Excellence: From Transaction to Trust

The core imperative of this work is to move the industry past a transactional model—where success is measured solely by revenue and throughput—into a relationship-centric model where success is measured by Trust and Experience. This is not a soft concept; it is the hardest, most economically vital strategy for longevity.

The authors astutely recognize that the solutions cannot be found by simply working harder or pushing teams further. The change must be systemic, starting with the internal ecosystem of the hospital, captured perfectly in the mantra that Culture Drives Tactics (Chapter 2). You cannot sustainably deliver world-class Client Experience (CX) if your team is operating in a state of psychological jeopardy. Empathy must be modeled and reinforced from the top down, first within the four walls of the practice, before it can be reliably extended to the waiting room.

The chapters dedicated to articulating What Pet-Owner Clients Want (Chapter 16) are revelatory in their simplicity and actionable in their specificity. The clients' desired feelings—to feel Valued/Appreciated, Known, Competently Supported, Partnered, and Affirmed—are the emotional currency of the modern practice. These desires are not extraneous demands; they are the fundamental conditions under which the client will consent to and invest in the high-level medical care their pets require. They are the prerequisites for compliance and the bedrock of retention.

This book provides the blueprint for designing a veterinary journey that intentionally generates these feelings. It is a wake-up call that every interaction—from the first call to the final farewell—is a critical touchpoint. Are we designing a system that makes clients feel known, or one that treats them like a number? Are we designing conversations that foster Partnership and inclusion, or ones that inadvertently communicate, "Trust us, pay the bill, and don't ask questions"? The answers to these questions determine the future solvency and sanity of every practice.

The Engine of Sustainability: The Veterinary Trust Flywheel

The true genius of this text lies in its presentation of the Veterinary Trust Flywheel (Part 2 of this book). This concept is not a quick fix or a linear process; it is a self-reinforcing system—an engine—designed to generate continuous, exponential momentum. It recognizes that the health of the organization is a holistic equation where internal welfare directly powers external success.

The Flywheel begins by confronting an undeniable truth: fair pay isn't optional. It's the floor. (Truth #1). This is a moral and economic necessity. A team stressed by financial instability cannot provide the focused, empathetic care required for premium CX. By establishing fair compensation and a foundation of financial well-being, the practice invests in the stability of its people, which immediately frees up their emotional capacity to engage the next element: Competency and Training.

The Flywheel demands a commitment to continuous professional development, ensuring that every team member—from the receptionist to the DVM—is equipped with not only the technical skills but, crucially, the communication and emotional intelligence required for high-stakes interactions. Competency builds confidence, and confidence is the fuel for the next crucial spoke: Empathy and Psychological Safety.

This book insists on a brave shift in leadership to foster a culture where team members feel psychologically safe to ask for help, voice concerns, and receive constructive coaching rather than criticism. This internal empathy is what allows the team to deliver genuine, unforced Empathy to the client, leading to the final spoke: Partnership. This is the ultimate goal—the collaborative relationship where the client is Heard and Included, feeling like an active, respected participant in their pet's care journey.

When this partnership is achieved, it directly generates Trust. Trust reduces conflict, increases client compliance and retention, and ultimately leads to greater business sustainability. This stability then allows the practice to reinvest in its team (the "Fair Pay" starting point), thus increasing the velocity and power of the Flywheel. This is the path out of the perpetual crisis cycle. This is the self-sustaining model for prosperity.

The Mandate for Courageous Leadership

To the veterinary leaders, managers, and practice owners who pick up this book, understand that this is not a manual for incremental improvement; it is a mandate for philosophical change. It asks you to stop viewing your team as a disposable resource and your clients as a necessary transaction, and instead to see both as the indispensable, relational assets they are.

Implementing the concepts outlined here will require courageous leadership. It demands that you:

1. Look Inward: Honestly assess the internal culture, acknowledging the Leadership Gap and accountability deficits that contribute to staff stress.

2. Invest Upfront: Recognize that investing in fair wages and high-quality communication training is not a cost, but a strategic investment with a measurable return on retention and CX.
3. Design, Don't Default: Shift from reacting to problems (angry clients, staff quitting) to proactively designing systems and touchpoints that are engineered to build trust and prevent crisis.

This book is a challenging read because it asks the veterinary profession to hold itself to a higher, more holistic standard—one that honors the business of providing care just as much as the science of providing care. It is a comprehensive roadmap for transforming the industry's default operating system.

The Future Awaits

The stakes could not be higher. If the veterinary profession continues on its current trajectory, driven by scarcity, burnout, and transactional interactions, it risks permanently fracturing the relationship with the very public it exists to serve. The result will be a diminished workforce, limited access to care, and a tragic decline in the health and welfare of companion animals.

However, the vision painted by this book is one of hope, prosperity, and enduring purpose. It is a vision where veterinary professionals are emotionally and financially sustained by the work they love. It is a vision where pet owners feel Partnership and Trust, allowing them to wholeheartedly pursue the best possible medical outcomes for their beloved family members.

With that in mind, keep in mind the following THREE ASSUMPTIONS that I present to audiences of friends, colleagues, veterinary team members, industry supporters, and anyone that will listen to me—whether by choice or by chance.

Assumption Number ONE—Companion Animal veterinary practices should consider themselves as a service industry provider FIRST and a healthcare provider SECOND.

Assumption Number TWO—We can't deliver healthcare, let alone service by ourselves. Veterinary medicine is a team sport, and we need a team to meet the needs and expectations of our clients and patients.

Assumption Number THREE—The ultimate determinant if numbers one and two are part of a practice vision, mission, and values is the leadership. If the leadership IS NOT fully committed to the above assumptions; they will not have the support needed to be successful. Leadership sets the tone.

This book is the essential tool for any leader who is tired of the struggle and ready to build a legacy of health, happiness, and true sustainability. It is a blueprint for the future. It is time to stop reacting to the crisis and start building the architecture of trust. Read it, embrace its principles, and become the architect of a better veterinary world.

Peter Weinstein, DVM, MBA
October 2025
PAW Consulting
Veterinary Ownership Advocates (www.voa.vet)
Simple Solutions for Vets (www.ss4v.vet)

Acknowledgments

This book came from real people, real struggle, real leadership, and real care.

To my family—you carried me when the load got heavy. I don't take that lightly.

To the CSRs, technicians, doctors, managers, and leaders who trusted me with their raw truths—you're the heartbeat of this profession. Every chapter of this book carries your fingerprints.

To the mentors and leaders who raised my standards and reshaped the way I think about leadership and service—this book exists because of your influence.

To the hospital teams who opened their doors and let me see the real work—the wins, the struggles, and the growth in motion—thank you for trusting me with your truth. This book was forged alongside you.

And to the reader—if you picked this up because you care about trust, culture, and doing right by people and pets—welcome. You're my people.

Part 1

Introduction

Introduction

Customer experience (or, CX) has been my obsession for years. And let me tell you something: it's not a buzzword, and it's not a "soft skill." It's often the difference between businesses that thrive and businesses that fade into irrelevance. I've spent my career teaching leaders how to blow past mediocrity, how to stop treating their customers like transactions, and how to deliver experiences that make people stop in their tracks and say, "Wow, these guys actually give a shit."

I cut my teeth helping big industries—banks, retailers, and consumer product companies—craft customer experience strategies as a CX consultant. And sure, it was fun. But helping rich banks chase richer clients so they could get even richer? That didn't light me up inside.

Then I found veterinary medicine, and everything changed.

Veterinary medicine is special. It's unique. When you're in this profession, you're not just "running a business." You're helping people make some of the most important decisions of their lives about the creatures they love most. You're giving families more time with their best friend. You're reducing suffering. You're extending joy. You're creating moments that people will never, ever forget. That's not business-as-usual—that's legacy work. And I felt it from the moment I worked with my first veterinary client as a CX consultant.

I've been lucky enough to live it from every angle: as a consultant, as the head of Client Experience and Innovation Strategy at VCA Animal Hospitals, and now as the VP of Business Development for Mission Pet Health, helping hospital owners plan for their and their hospital's future. In my almost 10 years in the industry, I've toured more than 600 hospitals. I've sat in on countless staff meetings. I've watched maybe 100 surgeries. I've listened to clients in the waiting room. And I'll tell you this: the hospitals that crush it—the ones with strong finances, happy teams, and pets that live healthier, longer lives—aren't the ones with marble countertops or the newest MRI machine.

They're the ones who *own* and *prioritize* client experience. They're obsessed with making pet owners feel seen, heard, valued, and cared for. They understand the most important truth about client experience in veterinary medicine: it's not about "making people happy" or simply "creating joy." It's about earning trust.

Because when clients trust you, they follow your advice. They don't ghost you on follow-ups. They don't nickel-and-dime you on price. They don't ignore your care plans. And that means healthier pets, more fulfilled hospital teams, and better business outcomes. Trust is the fuel that powers everything.

Why I Care So Damn Much

This isn't just theory for me. It's personal.

A Norfolk terrier named Buddy was my best friend for 15 years. He was with me through grad school, through almost a decade of life as a professional business consultant, through a cross-country move, through romantic breakups, through career highs and lows ... you name it. Buddy wasn't just a dog to me. He was family. He was my anchor. He passed peacefully in 2023, but he will forever be a part of me.

It was an experience with my Buddy that gave me such a deep appreciation for the veterinary industry—the industry that would later become my home.

The summer of 2011 began with a bang—specifically, the clunk, whirr, and final sputter of my car breaking down 18 miles from my destination: a subleased apartment in University City, Philadelphia. I had attempted the 229-mile drive from Ithaca, New York, with Buddy riding shotgun, excited (or more likely indifferent) about our temporary relocation. I was starting a summer internship at Johnson & Johnson as part of my MBA program at Cornell. I thought I was entering a big, new chapter in my professional life, but I arrived in Philadelphia in the back of a tow truck.

To make matters worse, for reasons I'll never understand, my AAA coverage only allowed my car to be towed to my final destination, not to a repair shop. So, there it sat, immobile, outside my summer apartment like a sad monument to broken dreams. Within *four minutes* of arriving (I'm not kidding), Philadelphia welcomed me with a hefty parking ticket. I pleaded with the officer, explaining that the car couldn't move. He gave me a look that screamed, "Not my problem," slapped the ticket on the windshield, and walked away. I had been in the city for less than 10 minutes and already owed it money.

That summer was a slow-motion train wreck: sweltering heat, a high-stress job, a failed mugging attempt on the subway, the successful burglary of my kitchen supplies by a cleaning crew I had hired, and—far and away the worst—Buddy's medical emergency.

I had left Philly for a quick weekend visit home to Boston, and while I was away, I left Buddy with a local dog walker I had been using that summer. She had a dog of her own named Max. The day I returned, she sent me a text I'll never forget:

"Max attacked Buddy. He'll be fine."

And that was it.

I returned to my Philly apartment to find Buddy lying on my bedroom floor, bleeding. He had a deep gash near his eye and another on his stomach. I didn't know how long he had been there, but the sight of him—barely conscious, his little body soaking the carpet with blood—shook me in a way I can still feel today. I dropped my bags, knelt beside him, and panicked. I was filled with guilt and fear and helplessness. I thought he might die right there.

The only thing that saved him was geography. Just five blocks away was Ryan Veterinary Hospital at the University of Pennsylvania. I scooped Buddy into my arms and ran. Full sprint. The kind of running you do when adrenaline kicks in and nothing else matters.

I burst through the hospital doors and was immediately met by Dr. Evelyn, a veterinarian I will never forget. She took one look at Buddy, grabbed him from my arms, and literally ran toward the surgical suite. As she disappeared down the hallway, she yelled over her shoulder, "We've got Buddy! We're going to do all we can, Ryan! He's going to be OK!"

It was the first moment I'd heard anyone say he might be OK. And even though I was still terrified, those words mattered.

While I waited, Carla, one of the client service representatives, sat with me in the lobby. She didn't try to rush my emotions or give me platitudes. She just *sat* with me. She reassured me that I had done the right thing bringing Buddy in so quickly. She told me it wasn't my fault and that I couldn't have seen this coming. I remember her kindness, her calm, and (somehow) even her humor. I don't recall the exact jokes, but I remember her making me laugh through my tears. It felt like a lifeline.

Eventually, Dr. Evelyn returned with the news: Buddy had made it through surgery. He was going to be OK. I hugged her, overwhelmed with gratitude and relief, only to pull back and see I had left a giant wet patch of tears on her shoulder. She smiled and said, "Hey, I'll take happy tears on my scrubs any day."

I don't remember how long the surgery took. I don't remember how much it cost. But I remember *them*: Dr. Evelyn and Carla. I remember the way they made me feel in one of the scariest moments of my life. I remember that they saved my Buddy.

(By the way, I'll also always remember that betrayal from the dog sitter, who blocked my number and disappeared. I've forgiven a lot of people in my life—I try to live by grace and second chances. But honestly? She's not on that list.)

That night at Ryan Veterinary Hospital opened my eyes to what it means, and what it takes, to work in veterinary medicine: not just clinical expertise, but the compassion, the humanity, and the instinct to meet fear with reassurance and pain with presence. The instinct to be strong for others when they're at their weakest and most vulnerable.

That experience would later inspire me to join the veterinary industry myself—to dedicate my life to empowering hospital teams like the ones that had once taken care of me and my best friend.

Maybe by some miracle, someone from Ryan Veterinary Hospital will read this. If so, thank you. I mean it with my whole heart. I'm sure you don't remember me—you see distraught clients and medical emergencies every day—but I'll always remember you and the miracle you performed that day. You saved Buddy—and me—that day, and you'll forever own a grateful place in my heart.

And that is what's so special about working in veterinary medicine, isn't it? The work that our teams do every day, the work that so often feels routine and "normal" and regular, can feel anything but routine and normal to our clients. What a special gift we have to be changing lives by the hundreds and creating memories that last a lifetime for our clients every single day. Clients that we may not see or even think about again, or clients that we don't remember from years and years ago—many of them still remember and think about us and the work that we do for them (especially if we do it well). It's amazing to think about. What a privilege.

And damn, what a heavy responsibility that is, too.

The hospital team at Ryan Veterinary Hospital, and the hundreds of animal hospital teams I've had the privilege to know, coach, and advise over the years, have consistently proven to me and reminded me of what I already believed: veterinarians and hospital teams are heroes. Full stop.

That's why I do this work. Every day I wake up and whisper, *"This is for you, Buddy."* He's my why. My fuel. And when things get hard—and let's be real, this work is hard—he's what keeps me going.

Why This Book Matters Now

Right now, as I write this in 2026, our industry is under pressure. Inflation, recession fears, pet owners cutting back. Consolidators and independents alike are scrambling for demand, too often chasing gimmicks that rarely work.

Here's the inconvenient truth nobody wants to admit: marketing tricks can't save you. Yelp stars won't save you. A shiny new building won't save you. The only thing that will? Delighting the shit out of your clients. Blowing them away with compassion, trust, and care. Turning them into raving fans who can't shut up about you.

That's the opportunity. That's how you win. That's how you future-proof your hospital.

This book is my playbook for doing exactly that. It's built on thousands of conversations with clients, teams, and leaders. It's fueled by data, stories, heartbreak, and triumph. And it's written with one goal: to help you build a hospital where clients trust you, teams love working for you, and pets live longer, healthier lives.

What really inspires me to get out of bed every day and work in this industry has also motivated me to write this book, and that's my deep conviction that we can do better, as an industry overall, in supporting our teams and our clients. There is so much opportunity and so many simple practices that, if we would just embrace them, would drive enormous benefits to our teams, our clients, our patients, and our hospitals. And if even one page of this book helps even one hospital up their game, creates a healthier culture that brings joy to their teams, creates more trust and delight for their clients, or gives one more pet a little better care, then it's worth every hour I've poured into this.

To every hospital team that has let me in, and to the heroes who cared for Buddy, this book is for you. You'll never fully know the impact you've had. But I promise you this: it's immeasurable, and it matters a whole damn lot.

The Science Behind the Veterinary Trust Flywheel

The ideas in this book aren't theory. They're not fluffy guesses or wild hunches from some random guy who likes pets. They're built from years in the trenches, testing, failing, learning, and proving what actually moves the needle in veterinary hospitals.

I've been obsessed with this work for over a decade. I've poured thousands of hours into studying what makes hospital teams tick and what makes pet owners trust, or walk away. I've sat in lobbies, exam rooms, treatment areas, ERs, and specialty hospitals in 49 states (Alaska, I'm coming for you). I've shadowed countless client interactions and poured over millions—literally millions—of surveys and online reviews from pet owners. I've run nearly 100 focus groups with clients, and dozens more with

CSRs, techs, assistants, doctors, hospital managers, and regional leaders, to understand what they need, where they struggle, and what lights them up.

For over six years at VCA Animal Hospitals, I had the privilege—and the pressure—of leading client experience strategy for over 1,000 hospitals across the country. We drove our net promoter score (NPS) up more than 13 points nationwide. I built five brand-new programs from the ground up: VCA's call center, telehealth, telemedicine, virtual scribe, and review management programs. Those weren't side projects; they became core engines because we built them around what hospitals and pet owners actually needed, not what looked good in a slide deck.

And to be clear: I didn't do it alone. One of my biggest wins was hiring and empowering incredible leaders who taught me every day what resilience in the veterinary industry looks like. I trusted them, I advocated for them, I fought for their growth. We had bumps, and we had ugly days, but we built cultures where people knew they mattered and where they could thrive. That's why the programs stuck. That's why the results lasted.

Since leaving VCA in 2025, I've doubled down on working directly with hospital owners and leaders planning their futures at Mission Pet Health. And if there's one thing I can tell you: every day I'm reminded that this industry is filled with some of the most passionate, talented, good-hearted humans on earth. Doctors, techs, managers—these people would bleed for their teams, their clients, and their patients. Getting to partner with them humbles me daily and fuels my fire even more.

I'm not rattling all this off to brag. I'm telling you because you need to know I'm not bullshitting you. I know my shit. My experience in fixing broken cultures and building healthy new ones, scaling hospitals, advancing CX, earning client trust, innovating new programs, and helping hospitals grow financially is real. This book is the culmination of that work—every lesson, every scar, every breakthrough—written for you: the hospital leaders and teams battling in the arena every day.

I wrote this because I believe in you. Because I believe CX isn't optional—it's necessary for survival. And because if you apply what's in these pages, your hospital won't just grow, it'll thrive.

And if all that still sounds too business-y, let me ground it for you. None of this is abstract for me. I've been on the other side of that exam table, scared out of my mind for my own dog, Buddy. I know what it feels like to sit in a lobby praying for good news, to hang on to every word from a doctor, and to put my trust—and my heart— in a hospital team. That's why this work matters. That's why I'm obsessed. Because for every Buddy out there, and every family who loves them, client experience isn't some fluffy metric. It's the difference between fear and trust, between despair and hope. That's why I wrote this book.

Who This Book Is For

When I first sat down to outline this book, I thought I was writing it for hospital owners and practice managers. The people who sign the checks, set the schedules, and carry the weight of the P&L. And yes, if that's you, this book is absolutely written with you in mind.

But here's what I've learned after years in this industry: leadership doesn't come with a title. It comes with mindset. It comes with hunger. It comes with the willingness to raise your hand and say, "We can do better."

I've seen CSRs at the front desk become the heartbeat of an entire hospital. I've seen techs lead culture shifts that managers couldn't. I've seen associates step up and inspire their teams just by the way they carried themselves in exam rooms. And I've seen hospitals change because one person—one voice—decided they weren't OK with "good enough."

So, let me be crystal clear: this book is for anyone in veterinary medicine who gives a damn. Anyone who wants to take the initiative to champion a healthy hospital culture. Anyone who wants to make client experiences not just transactional, but trust-building. Anyone who wants to improve patient outcomes, elevate the team, and grow a hospital that doesn't just survive, but thrives.

I don't care if you're an owner, a manager, a doctor, a tech, a CSR, or the brand-new assistant learning how to hold your first patient. If you've got the ambition and the drive, you can lead. You can spark change. You can make a difference.

This book is your playbook.

Chapter 1
A Crisis of Trust

Something's breaking in veterinary medicine. You can feel it.

It's in the tension at the front desk when a client argues about a bill.
It's in the rushed explanation of rising costs that doesn't land right.
It's in the burnout hiding behind a tech's forced smile.
It's in the heavy silence of a team huddled up after another brutal day.

At its core, this is about one thing: trust.

Trust between clients and hospital teams. Trust between teams and their leaders. Trust in the profession as a whole.

And the scary part? The trust that used to be the bedrock of veterinary care? It's eroding. Fast. Clients can feel it. Teams can feel it. Everyone can.

The New Client Reality

Today's pet owners are not the same as they were 10—or even 5—years ago. They're more informed, more emotionally invested, and more outspoken. They're Googling symptoms, watching vet influencers on TikTok, and treating their pets as full-blown family members.

U.S. pet ownership now spans more than 65% of households, and annual pet industry spending exceeded $150 billion in 2024 alone—with veterinary care accounting for nearly $40 billion of that total.

Their expectations are sky-high. They want collaboration. They want transparency. They want to feel like partners in their pet's care, not passive bystanders. And when those expectations aren't met, trust breaks.

And here's the kicker: broken trust doesn't just fade quietly. It explodes—through nasty online reviews, angry voicemails, and stories they retell at dinner parties about "that terrible vet visit."

The Money Problem

Then there's the elephant in the room: costs.

Veterinary care costs are climbing, especially post-pandemic. Pet owners are spending more than ever before, but many feel like their friendly neighborhood clinic has turned into a business first, care team second.

Over the past two decades, the cost of veterinary care has risen more than 60% faster than general inflation. Today, the average routine vet visit now runs roughly $214 for a dog and $138 for a cat—before diagnostics, medications, or procedures are added.

And it's not always about the number on the bill—it's the surprise of the bill. Clients feel blindsided, confused about line items, and frustrated by quotes that weren't fully explained. The American Pet Products Association reports that pet care spending is at an all-time high, but most clients still say they don't understand what they're paying for. That's a recipe for suspicion, resentment, and eventually withdrawal.

In recent national surveys, more than HALF of U.S. pet owners report they have skipped or delayed veterinary care due to cost in the past year alone.

When trust is shaky and bills are high, the emotional math stops adding up.

The Pressure Cooker Inside Hospitals

You want to know what trust erosion *actually* looks like? It's not some giant PR crisis. It's a Tuesday morning at Haven Veterinary Hospital.

Amanda is at the front desk, juggling three ringing lines and a client who showed up 10 minutes late but still expects to be seen "right now." Her eyes are darting between the phones, the clipboard, and the lobby door that just opened again. On call three, a woman named Kelly launches in, voice already hot:

"I requested Rufus's refill three days ago and nobody called me back!"

Amanda stiffens. She *knows* that refill was approved yesterday, but she can't find the note in the system. Kelly keeps talking, faster, louder.

Meanwhile, a tech walks by and mutters, "Here we go again," under her breath. Everyone hears it. Amanda's face turns red. She promises to "look into it," hangs up, and exhales hard.

Now pause that moment. No one died. No one cursed. But trust *just cracked*.

Kelly hung up thinking the clinic doesn't care. Amanda walked away thinking her team doesn't have her back. The doctor down the hall just heard the tension and silently added "another fire" to his list of reasons he's exhausted.

That's how trust erodes—drip, drip, drip. Not in the big blowups, but in the micro-misses that pile up.

If you want to rebuild trust, start here: fix the small breaks. Simplify the damn refill process. Give Amanda a system that actually supports her. Because no amount of marketing will save you if your team can't deliver the basics with empathy and consistency.

Inside too many hospitals, things are falling apart. Teams are being squeezed to fit in more (and often shorter) appointments, often while understaffed. Teams are thereby slammed and often feel like they're ill-equipped with the time and resources they need to practice quality medicine. Morale tanks.

Veterinary visit frequency has dropped in recent years, while the time between visits has increased by nearly 50%. At the exact same moment demand is rising, staffing levels are collapsing.

As a result, details and follow-ups get missed. Empathy fades when you're four patients behind and two team members called out. Communication becomes transactional. Comfort goes out the window. Clients expect more, but the experience is often worse.

For clients, that leads to disappointment.
For teams, it leads to exhaustion.
For everyone, it leads to the slow erosion of goodwill.

It's Not Because We Don't Care

Here's the part that hurts: it's not because our people don't care. If my 10+ years in the veterinary industry have taught me anything, it's this: our industry does a fantastic job of attracting well-intentioned people and leaders who authentically want to do good in the world—for both animals and their owners. What our industry doesn't tend to do very well is equip our teams and leaders with the necessary support they need to act on those genuine intentions effectively. But here's the blunt truth: good intentions aren't enough if the system doesn't support them. And right now, the system is failing.

As a result, our teams are quietly falling apart inside: between 30 and 40% of veterinarians report high levels of burnout. Average staff turnover in veterinary hospitals now runs between 15 and 20% annually—nearly double what is considered "healthy." The estimated annual cost of burnout to the veterinary industry? About $2 billion per year.

Our teams are overwhelmed, overworked, and underappreciated. They're told to do more with less: squeeze in one more patient, calm one more angry client, and deliver compassion at record speed with fewer resources. They're absorbing the emotional weight of an industry under stress, and it's crushing them. Burnout is rampant. Turnover is brutal. Mental health struggles are everywhere. And this is happening even though the teams showing up every day are doing it with the most genuine intentions. Nothing frustrates or saddens me more than seeing an animal hospital team struggling with overwhelm or seeing their intentions questioned by frustrated clients yelling at them in a crowded lobby ... When behind the scenes those team members get out of bed, every morning, simply trying to do as much good as possible for animals and their owners, often at great personal sacrifice.

The Training Gap

Another part of the problem? Training. Or more accurately, the lack of it.

Too many hospital teams are thrown straight into the fire without any real education on how to manage client experiences (CXs): how to build trust, communicate about costs, or show empathy when emotions run high.

The vast majority of veterinary professionals report receiving little to no formal training on conflict resolution, emotional intelligence, or client communication before being placed in high-stress client-facing roles.

And yet, the reality in our industry is that client trust is decreasing. Too often, both clients and teams feel like the other side just doesn't care about or understand them. They feel unseen, unheard, and unappreciated. They speak seemingly different languages and too often assume the worst of each other.

The Accountability Problem

Right now, CX—client experience—isn't treated as a core priority. It's treated as extra credit. Something you'll get to if there's time. And because CX and client-team trust building isn't always treated as a core function or hospital priority, there's often no accountability for it. "It's not my job," some say. "I have more urgent things to worry about." And in many ways, they're right: it feels like a luxury. But in reality, it's the foundation.

When teams are depleted, they can't go above and beyond. Clients feel that detachment. They leave disappointed, or angry. They complain. That complaint lands on the front desk or on a technician already running on fumes. And the cycle begins again: clients are unhappy, so teams grow defensive, and empathy fades.

"I hate people. I love animals." You hear that phrase more often now in our industry. But let's be real: that's not hate. It's grief. It's exhaustion borne from increasingly stressful interactions with clients. Or it's a coping mechanism, stemming from compassion fatigue. But behind it is often grief: grief over what this work used to feel like and what it's becoming.

The Leadership Gap

Behind it all is another issue: leadership.

It's not that our leaders don't care. They do! But most haven't been equipped with the right tools. CX is treated like fire control instead of fire prevention. A way to put out complaints, not a strategy to build trust.

Most leaders in hospitals were never trained on how to build joyful, inclusive cultures. Or how to train teams on communication and empathy. Or how to retain talent and inspire pride in the work and in the hospital's mission. They're doing the best they can with what they have, but what they have isn't enough.

And the ripple effects are massive. Clients come less often. Pets miss treatment. Word-of-mouth dries up. Staff churn accelerates. Revenue dips, prices rise, and clients get angrier. The cycle keeps spinning.

Here's the Good News

I don't believe it has to stay this way. I've seen hospitals turn things around. I've watched leaders embrace real strategies—not band-aids—and rebuild trust within their teams and between staff and clients, from the ground up.

I'm not going to sell you some magic "cure all" for everything wrong in veterinary medicine. That doesn't exist. But I can tell you this: the systems, strategies, and exercises in this book *work*. They've improved team morale and retention. They've increased client trust. They've boosted hospital performance. They've led to better pet outcomes.

And none of that is coincidence. It's all connected.

This book isn't about quick fixes. It's not about posters on the wall or chocolate chip cookies in the break room. It's about equipping leaders, at every level, to rebuild trust. To create places where clients and teams feel safe, seen, and valued.

Where We're Headed

So, here's our road map.

We're going to start by first describing what NOT to do: jumping straight to CX training and forcing tactics or behaviors on your team without first establishing a foundation and clear "why."

Then I'll show you the Veterinary Trust Flywheel—a model that proves how successful CX strategy starts with a focus on your team's culture, clarity, and safety and how a better team experience drives better CX, better team retention, and better outcomes, all of which drive better financial health for your hospital.

Then we'll get tactical. We'll talk about what pet owners really want from you and your team. Then, I'll outline a six-step process you can put into play in your hospital tomorrow. We'll talk leadership. Then, we'll talk about CX strategies and practices that actually work for clients, based on their deepest needs and expectations of your hospital team. We'll talk specific roles—doctors, techs, and Client Service Representatives (CSRs). We'll even talk about how to repair trust in complex environments like specialty hospitals.

And because I don't believe in fluff, I've loaded the appendix with practical tools and guides you can actually use. Not theory. Not slogans. Tools.

This isn't just a book. It's an invitation.

To lead.
To care.
To rebuild trust.
To create a hospital where both your team and your clients *want* to be.

Buckle up.

Summary

Without trust, veterinary medicine breaks. With it, everything thrives. Let's set this profession back in motion.

Veterinary medicine is in a trust crisis. You feel it at the front desk when a client blows up over a bill. You see it in your tech's eyes when burnout hides behind a forced smile. You hear it in the silence of a team that's just been through another exhausting day. At the root of it all? Trust is breaking.

And here's the blunt truth: without trust, nothing works. Not your medicine, not your client relationships, not your business. Trust is the oxygen of this profession. And right now, too many hospitals are suffocating.

But here's the part that should fire you up: this is fixable. The good news is that trust isn't some mystical unicorn we can't define. It's practical. It's learnable. And it can be rebuilt. I've seen it happen. Hospitals that were falling apart have turned the ship around by committing to trust as their core strategy.

That's what this book is about. Not Band-Aids. Not gimmicks. Real, repeatable systems that give your people the support they deserve, your clients the experience they crave, and your business the momentum it needs to thrive.

Later in this book, I'm going to hand you the blueprint: the Veterinary Trust Flywheel. It's the engine that shows exactly how investing in your team sets off a chain reaction: better CXs, better medicine, stronger business results, and reinvestment right back into your people. Push after push, the wheel starts spinning. And once it's spinning? Good luck stopping it.

So, buckle up. Chapter 2 is where we start turning the wheel.

Suggested Readings

American Animal Hospital Association (AAHA). *Cost of Care Cited as Primary Reason Pet Owners Skip Veterinary Visits.* 2025, https://www.aaha.org/trends-magazine/publications/labby-digs-into-the-data-cost-of-care-cited-as-reason-pet-owners-skip-vet-visits/

American Animal Hospital Association (AAHA). *There's a Disconnect When it Comes to the Lifetime Cost of Pet Care.* 2024, https://www.aaha.org/trends-magazine/publications/theres-a-disconnect-when-it-comes-to-the-lifetime-cost-of-pet-care/

American Pet Products Association (APPA). *U.S. Pet Industry Market Size & Ownership Statistics.* 2024, https://www.americanpetproducts.org/industry-trends-and-stats

Cornell University College of Veterinary Medicine, Center for Veterinary Business and Entrepreneurship. *Burnout Takes a Heavy Financial Toll on Veterinary Medicine.* 2022, https://www.vet.cornell.edu/about-us/news/20220829/burnout-takes-heavy-financial-toll-veterinary-medicine

DVM360. *The Rising Costs of Veterinary Care: Challenges and Pathways to Greater Access.* 2024, https://www.dvm360.com/view/the-rising-costs-of-veterinary-care-challenges-and-pathways-to-greater-access

DVM360. *Veterinary Visits Decline as Clients Face Rising Costs.* 2024, https://www.dvm360.com/view/veterinary-visits-decline-as-clients-face-rising-costs-data-reveals

Forbes Advisor. *Pet Ownership Statistics and Veterinary Spending Trends.* 2025, https://www.forbes.com/advisor/pet-insurance/pet-ownership-statistics/

Pawlicy Advisor. *Average Cost of a Vet Visit in 2025.* 2025, https://www.pawlicy.com/blog/vet-visit-cost/

U.S. Bureau of Labor Statistics (BLS). *Consumer Price Index: Veterinary Services Inflation.* 2024, https://www.bls.gov/cpi/

Chapter 2
Culture Drives Tactics

Back in the 2000s, Cleveland Clinic, today one of the most respected healthcare brands in the U.S., was facing a serious problem. Their reputation for delivering world-class medical outcomes was solid, but patient satisfaction was falling apart. Patients routinely described their care as "cold, impersonal, and dismissive." They trusted the medical skill, but they didn't feel cared for as people. Many reported feeling like numbers, not people.

When the first HCAHPS survey (the Hospital Consumer Assessment of Healthcare Providers and Systems—a national survey that measures patients' satisfaction of their hospital experience) dropped in 2007, the results were brutal: only 63% of inpatients rated their stay a 9–10. That placed the Clinic at the 55th percentile nationally—middle of the pack at best. By 2009, CEO Toby Cosgrove admitted publicly that patient satisfaction scores were "terrible" and that, frankly, "patients didn't like us very much." Inside the organization, morale tanked.

The timing couldn't have been worse. Patients were beginning to shop for care, comparing both outcomes and experience. Hospitals like Cleveland Clinic risked losing patients to competitors who delivered excellent medicine AND superior service. And to make things worse, the Centers for Medicare and Medicaid Service (CMS) was preparing to tie reimbursements to patient experience scores. This wasn't just about reputation anymore; it came with financial consequences.

Cleveland Clinic responded by introducing what I would consider an empty, "quick fix" patient experience strategy. They rolled out surface-level fixes: rules about making eye contact, "smiling guidelines," and scripted phrases like, "Is there anything else I can do for you today?" On paper, it looked like a plan. In reality, it landed with all the authenticity of a telemarketer script.

Staff felt demeaned. Patients felt patronized. Doctors and nurses—people trusted with life-and-death decisions—were suddenly being measured by whether they followed a "smile checklist." Staff felt that the scripting felt really superficial, that they were being forced to perform "fake niceness" rather than feeling empowered to actually connect with patients. And without any clear mission or explanation from leadership about why patient experience actually mattered—beyond "the government is measuring it" or "we want better scores"—staff became resentful. There was no genuine or authentic focus on healing the human experience, only "rules." And in an organization long lauded for its technical brilliance and medical outcomes, these new required behaviors felt "bolted on," not truly integrated into the institution's identity. The culture, in other words, didn't yet recognize that empathy and patient emotional needs are core to patient healing or quality of care.

And here's the kicker: patients noticed. They could feel the lack of authenticity. Instead of warmth, they got empty gestures. Instead of connection, they got a performance. Patients still felt like numbers. And scores didn't improve. Morale tanked further.

Cleveland Clinic learned a hard but vital truth: patient experience isn't a tactic. You can't fake it with scripts and checklists. Without a culture that values empathy and true connection with customers, tactics come across as hollow ... and don't work.

Happily, Cleveland Clinic learned its lesson and in 2009 began implementing a more genuine shift toward embedding patient experience into its culture and priorities. It established a Chief Experience Officer role, one of the first organizations in healthcare to do so. It created and shared its new CX mission statement, "Every patient, every time, treated with empathy and compassion."

The organization trained every employee—from janitors to surgeons—in empathy skills, communication, and emotional intelligence. Staff were encouraged and empowered to show genuine empathy and compassion in ways that felt authentic to them, rather than being given scripts and rehearsed talking points. Patient experience was redefined as a cultural value, not just a bolted-set set of customer service tactics. And not only did HCAHPS scores improve dramatically, but so too did employee engagement and morale. Ever since, and still today, Cleveland Clinic is a highly respected, national model for patient-centered care.

The lesson is this: culture must precede tactics, because a healthy culture will drive the behaviors that result in improved client trust.

It's no surprise that both employee morale and patient satisfaction were both simultaneously low. It's no surprise that both employees and patients independently came to the same opinion that Cleveland Clinic's "quick fix" tactics felt empty, forced, and inauthentic. Employees felt demeaned, while patients continued to feel like numbers. But it's also no surprise that when Cleveland Clinic made patient experience an authentic priority that became genuinely embedded into its culture, staff morale and patient satisfaction scores increased in lockstep. It almost suggests that team morale and empowerment might be linked to patient or client experiences (CXs), right?

In this book, I will argue, in fact, that they are. And because they are, creating authentic pet-owner CXs (that keeps clients coming back for their pets' care and that inspires clients to rave about your animal hospital to their friends and family) must begin with a genuine strategy and effort to embed CX into your animal hospital's culture. And that starts with building trust and safety within your team.

We don't need to choose between client satisfaction and team well-being, in other words. The best kind of veterinary experience is one where both are lifted together.

I've always had a deep passion for the CX. For me, it's never felt like a "strategy." It's fun. It brings me joy. Creating experiences for veterinary hospital teams and clients is the reason I get out of bed in the morning. Making our teams and clients feel seen, heard, and cared for is deeply fulfilling work. I'd even go so far as to call it my life's work.

That passion has led to me having the opportunity to advise hundreds of animal hospital teams over the past eight years. In that time, I've found that too often, like at Cleveland Clinic in the 2000s, CX is misunderstood. In many hospitals, it's reduced to smiley face posters, generic training modules, mandatory scripts, or worst of all—used only as damage control when a client gets angry. That's not CX. That's optics. And it does a disservice to the powerful, human-centered work we're capable of in this industry.

A healthy focus on CX doesn't just drive better Yelp reviews. It creates a workplace where gratitude flows freely. Where the small thank-yous from clients land with more weight. Where the joy of saving a life, or easing a passing, is shared more fully. It reminds teams *why* they chose this work in the first place. And it all starts with empowering your team.

In the next few chapters, I'll walk you through my *Veterinary Trust Flywheel*. It's simple: when you retain your team, you retain your clients. When you care for one, you care for the other. But if you fail one, the other follows. These two experiences—client and team—are inextricably linked.

Summary

Tactics might get you a smile, but only culture earns you trust.

Here's the punchline: you can't duct-tape scripts and smile checklists onto a broken culture and expect magic. Clients smell inauthenticity a mile away. Teams feel demeaned. Everyone loses. Cleveland Clinic learned that the hard way—and so have too many veterinary hospitals.

The real win comes when culture and tactics line up. When empathy, trust, and connection aren't just rules but values, your whole team actually believes in and lives every day. That's when morale rises. That's when CXs improve. That's when the whole place starts to feel alive again.

And here's the kicker for us in veterinary medicine: you don't have to choose between client happiness and team well-being. They rise and fall together. Build a culture where your people feel empowered, trusted, safe, and proud, and your clients will feel it too.

Suggested Readings

Berry, Leonard L., Lewis P. Carbone, and Stephan H. Haeckel. "Managing the Total Customer Experience." *MIT Sloan Management Review*, vol. 43, no. 3, 2002, pp. 85–89.

Beryl Institute. *Defining Patient Experience: Culture, Leadership, and Systematic transformation*, 2012, https://www.theberylinstitute.org

Centers for Medicare & Medicaid Services (CMS). *Hospital Consumer Assessment of Healthcare Providers and Systems (HCAHPS): Overview and Survey Methodology*, 2007, https://www.cms.gov/Medicare/Quality-Initiatives-Patient-Assessment-Instruments/HospitalQualityInits/HospitalHCAHPS

Centers for Medicare & Medicaid Services (CMS). *Hospital Value-Based Purchasing Program: Linking Patient Experience to Reimbursement*, 2011, https://www.cms.gov/Medicare/Quality-Initiatives-Patient-Assessment-Instruments/Hospital-Value-Based-Purchasing

Cleveland Clinic. *Every Patient, Every Time: Embedding Empathy into Healthcare Culture*. Cleveland Clinic Office of Patient Experience, 2010.

Cosgrove, Toby J. *Cleveland Clinic Transformation and the Role of Patient Experience*. Cleveland Clinic Health System Annual Report, 2009.

Goleman, Daniel. *Emotional Intelligence: Why it can Matter more than IQ*. Bantam Books, 1995.

Kotter, John P. *Leading Change*. Harvard Business School Press, 1996.

Press Ganey Associates. *The Rise of Patient Experience as a Strategic Healthcare Priority*, 2013, https://www.pressganey.com

Chapter 3
A Case Study in Veterinary Client Experience

I once worked with a regional operations leader—we'll call her Linda—who oversaw 16 hospitals for a large veterinary consolidator. Linda cared deeply about client experience (CX). She wanted her region to lead the company in satisfaction scores.

She studied monthly survey results and saw two big issues: clients didn't feel welcomed or acknowledged, and her hospitals were struggling to generate positive reviews online.

Armed with that intel, Linda went to work to create a new "premium, high-touch service" at her hospitals. As part of her new strategy, Linda:

1. Introduced new guidelines for her hospital teams, listing specific tactics that she expected her hospital managers to strictly enforce
2. Developed and distributed simple guidebooks and video trainings that walked through each of these tactics in detail

3. Hired secret shoppers to visit her hospitals and report their findings back to her
4. Introduced incentives like quarterly pizza parties to reward hospitals in her region that showed the highest survey score improvements and that performed best during the secret shopper visits

The tactics that Linda sought to introduce and enforce were certainly practical. They included rules like:

- Greet every client and pet within 20 seconds
- Offer water and treats in the lobby to every client waiting more than 10 minutes
- Say to every client "We're so happy you're here."
- Use clients' and pets' names at least twice per visit
- Always ask for online reviews at checkout

Six months after launching her strategy, Linda noticed that the secret shopper scores were actually pretty high—the teams were following the tactics she had mandated—but her CX survey scores weren't improving at all. She was a bit perturbed, to say the least. After all, the practices she introduced seemed practical enough, right? What clients wouldn't want to be greeted by name and given treats? Something was amiss.

So, I went undercover. I brought my dog Buddy to one of Linda's lowest-performing hospitals during a busy hour, hoping for a long wait so I could observe. The team followed the rules exactly. And yet, the experience felt flat, mechanical, and at times, absurd.

What I found was that the team was, in fact, sticking steadfastly to the rules that Linda had introduced. But not surprisingly, this list of rules and tactics were not actually improving things. Much like what initially happened at the Cleveland Clinic, the team was going through the motions and treating CX like a list of rules to be followed. And since it was truly engrained into the hospital culture, things were running amuck. This was a textbook case of how NOT to do CX. I'll share some examples of some especially cringe-worthy moments:

As one client, Liz, walked out the door with her dog, I think the team realized they had only said her name once during the visit, which would constitute breaking the rule that every client should be addressed by name at least twice. So in a last-ditch effort to remedy that, in a moment that I thought was both comical and cringe-worthy, the Client Service Representative (CSR) literally chased the client out the door, and as she sprinted across the parking lot, yelled several times, "Have a wonderful day, Liz!"—rule satisfied, authenticity destroyed.

Another client who had grown frustrated by a long wait time, a rushed appointment, and an unexpectedly hefty bill for what she felt were "routine services" for her dog. A lot had gone wrong. And while not exactly rude to the CSR during the checkout process, she did make her frustrations very clear. The CSR, clearly untrained for real conflict, apologized "for the inconvenience," but she clearly didn't do enough to make the client feel heard or understood. And in yet another cringe-worthy moment, that same CSR locked eyes with the frustrated client just as she was turning to leave and said with a forced smile, "Please be sure to leave us a review on Yelp!" Oh, that client left a review, all right ... But it wasn't exactly five stars.

Now it was my and Buddy's turn. I had brought Buddy in under false pretenses that he was scratching himself a lot. We were offered water and treats during our wait in the lobby, which was a nice touch. And I did appreciate the Technician greeting Buddy and me by name. The scripted tactics weren't terrible.

What I didn't appreciate was both the Technician and then the Doctor asking me "what brought me in today"—information I had also already shared with the CSR. The Doctor—we'll call him Dr. Jones—then asked me to confirm whether the Technician had already taken Buddy's weight. He barely looked at Buddy as he entered the exam room, getting straight to work with his scripted questions, which I knew were an attempt to determine whether Buddy's scratching was from allergies, parasites, or an infection, and then offered his prognosis and recommended treatment—a Cytopoint injection and an Apoquel prescription. The "conversation" felt like anything but. It felt more like a rushed interview, made worse by Dr. Jones checking his watch (yes, I was counting) at least six times in the four minutes he was with us. As he turned to leave the exam room, thereby facing away from me and Buddy, Dr. Jones said inauthentically and with zero emotion, "We're so happy you're here, Ryan." Hey, two rules checked off at once! Dr. Jones said "we're so happy you're here" AND addressed me by name! Success!

Later that week, during dinner at the Olive Garden (don't judge me because I'm not even sorry—those breadsticks!), I reported back to Linda that her "strategy" had flopped harder than a fish on a hot dock. We read through some of the client reviews and survey responses from the past six months, which included:

- "They're trying too hard."
- "It's all for the reviews."
- "I'd rather they spent time explaining my dog's bloodwork than asking me three times if I want water."

As a common theme, online reviews mentioned surface-level friendliness but a lack of real connection or transparency. One even mentioned that she was greeted by name TOO MANY times, and that it had started to feel unnatural: "It was obvious that the team has been instructed to use my name as much as possible, and it was overkill."

With Linda's permission, I then held a focus-group style meeting with her 16 hospital managers and some select other team members from across her hospitals—a mix of Doctors, Technicians, and CSRs. There were about 40 of us in the room total. Linda wasn't present, so the group could share feedback openly and without pressure.

The feedback bore a lot of similarities to what Cleveland Clinic's staff had reported in the 2000s. The team felt pressured to follow Linda's directives rather than trusted to use their own judgment, which left them feeling restricted and undervalued. While they generally believed Linda's intentions were positive, they were frustrated by the lack of explanation for *why* improving the experience mattered—for clients, patients, or the team. The initiative felt more like a superficial push to artificially boost scores than a sincere effort to enhance care and take better care of clients and patients.

Many team members genuinely wanted to create warmer, more authentic experiences, so the mismatch was disheartening. When asked to describe the strategy, they used words like "tone-deaf," "corporate," "disconnected," "robotic," "inauthentic," and "superficial." The strain even led to one hospital losing a CSR and a long-tenured Technician.

I asked the team what a better rollout would have looked like. Interestingly, after some discussion and debate, the team agreed that before a new strategy was introduced and rolled out, they would benefit from two things: stronger team support and a clear "why." We then defined these things together.

I loved that the team wanted to start there. It aligned exactly with everything I've always believed about effective leadership in the midst of change—that portraying a compelling vision and then motivating the team toward that vision by articulating benefits must come first.

And that's the truth: effective CX can't start with tactics. It has to start with culture, vision, and a clear purpose. Tactics come last, not first.

Again, culture drives tactics.

So, let's dig into what DOES work. I'm excited to introduce my *Veterinary Trust Flywheel*, which articulates not only why we should prioritize CX, but on how an authentic focus on both client and team experience together improves team retention and happiness, client retention and trust, pet medical outcomes, and hospital financial fitness.

Let's hop in.

(By the way, Linda's story returns later with a turnaround using these principles.)

Summary

Checklists don't build trust. People do.

Linda's playbook looked good on paper. She thought through details. Secret shoppers. Rulebooks. Pizza parties. A checklist for friendliness. But once it was executed? Brutal. Teams felt micromanaged. Clients felt like they were part of a skit. And the whole thing backfired.

Because here's the truth: you can't checklist your way into trust. You can't fake warmth with scripts. You can't bribe culture with breadsticks and gift cards. Clients want to feel heard. Teams want to feel trusted. And when they don't? Everyone smells the BS.

What Linda's case proved, painfully, is that CX tactics without culture are hollow. A forced smile, a forced "we're so happy you're here," or a forced Yelp request is worse than nothing at all. It's inauthentic. And it burns more trust than it builds.

The good news? The teams themselves already knew the answer. They didn't want to be robots. They wanted vision. They wanted to understand the "why." They wanted freedom to actually connect with pet owners like humans, not live by checklists.

Suggested Readings

Adams, Stacy J. Inequity in Social Exchange. In Leonard, Berkowitz (Ed.), *Advances in Experimental Social Psychology*. Academic Press, 1965, Vol. 2 pp. 267–299.

Beryl Institute. *Defining Patient Experience: A Shared Understanding*. 2012, https://www.theberylinstitute.org

Collins, Jim. Good to Great: Why Some Companies make the Leap… and Others Don't. *HarperBusiness*, 2001.

Colquitt, Jason A., Donald E. Conlon, Michael J. Wesson, Christopher O. Porter, and Yee K. Ng. Justice at the Millennium: A Meta-analytic Review of 25 Years of Organizational Justice Research. *Journal of Applied Psychology*, vol. 86, no. 3, 2001, pp. 425–445.

Edmondson, Amy. *The Fearless Organization: Creating Psychological Safety in the Workplace for Learning, Innovation, and Growth*. Wiley, 2019.

Gallup, Inc. *State of the Global Workplace Report*. 2023, https://www.gallup.com/workplace

Goleman, Daniel. *Working with Emotional Intelligence*. Bantam Books, 1998.

Greenleaf, Robert K. *Servant Leadership: A Journey into the Nature of Legitimate Power and Greatness*. Paulist Press, 1977.

Kotter, John P., and James L. Heskett. *Corporate Culture and Performance*. Free Press, 1992.

Locke, Edwin A., and George P. Latham. Building a Practically useful Theory of Goal Setting and Task Motivation. *American Psychologist*, vol. 57. no. 9, 2002, pp. 705–717.

Sinek, Simon. *Start with Why: How Great Leaders Inspire Everyone to Take Action*. Portfolio, 2009.

Part 2

The Veterinary Trust Flywheel

The Flywheel Starts by Focusing on Your Team

Okay, we've laid the groundwork. We've dug into why this work is so damn urgent in our industry right now. We've talked about the lack of trust dynamics in the veterinary space and the consequences of ignoring them. I've given you case studies and examples that prove one thing: scripts and quick fixes don't work. Mandating tactics without a foundation is lipstick on a pig.

Here's the problem: most people completely misunderstand client experience (CX). In fact, they butcher it.

Either they jump straight into tactics—which as we've talked about is the kiss of death—or they oversimplify or minimize CX until it's meaningless. How many times have you heard leaders attempting to "champion client experience" who toss out feel-good slogans like, "Just be nice," "Deliver joy," "Treat others how you want to be treated," or "Create smiles"? These sound good on a poster. They might look nice on a wall. But they definitely don't move the needle.

Now, don't get me wrong. There's nothing inherently bad about "delivering joy" and some of these other ideas. And it's absolutely true that CX doesn't need to be complicated. But when you reduce it to platitudes, you send the message to your team (and clients) that it's a "nice to have" or so commonsensible that it doesn't *really* matter or warrant any attention. And if your team hears or senses that, they'll treat it the same way: as an optional side dish, not the main course.

In veterinary medicine, creating a best-in-class pet owner experience doesn't start with tactics or cute phrases. You also don't start with gimmicks or marketing tricks.

True change starts deeper. You start with your team, because their experience inside the hospital sets the tone for everything else. You invest in your hospital's culture and give them the respect of portraying a clear vision and "why" for your hospital. Suddenly, your staff shows up energized, your clients feel seen and cared for, pets get better medicine, and your business finally breathes. That momentum compounds. One good push feeds the next.

That's the heart of the Veterinary Trust Flywheel. It explains how when you put your people first, everything else falls into place. You invest in your team, trust skyrockets, clients feel it, medicine gets better, the business grows, and you've got more fuel to reinvest right back into your people. When the team culture and identity are strong, and the team feels safe and appreciated, it fuels an amazing CX. That momentum keeps building, creating better results for the team, clients, patients, and the hospital itself. It's compound interest for culture. Push after push, the wheel spins faster until momentum takes over—and once it's moving, nothing can stop it. And here's the kicker: effective leadership is the grease. It's what keeps this whole machine moving smoothly. The model is simple, but the effects are massive.

If the term "flywheel" sounds new to you, don't worry: here's the quick and dirty. A flywheel is a heavy wheel that stores energy. Hard to get moving at first, but once it spins, momentum takes over. Jim Collins made it famous in his book Good to Great, where he argues that success isn't about onc big push, it's about consistent pushes in the same direction until *growth reinforces growth.*

That's what this is all about.

I'm fired up to share the Veterinary Trust Flywheel with you, because it's not theory. It's real. It shows you how investing in your team's morale and culture pays out in spades: higher retention, stronger client trust, better pet medical outcomes, and yes—bigger hospital profitability.

So, it's not just a win-win. It's a win-win-win-win. Your team wins. Clients win. Pets win. The hospital wins.

Let's kick it.

What "Starting with Your Team" Actually Looks Like

So hopefully at this point you're asking, *"Okay, but how the hell do I actually get this thing spinning?"* In other words: *"What do I, as the leader, have to actually* **do** *to turn this from a cool idea into a hospital where my team thrives, my clients stay loyal for life, my medical standards stay untouchable, and the business generates real money instead of scraping by?"*

In truth, step 1 of the Flywheel starts with you. Not your team. Not your client service representative (CSR). *You.*

To even **earn the right** to build culture, perfect your CX, and get the results you and I both want for your hospital, three things must be locked in first. If they're not, you're basically trying to pour concrete on a trampoline. Nothing holds. This is step 1 of the Flywheel.

1. *Fairness*

Let's get this out of the way right now: if your team doesn't believe they're being treated fairly—compensated fairly, scheduled fairly, recognized fairly—you are done before you even start.

You cannot build culture on resentment. You cannot build trust on suspicion. You cannot rally a team that's quietly thinking, *"Why am I giving extra effort when the system feels rigged?"* Fairness isn't a "nice-to-have." It's not a perk. It's not culture frosting.

Fairness is oxygen. If people don't feel it, nothing else will breathe.

2. *Clarity*

Shared Identity

Everybody loves to dunk on mission and vision statements.
"They're corporate."
"They're fluffy."
"They're pointless."

That can be true—when they're written by a committee, plastered on a wall, and never mentioned again. That's not direction. That's décor.

But a hospital with a crystal-clear understanding of what it stands for, what it's aiming toward, and what it refuses to compromise on? That's a hospital that becomes unstoppable. That's a team that works with purpose, not pressure. That's where daily work becomes meaningful, not mechanical. And clients can feel it. They can sense when a hospital is aligned—and when it's just winging it.

Direction doesn't just make the hospital better. **It makes the team's daily life better.** Clarity reduces stress. Clarity builds unity. Clarity accelerates excellence.

Culture of Standards and Accountability

Culture isn't just how people feel at work. It's the operating system your entire practice runs on. It shows up in who you hire, how you onboard, how you handle conflict, how consistently care is delivered, how confidently your team advocates, and whether clients feel like they're being given an appointment or a healthcare experience. Those are not the same.

One is a transaction—rushed, reactive, check-the-box. The other is intentional—proactive, guiding, educational, connected.

Clients don't come to you for rabies shots and X-rays. They come to you for peace of mind. They come for meaning. They come for someone to help them keep the heartbeat on the floor next to them alive longer. Nike sells shoes. Chipotle sells burritos. You sell maximizing vitality while minimizing suffering for their pet. When you forget that, your culture drifts into "treating cases" instead of serving lives.

A healthy hospital culture is established when hospital leaders intentionally champion clarity: standards, shared accountability, clear communication.

3. *Servant Leadership*

If you're leading from ego—clinging to control, chasing credit, micromanaging tasks, or optimizing only for short-term output—you're not leading. You're draining.

Servant leadership isn't soft. It's not submissive. It's not rainbows and kumbaya.

It's the discipline of removing roadblocks for your team instead of creating them. It's the courage to develop people who might someday surpass you. It's the humility to make the hospital the hero—not yourself. And it's the only leadership style that sustains a strong culture instead of burning it out.

When you do this well, people don't just work for you; they work **with** you. They don't comply; they commit. They don't clock in; they buy in.

(For more tangible guidance on strategies you can undertake to show servant leadership, see Appendix B.)

These three elements—**fairness, clarity, and servant leadership**—aren't optional. They're the bedrock of the Veterinary Trust Flywheel. Without them, nothing spins.

In the next three chapters, we'll break each one down. Because once those foundations are in place, we'll get into the real magic: how to create psychological safety within your team that lights the Flywheel on fire and gains momentum month after month, year after year.

Chapter 4
Fairness First

As I mentioned, Step 1 of the Flywheel is to invest in your team. That starts with ensuring that your team is being treated fairly. That's a nonnegotiable first step and the focus of this chapter.

I'll be honest: one of my guilty pleasures is the TV show *Kitchen Nightmares*. If you've watched Gordon Ramsay walk into some half-dead restaurant, chew a frozen "signature dish," spit it out in disgust, and verbally body-slam the staff, you know the formula. The food sucks, the kitchen's filthy, leadership's in denial, and the staff is checked out. Then Gordon does what great leaders do—he strips everything down to the basics: fresh ingredients, tight menu, real standards, real training, and actual leadership.

And the part he never sugarcoats? If the staff is treated unfairly—if they're underpaid, disrespected, burned out, or ignored—nothing else matters. You can't build greatness on exploitation. Period.

Vet med isn't a restaurant, but the lesson is identical: you can have elite medicine, the best tools, gold-standard protocols ... But if your team feels screwed, overlooked, or underpaid, it's game over. They leave. And when they leave, your culture collapses, your client experience tanks, and your hospital bleeds out.

That's why before we talk about Client Experience (CX), psychological safety, retention, or "empowering your team," we have to start with **fairness**. Not as a slogan. As a nonnegotiable.

"Customers will never love a company until the employees love it first."

Simon Sinek didn't say that for fun. He said it because it's the truth every great business is built on. And in veterinary medicine, it's 10 times more real. If you want a hospital that clients rave about ... if you want elite medicine delivered consistently ... if you want a practice that actually *lasts* ... then let me be crystal clear:

Your team is the engine.
Your team is the brand.
Your team is the experience.
Your team is the outcome.

Everything else—the equipment, the décor, the marketing—is window dressing. None of it matters if your team is exhausted, undervalued, unclear, or unsupported.

The foundation of the Veterinary Trust Flywheel is brutally simple: you invest in your team first. Before strategy. Before client experience. Before anything. And your first, pivotal, nonnegotiable, mandatory step in investing in your team? Ensuring that they feel that they're treated fairly.

The Data Doesn't Lie

AAHA's 2024–2025 Stay, Please study made this painfully clear. They broke workplace factors into:

- Attrition Factors: the minimum table stakes. Screw these up and people bounce. Fast.
- Retention Factors: the things that keep great people around once the basics are met.

And here's what the study found:

The biggest Attrition Factors? Fair pay. Career development. Believing leadership actually cares.

The strongest Retention Factors? Meaningful work. Feeling equipped. Quality medicine. Team collaboration. Culture.

Translation? Compensation mistakes push people out. Strong culture, medicine, and teamwork pull people deeper in. Your team wants to do good work, with the right tools, the right standards, and the right people beside them. When they can? They stay.

Fairness Isn't a Luxury. It's the Floor

If you want retention, trust, momentum—hell, if you want basic stability—meet your team's baseline needs. It's not complicated:

Pay people what they're worth. Full stop.
Give them clear roles and expectations.
Show them you care—loudly, consistently, emotionally.
Build staffing that doesn't set them up to fail.

You cannot build psychological safety on top of resentment.
You cannot demand excellence from people who feel exploited.
You cannot run a human business with people who feel unseen, unheard, and underpaid.

Vet med is a service industry wrapped in medicine. Humans deliver service. Humans deliver care. And humans cannot deliver greatness when they feel screwed.

Fair Pay Isn't the Finish Line. It's the Starting Line

Too many owners act like fair compensation is a bonus. No.
Fair pay doesn't motivate greatness—it removes the injustice that blocks greatness.

If your team *feels* underpaid or undervalued, you're already done.
Culture? Dead.
Retention? Gone.

The numbers back it up: **37% of vet staff quit because of compensation and benefits.** Fall below market wages, and most of your team will walk, sooner or later, guaranteed.

And don't think that pizza parties, a random bag of chips, or a "we appreciate you!" post-it note fixes unfair pay. It doesn't. It's an insult.

And it's not just money.
Your people need respect.
They need clarity.
They need to not be short-staffed into oblivion.
They need to feel set up to succeed.

If they feel set up to fail? They will leave, before or after burnout. Either way, they're gone.

Stop Using Excuses as a Business Strategy

"Ryan, I can't afford to pay more."
"Ryan, I can't afford to staff up."

Yes, you can. In truth, leaders must take the risk first. Leaders bet on their people first. Leaders sacrifice first. If you want your team to go the extra mile for your clients, go the first 10 miles for *them*.

The two strategies guaranteed to sink you:

1. **Underpaying and running skeleton crews** hoping that "one day" you'll magically save enough to fix it. You won't.
2. **Jacking up prices until clients resent you.** Price yourself out of the local market and those clients will find another hospital fast.

If your entire model is built on squeezing clients or squeezing staff, you're finished.

The Only Bet That Works? Betting on Your Team

If you can't keep your team, stop guessing why and just ask:
"Do you feel treated fairly?"
"Do you feel compensated fairly?"

If they hesitate—or worse, say no—you have to pivot immediately. Unfairness spreads like cancer. It kills morale, kills pride, kills enthusiasm, and kills culture from the inside out.

Fairness isn't optional.
It's foundational.
It's the concrete slab you build everything else on.

Try building culture, loyalty, psychological safety, teamwork, retention, or client trust on top of unfair pay and unfair treatment and you'll get the same result every time: A skyscraper built on quicksand. It might look impressive for a while. Then it sinks. Every. Single. Time.

Lessons in Fairness

Emily the CSR

Take Emily, for example. She was a Client Service Representative (CSR) at one hospital I worked with. Smart, sharp, the kind of person clients adored. She knew every pet by name, remembered clients' kids, and could calm down even the most furious owner. But Emily was making $13.25 an hour. One day she pulled me aside and said, *"Ry, I love this job. I love the clients, the pets, the team. But Starbucks up the road is paying $16 an hour to start, plus health insurance, tuition reimbursement, free coffee, and I'd get weekends off. How am I supposed to say no to that?"*

She wasn't being dramatic. She was exhausted, overworked, covering callouts, and barely keeping up with her rent. And soon, she left—not because she didn't care about the hospital, but because she couldn't afford to stay. And immediately, clients noticed the turnover. Service slipped. Trust eroded. The front desk turned into a revolving door.

Now contrast that with another hospital I worked with just down the road, led by a manager named Mark. He'd been burned by turnover before and decided to fix it at the root. He started benchmarking pay and adjusted ranges to match real-time market rates. He built clear pay bands for every role. And raises weren't random. If you got a certification, hit tenure milestones, or crushed performance reviews, you *knew* what that meant for your paycheck. No secrets. No favoritism.

Then he upgraded benefits. Better health and dental, a 401(k) match, bigger CE stipends, licensing reimbursements, uniform stipends, and even mental health support. But here's the kicker: he asked his team first. Benefits nobody used got cut, and those dollars went into the ones they actually valued.

Most importantly, Mark was transparent with his team, "We benchmark pay every year. Here's your total comp statement—your salary plus the dollar value of benefits—so you can see the full picture. Here's how raises happen." No mystery. No favoritism.

The result? Zero turnover that year. Clients noticed the same faces every visit. Referrals doubled. Margins dipped for a few months, but the hospital ended up more profitable than ever thanks to efficiency gains, higher retention, and stronger client loyalty.

That's the difference. Emily's hospital treated pay like a cost to be contained and lost her to Starbucks. Mark's hospital treated pay like a strategy and built a team nobody wanted to leave.

Northwest Pet Care's Pay Gap

At Northwest Pet Care, Dr. Lopez thought everything was fine. Great medicine, good reviews, solid revenue. Then her manager, Tasha, ran a quiet internal pay audit. Just curiosity—or maybe intuition. What she found made her stomach drop.

Two senior techs. Same tenure. Same certifications. Same responsibilities. Four-dollar-per-hour pay gap.

No bad intent—just years of inconsistent raises and "we'll fix it later." But here's the thing: the team *knew*. You can always feel unfairness in the air. It leaks out through eye contact and side comments and the way people volunteer (or stop volunteering).

When Tasha showed the data to Dr. Lopez, she didn't spin it or justify it. She owned it.
Within a week, pay was corrected and back pay was issued. They held a team meeting—short, honest, and raw.

"We discovered something that wasn't right," Dr. Lopez said. "We fixed it. And we're committed to checking this every year."

You could feel the sigh in the room. People straightened up. Smiles cracked. One of the techs said quietly, "Thank you for not pretending it was nothing."

Within three months, turnover dropped to zero. Engagement scores shot up. Clients even noticed: "Your team just feels happier lately."

Fairness isn't a *nice-to-have*. It's a trust accelerant. You can't preach transparency to clients while hiding inequity from your own people. So, you want loyalty? Start by paying people what they're worth— and *proving* it.

How to Ensure Fairness in Your Hospital

So as we transition into the *how* part of this book, here are the strategies behind Mark's ensuring fairness in your hospital.

Benchmark

When it comes to pay and benefits, you can't wing it. This stuff has to be systematic, and it has to be competitive. Don't just guess at what "fair" looks like; pull real data. Tap into Veterinary Hospital

Managers Association (VHMA), American Veterinary Medical Association (AVMA), American Animal Hospital Association (AAHA), and your regional association surveys. Then, back that up with real-world intel: job boards like Indeed, ZipRecruiter, LinkedIn, and even local classifieds. That's where you'll see what people in your area are *actually* getting paid today. And don't ignore cost of living. If inflation and housing costs have spiked, you need to adjust your ranges. Otherwise, you'll lose people to the Starbucks down the street.

Pay Structures

Every role in your hospital—CSRs, techs, assistants, managers, DVMs—needs updated pay bands with clear entry, mid, and senior levels. Raises shouldn't be random. Tie them to objective criteria like certifications, tenure, and performance reviews. And for the love of God, check for pay equity. If two techs are doing the same job and one's making way less, you're sitting on a culture bomb waiting to go off.

Benefits

Then there's the benefits package. This is where hospitals get lazy and fall behind. Audit your health, dental, vision, disability, and life insurance options. Are they affordable and relevant? Check your retirement plans too: 401(k) with a match, SIMPLE IRA, whatever you're offering, make sure it's competitive. Look at PTO and holidays; stack them up against industry averages. Don't forget continuing education stipends, licensing reimbursements, and training opportunities. And yes, the "soft benefits" matter too. Things like pet care discounts, scrub or uniform stipends, wellness perks, or access to mental health resources. These little touches build loyalty.

Feedback Loops

You also need feedback loops. Run anonymous staff surveys to find out what benefits actually matter most. Then hold at least one open Q&A where people can ask about compensation and benefits directly. If nobody's using a certain benefit—like an insurance plan you're offering—you can consider reallocating that money into something your people are telling you they'd value more, like perhaps bigger CE stipends. It's a great way to apply your team's feedback to create more impact without raising costs.

Communication

Don't just do all this behind the scenes. Tell your team you benchmark pay and benefits every year against local and industry data. Provide a total compensation statement so they can see the full picture: not just salary, but benefits value too. And keep reinforcing how raises tie back to performance, certifications, or tenure.

Annual Cycling

Finally, make it a cycle. This review should be built into your annual budget planning every single year. Document updates. Keep records. Repeat the process. Staying competitive isn't one-and-done: it's an ongoing effort.

Treat Your Team Like Volunteers, Because They Are

Outside of working in the veterinary industry, there's one commitment that I make every year that I'm really proud of: I'm part of a small team of leaders who organize an annual Thanksgiving event for people experiencing homelessness or similar difficulties in Santa Monica, CA—the area I'm proud to call home. Each year, our event attracts over 1,000 mostly homeless "guests," to whom we provide a full Thanksgiving meal; a "boutique" of new and used clothing, sleeping bags, backpacks, thermal underwear, and toiletries. We also offer them free haircuts and access to third-party services like career coaching, medical services, housing, and reunification with their families. The day is so happily exhausting and wonderfully rewarding. It's my favorite day of the year, every year. And it works because we attract, train, and support over 400 volunteers to make it happen. Together, these volunteers cook hundreds of turkeys, cook hundreds of pounds of other food items like stuffing and mashed potatoes, fundraise and collect item donations months in advance, sort and distribute clothing, deliver food off campus to disabled guests who can't make it to the event, etc. It's the energy of those volunteers that makes that day not only possible, but so incredibly impactful. They give their all, work tirelessly, giving all the energy and kindness they can muster to make every guest feel special and welcome. And the result is a tear-jerking day that inspires and impacts not only our guests, but also the volunteers.

These volunteers work so hard despite receiving zero compensation. And damn, they give their ALL. No task is beneath them; no amount of initiative or effort or passion is too much. Their energy, their passion, and their initiative are just so inspiring. And most of them tell you that they get just as much from the day as our guests do. These volunteers could all easily be spending their time doing literally anything else, including working in their normal everyday jobs and thereby earning money—but they elect to instead volunteer for this incredible event. Why? Because it just feels really friggin good to work in support of a cause that you believe in, that you believe is adding value and goodness to the world. Teams go above and beyond when they're aligned toward a mission.

I bring this up not to impress you with my volunteerism or organization skills, but because I see so much parallel between the volunteers for this Thanksgiving event and the staff in our hospitals.

The reality is that our hospital team members are volunteers, and it would behoove us to see them as such and always remember that. Here's what I mean: in a typical town, there are several animal hospitals vying for employees. CSRs, Technicians, Veterinary Assistants, and Doctors—all of our team members—could easily pack up and bring their talent to another veterinary hospital and very easily get hired. There's no shortage of short-staffed hospitals out there ready to take whatever quality talent they can find. In other words, anyone qualified for a job in your hospital is just as qualified for a job at the same pay scale—and sometimes more—elsewhere.

So, as we transition to the Veterinary Trust Flywheel and really start to dig into how to retain our team members, remember that: our team members are volunteers. They're working for us voluntarily. They are gifting us their talents in an environment where they could very easily go elsewhere.

We have a responsibility to acknowledge and reward that loyalty by creating a hospital work environment that's worth sticking around for.

Fair pay and basic decency are the floor, not the ceiling. Your volunteer employees won't stick around just because you have these things in place. The real magic happens when you give your people something bigger to believe in—when you create a culture where they feel valued, energized, and proud to wear your logo on their chest. That's when a job turns into a mission. And that's what we're aiming for with the Veterinary Trust Flywheel—a culture that makes people say, "Hell yes, I want to be here. I can't imagine going anywhere else."

Establishing Fairness, In Summary

If you treat fairness as if it's optional, don't be surprised when your best people treat your hospital the same way.

Let's not sugarcoat it: if you're underpaying your people, hiding behind vague promises, or treating fairness like an afterthought, you're bleeding trust and you're bleeding talent. And no shiny strategy, no new tech, and no marketing gimmick is going to cover that up. Passion doesn't pay the bills. Loyalty has limits.

Emily's story proves it: a rockstar CSR walked out the door for Starbucks because she couldn't afford to stay. Mark's story proves the opposite: transparency, fair pay, clear standards, and benefits people actually valued created zero turnover and booming loyalty. One hospital treated pay as a cost. The other treated it as a strategy. Guess who won?

Here's the truth: your team members are volunteers. Not literally, but close enough. They could walk out tomorrow and get hired at another clinic down the street. They *choose* to bring their energy, their heart, and their skill to you. That's a gift. And if you don't honor that, someone else will.

So, this is the foundation: fair pay, clear roles, and visible care from leadership. That's the floor. Miss it, and nothing else matters. Nail it, and you unlock the chance to build something bigger: a culture that doesn't just keep people but inspires them. A place where your team isn't just showing up for a paycheck, but for a mission.

And that's where we're headed next. Because once fairness is in place, the Veterinary Trust Flywheel has the initial foundation it needs to actually spin. And when it spins, it doesn't just retain teams—it creates pride, energy, trust, and momentum you can't fake.

Suggested Readings

Adams, J. Stacy. "Inequity in Social Exchange." In Leonard Berkowitz (Ed.), *Advances in Experimental Social Psychology* (vol. 2, pp. 267–299). Academic Press, 1965.

American Animal Hospital Association. *Stay, Please: Phase 2 — Retention and Relational Dynamics in Veterinary Medicine.* AAHA, 2024–2025, www.aaha.org/resources/stay-please-phase-2

American Veterinary Medical Association. *Economic State of the Veterinary Profession.* AVMA, 2024, www.avma.org/resources-tools/reports-statistics

Bureau of Labor Statistics, U.S. Department of Labor. *Occupational Employment and Wage Statistics: Veterinary Technologists and Technicians.* BLS, 2024, www.bls.gov

Colquitt, Jason A., et al. "Justice at the Millennium: A Meta-Analytic Review of 25 Years of Organizational Justice Research." *Journal of Applied Psychology*, vol. 86, no. 3, 2001, pp. 425–445.

Cornell University College of Veterinary Medicine, Center for Veterinary Business and Entrepreneurship. "Burnout Takes a Heavy Financial Toll on Veterinary Medicine." *Cornell Vet*, 29 Aug. 2022, www.vet.cornell.edu/about-us/news/20220829/burnout-takes-heavy-financial-toll-veterinary-medicine

Gallup, Inc. *State of the Global Workplace 2023 Report*. Gallup, 2023, www.gallup.com/workplace

Greenleaf, Robert K. *Servant Leadership: A Journey into the Nature of Legitimate Power and Greatness*. Paulist Press, 1977.

Sinek, Simon. "Customers Will Never Love a Company until the Employees Love It First." *Start with Why*, Portfolio, 2009.

Sinek, Simon. *Leaders Eat Last: Why Some Teams Pull Together and Others Don't*. Portfolio, 2014.

Veterinary Hospital Managers Association (VHMA). *Biennial Compensation & Benefits Survey*. VHMA, 2023, www.vhma.org

Chapter 5

Mission, Vision, and Values—The Clarity That Makes Everything Else Possible

Once fairness is in place, the real work begins. Because let's cut straight to the truth most veterinary hospitals never slow down long enough to face:

You can have the best medicine in town.
You can have brand-new equipment, Fear Free certifications, great intentions, and a lobby that smells like eucalyptus and hope.
But if your team lacks clarity on what they're working so hard for and has no clarity on what you stand for and are striving toward, they're playing a guessing game.

And guessing is the most expensive operational model in veterinary medicine.

The biggest myth in our profession is the idea that culture "just happens" if you hire the right people or work really hard. Nope. Culture doesn't appear. Culture is built intentionally and strategically.

In Chapter 6, we'll talk about what culture truly means, particularly in veterinary medicine. But the foundation of culture-building for any hospital—which we'll address here in this chapter—is clarity. That is: **Mission, Vision, and Values**. Not the cutesy Pinterest kind. Not the "we did this on a staff retreat and then never looked at it again" kind. Not the copy–paste from Google that looks like every other hospital's poster in every breakroom across the country. I'm talking weaponized clarity. Clarity so sharp that your team can operate when you disappear for a week. Clarity so detailed that a new grad can walk into your building and know exactly what "good" looks like by lunchtime. Clarity so embedded that no client, no doctor, no tech, and no Yelp warrior can push your culture off its rails.

Mission, Vision, and Values are not corporate fluff. They're the **operating system** that determines how your hospital thinks, moves, communicates, treats patients, and shows up for clients.

Let's get into it—the real version.
Not the Pinterest version.
Not the break-room-poster version.
The version that actually transforms a hospital.

VISION: The Decision That Defines Everything

Vision is a line drawn in the sand that says:

"This is the kind of veterinary hospital we are building, and everything we do needs to reinforce that future."

Vision is not a slogan. Vision is a freaking decision. What are you building? A boutique, relationship-driven primary care clinic with

Nordstrom service vibes? A dentistry powerhouse with recheck discipline and pain scoring tighter than Taylor Swift's tour choreography? An urgent-care-forward, access-driven machine that gets same-day appointments done with humanity and speed?

Pick. A. Lane.

If your vision is "we do everything for everyone," congratulations— you built confusion, not a brand. And you can't scale fog. Vision is saying: "THIS is who we are. THIS is who we are not." It's trade-offs. It's discipline. It's choosing excellence over comfort every single day.

A few examples from real veterinary life:

- Are you a gold-standard dentistry hospital, where every patient gets full-mouth radiographs, pain scoring, and tailored prevention? If yes, then everything—training, scheduling, recheck systems, pricing, and client education—should reflect that.
- Are you an access-driven, same-day-service hospital, built to reduce community overwhelm? If yes, you design workflows around speed, clarity, and predictable triage.
- Are you a relationship-first primary care practice, where every appointment is about trust, communication, and long-term partnership? If yes, then maybe you build longer appointment blocks, champion advanced client communication training, and develop a continuity-of-care model.

The wrong vision is "We do everything for everyone." That's not a vision—that's a fog machine.

Fog doesn't scale.
Fog doesn't attract talent.
Fog doesn't build client loyalty.
Fog doesn't create consistency.

Your hospital's Vision is the North Star your team aligns around— the filter for decisions, the anchor for standards, the story you tell clients, and the direction your practice grows.

MISSION: The Emotional Machine of the Hospital

Let's talk Mission, and not the fluffy version. Not "we strive to provide compassionate care." We get it. You like pets. Everyone here likes pets. That's not a mission.

Mission answers one raw question: "Why the hell do we grind this hard?" And if your team can't answer it? They don't work for a purpose. They work for appointments and chaos. And chaos burns people out faster than Cerenia will stop vomiting. You want talent to stay? Give them meaning, not pizza parties.

Your Mission is not "providing compassionate care."
Every veterinary hospital on planet Earth could say that.
It's so generic; it barely means anything anymore.

A Mission is why this hospital exists, in this community, with these people, serving these pets.

Veterinary medicine is hard.
It's emotional.
It's unpredictable.
And when your team is in the trenches, they need more than "be nice to animals." They need purpose.

Real mission sounds like:

- "To strengthen the bond between pets and families through proactive, relationship-centered veterinary care."
- "To elevate oral health and quality of life through dentistry delivered with precision, empathy, and excellence."
- "To create accessible, same-day veterinary care that combines speed with humanity."

Mission is what keeps your team grounded when caseload spikes.
Mission is what keeps your team steady when they're delivering hard news.

Mission is what makes a CSR say, "Let's see how we can help," instead of "We're booked."

Mission is what gets you up when a client sobs to you over the phone at 10 p.m. Mission is what carries you through a euthanasia where a kid whispers "thank you for helping my best friend."

Mission gives meaning to the grind. And meaning is the antidote to burnout.

VALUES: The Behavioral Rules of the Game

Values are not posters. Values are rules. They are the difference between culture and daycare.

Values are behaviors you can see, coach, hire for, fire for, and reward. If your values don't influence who you hire, who you fire, what behaviors you reward, how you talk to clients, how you coach new grads, and how you handle conflict, then they're not values—they're wall art. And wall-art values build resentment and turnover. Values with teeth build culture that prints trust, retention, and profitability on repeat.

Another way to think about it: values are how you want people to act when no one is watching and things are chaotic.

Good values don't sound like corporate jargon. Real values sound like:

- "We explain medicine in clear, human language—no jargon, no ego."
- "We close loops—with clients, with each other, and with every patient handoff."
- "We treat each other with respect, even on hard days."
- "We advocate for pets boldly and consistently, even when conversations are uncomfortable."

- "We train kindly and correct directly."
- "We own mistakes without hiding them and fix them fast."

Values with teeth change everything. They shape:

- how rechecks are handled
- how conflicts are resolved
- how clients are educated
- how technicians step into leadership
- how Client Service Representatives (CSRs) communicate estimates
- how onboarding is done
- how doctors align on standards
- how the team advocates for care
- how psychological safety is built
- and so much more.

Values aren't what you say. Values are what you enforce.

They're the backbone of trust. They're the backbone of consistency. They're the backbone of your hospital's identity.

Why This Matters So Much More than People Think

Mission, Vision, and Values create predictability and clarity, which create trust—internally and externally.

Here's what happens when you get this right:

- Your team stops guessing and starts executing.
- New hires become confident faster.
- Doctors stop practicing in silos.
- Techs anticipate next steps instead of waiting for instructions.
- CSRs speak with authority instead of hesitating.
- Client trust skyrockets because your hospital feels unified.
- Efficiency improves because alignment reduces friction.
- Mistakes go down because everyone knows "how we do things here."

- Medical consistency improves across every doctor and shift.
- Psychological safety increases because people feel anchored.
- The hospital becomes easier to lead, not harder.

When a team knows *who they are*, they perform like it.

Mission = meaning
Vision = direction
Values = behavior

Together, they form the **infrastructure of a healthy, powerful, unified veterinary hospital**.

The Gold Is in the Process

The real value in defining Mission, Vision, and Values lies in the process of having your team define them collaboratively. Defining these things doesn't mean a hospital leader sitting on a beach in Bermuda and returning to inform the team what the hospital's Mission, Vision, and Values are, because your team will look at them and go, "Well, looks like you had fun on the beach. But those are not my values."

Your team needs to be involved in the process. And in my experience helping hundreds of hospitals through these exercises, here's what I can promise you: your team will never pick a bad value, I promise. You'll hear words like trusted, valued, empowered, integrity, etc. And when your team is intimately involved in defining their hospital's Mission, Vision, and Values, they'll stay much more committed to them.

Later in this book, I'll walk you step-by-step through how to build these with your team. And in the Appendix, I'll give you the exact facilitation guide I use for my Veterinary Hospital Identity Workshop with practices across the country—the one that transforms culture from "accidental" to "intentional" in a matter of weeks.

Because once you get this right? You're off to the races. Everything—and I mean *everything*—gets easier.

Suggested Readings

Collins, Jim, and Jerry I. Porras. *Built to Last: Successful Habits of Visionary Companies.* HarperBusiness, 2004.

Cotton, John L., et al. "Employee Participation: Diverse Forms and Different Outcomes." *Academy of Management Review*, vol. 13, no. 1, 1988, pp. 8–22.

Deci, Edward L., and Richard M. Ryan. *Intrinsic Motivation and Self-determination in Human Behavior.* Plenum Press, 1985.

Edmondson, Amy C. *The Fearless Organization: Creating Psychological Safety in the Workplace for Learning, Innovation, and Growth.* Wiley, 2019.

Gallup, Inc. *State of the Global Workplace 2023 Report.* Gallup, 2023, www.gallup.com/workplace.

Hackman, J. Richard, and Greg R. Oldham. "Motivation through the Design of Work: Test of a Theory." *Organizational Behavior and Human Performance*, vol. 16, no. 2, 1976, pp. 250–279.

Kanter, Rosabeth Moss. *The Change Masters: Innovation for Productivity in the American Corporation.* Simon & Schuster, 1983.

Kotter, John P. *Leading Change.* Harvard Business School Press, 1996.

Latham, Gary P., and Edwin A. Locke. "New Developments in and Directions for Goal-Setting Research." *European Psychologist*, vol. 12, no. 4, 2007, pp. 290–300.

Maslow, Abraham H. "A Theory of Human Motivation." *Psychological Review*, vol. 50, no. 4, 1943, pp. 370–396.

O'Reilly, Charles A., Jennifer A. Chatman, and David F. Caldwell. "People and Organizational Culture: A Profile Comparison Approach to Assessing Person–Organization Fit." *Academy of Management Journal*, vol. 34, no. 3, 1991, pp. 487–516.

Schein, Edgar H. *Organizational Culture and Leadership.* 5th ed., Wiley, 2016.

Sinek, Simon. *Start with Why: How Great Leaders Inspire Everyone to Take Action.* Portfolio, 2009.

Wrzesniewski, Amy, et al. "Jobs, Careers, and Callings: People's Relations to Their Work." *Journal of Research in Personality*, vol. 31, no. 1, 1997, pp. 21–33.

Chapter 6
Establish Actual Culture

Mission, Vision, and Values are the blueprint of the entire damn building. They're the bedrock upon which you build culture: you can't build a culture on vibes and hope. If you skip this step, your culture becomes whatever the loudest tech, grumpiest doctor, or most stressed-out manager decides it is that day. But when your team knows why you exist, where you're going, and how you operate, you finally create a shared truth everyone can rally around. That clarity becomes the filter for who you hire, who you coach, what you tolerate, and what you shut down instantly. And once every decision and behavior ladders back to those three anchors, culture stops being an accident and starts becoming a weapon. That's the foundation that actually lets the Veterinary Trust Flywheel catch fire and spin with force.

Culture is the discipline to bring your Mission, Vision, and Values to life. Culture is systems. Culture is clarity for your team. Culture is performance psychology.

When a hospital team lacks the clarity that a Mission and Vision create and guidance of values and a true culture, it's an emotional free-for-all:

- Every doctor has their own idea of "good medicine."
- Every Client Service Representative (CSR) explains care differently.
- Every tech prioritizes tasks based on who trained them last.
- Every new hire spends six months trying to decode "how we do things here."
- Every tough moment becomes a tug-of-war instead of a unified response.

Not because people don't care—but because the hospital never defined who it is. And teams can't align around a ghost.

So, let's talk about culture and what it really means. If you find it to be a bit of an ill-defined buzzword that's thrown around in a lot of different contexts, you're not alone. But culture is real and does mean something concrete. Understanding what culture is and how it needs to be applied is crucial toward setting the Flywheel in motion.

Why Culture Matters

I'll start by giving you some well-deserved grace: if you're tired, overwhelmed, frustrated with team drama, buried in "urgent but not important," and secretly wondering whether you're running a practice or babysitting adults in scrubs, you're not broken—you're normal. I've walked into more veterinary clinics than I can count—specialty centers with MRI machines and granite countertops, strip-mall clinics with duct tape on exam tables, global flagship hospitals in cities where a latte costs $14, and rural clinics where you have to ask three times if this road is actually a road. And across all of them, everybody thinks their chaos is unique. It isn't. The same patterns exist in Milan and Miami and Stockholm and Seattle. When there's a human–animal bond and veterinarians trying to care for patients, you see the same friction points, the same emotional load, the same belief traps, the same "we're doing pretty good, all things considered" energy, and the same excuses.

That's exactly why this chapter matters. Because the difference between a hospital that thrives—where clients are loyal, teams stay, doctors are energized, revenue grows, and you feel proud walking in—and a hospital that survives—where the days blur, people snap, standards slip, and leaders feel like walking conflict-management machines—is culture. Not medicine. Not equipment. Not your CE portfolio. Culture. Period.

So, let's start where most veterinary conversations don't: with the truth. Not the polite version. Not the conference-stage version. The actual truth the profession whispers in break rooms and parking lots and therapy offices and in the quiet moments alone with the clinic lights off after a hard day.

Veterinary medicine isn't broken because of clients. It isn't broken because of the economy. It isn't broken because of "kids today" or online pharmacies or Dr. Google or student debt or staffing shortages.

Those are pressure points, not root causes.

The real fracture? The core fracture?

We built a profession on compassion and science and forgot the operating system that sustains both: culture.

When culture works, everything else compounds: medicine, compliance, case acceptance, client trust, team retention, and joy. When culture breaks, everything else becomes heavy: recruiting, conversations, case progression, referrals, revenue, reputation, and you name it.

Culture isn't seasoning. Culture is the damn foundation. And if the foundation isn't poured right? Everything on top cracks eventually—no matter how pretty you make the lobby.

Beliefs That Sabotage Veterinary Hospital Culture

If We Just Do Good Medicine, Everything Else Will Follow

There is a lie baked into this industry so deeply that people repeat it like gospel, which I believe have cost our industry billions of dollars:

"If we just do good medicine, everything else will follow."

Hard stop. No. False. Wrong century. Wrong economy. Wrong psychology. Wrong operating model. Just ... wrong. That may have been true in 1972 when pet care was transactional and expectations were low, and there weren't a thousand voices online telling clients how to think about you before they ever walked through your door.

Today? Clients expect excellence. Clients expect partnership. Clients expect advocacy with empathy. Clients expect follow-through, clarity, guidance, and actual communication—not a rushed, exhausted lecture delivered mid-sentence while someone else is knocking on the exam room door asking how many more patients you can squeeze in that day.

Good medicine is, of course, extremely important, but it is the price of admission. It's the baseline. It's expected. If good medicine alone built great practices, the most technically talented vets would be running empires. They aren't. Plenty are burned out, frustrated, under-earning, and quietly resentful of the weight they carry. Because great medicine without great culture is a Ferrari with no brakes. Looks impressive, but doesn't get far. And ... Crashes often. Good medicine is like brakes on a car. Nobody buys a car because the brakes work. Likewise, veterinary clients don't return to your hospital just because of solid medicine. They return because of trust, experience, relationship, consistency, emotional safety, clarity of communication, and the belief that you care as much as they do.

They return because they can *feel* your hospital's culture.

When you cling to "good medicine alone is enough," you unintentionally create a silent expectation that everything else should magically fall into place. And when it doesn't—because magic isn't a business model—you get bitterness, exhaustion, "no one cares like I do," and the slow erosion of the joy that brought you into this field in the first place.

Culture isn't the soft stuff. It's not the team-building pizza party crap people talk about to sound progressive. **Culture is discipline. Culture is the system. Culture is performance psychology**. It's the environment that either unlocks excellence or chokes it out. When culture is strong and the Flywheel gains its momentum, the medicine naturally levels up, clients feel it, your staff advocates instead of avoids, your revenue rises without you begging for compliance, and the practice becomes a place where talent wants to work. When culture is weak, everything falls on your shoulders, every decision is a negotiation, people start hiding mistakes instead of solving them, and medicine becomes a coin flip—who's in the room, what mood they're in, and whether the client "looks like someone who can afford it."

If that hits a nerve, good. That's the point. Because change doesn't start with new software, new DVMs, or new exam tables. Change starts with new beliefs. Most veterinary practices aren't held back by competition or the economy or "client compliance." They're held back by invisible ceilings of belief—leaders who think clients won't pay, teams who think advocacy equals being pushy, and owners who think "we're like family" is a flex when really it's code for blurred boundaries, inconsistent accountability, and emotional landmines disguised as teamwork.

We're Like Family

Okay, we've addressed the "If we just do good medicine, everything else will follow" myth. Now, let's go right after our other sacred cow: "We're like a family here."

The number of practices I've walked into where the owner proudly says, "We're like family here," and my gut instantly goes, *"Oh God, here we go again,"* is staggering.

Here's the truth that might make you uncomfortable: **Your practice is not a family**.

To be clear—I love my family, a lot. And I get it: family is wonderful. Family is beautiful. Family means loyalty and love and unconditional support. But family can also mean unspoken resentment, emotional landmines, "we don't talk about that," and a permission structure for behavior that would get you fired anywhere else.

In the real world? Family is where standards go to die if you're not careful.

Families tolerate dysfunction. High-performance teams eliminate it.

Families overlook accountability. High-performance teams demand it.

Families protect familiarity. High-performance teams protect standards.

At one hospital I worked with—let's call it Redwood Animal Health—the owner loved to say, *"We're family here."* And on the surface, it looked true—birthday cupcakes, baby showers, and group selfies in matching Christmas scrubs.

But behind the sugar frosting was resentment. One tech kept showing up late, and no one corrected her because she had "been here forever." A doctor routinely snapped at assistants, but *"that's just how she is."* Everyone tiptoed around conflict.

Then the practice manager quit. In her exit interview, she didn't cry. She didn't yell. She simply said: *"I love these people. But loving people and being able to grow with them aren't always the same thing."*

Redwood didn't need more cupcakes. They needed accountability—and clarity—and leadership with the guts to protect culture, not nostalgia.

Great teams aren't families. Families protect comfort. A hospital runs on **shared identity, shared standards, and shared accountability.** Calling your clinic a family is often a permission slip for drama, resentment, and sweeping issues under the rug. It's time to grow out of that. You are a professional organization serving medical needs—with empathy, yes—but also with clarity, systems, expectations, and purpose.

Our Hospital Is the Exception

Let's get brutally honest: the single most expensive problem in veterinary medicine isn't payroll, drugs, equipment, or rent. It's **belief-based revenue loss**. This is the silent assassin killing patient outcomes and killing your profitability while smiling politely at the front desk. So many hospitals are bleeding out not because clients don't care, but because too many teams walk into exam rooms already convinced they know what clients won't do.

Flawed beliefs sabotage client interactions in exam rooms every day:

"These clients don't want diagnostics."

"This community can't afford dentistry."

"Nobody will pay for prevention."

They're total fiction, confidence without data, myths repeated so often people think they're true. Meanwhile, pets suffer, revenue evaporates, team pride erodes, and everyone wonders why burnout keeps climbing. Spoiler: because **beliefs run behavior**. And your beliefs about clients are shaping your medicine more than your medical training is.

Let's call it what it is: self-sabotage disguised as humility.

Every time someone on your team—doctor, tech, CSR, kennel kid, doesn't matter—walks into a room and decides in their head, *"These people won't go for diagnostics,"* they aren't being empathetic.

They aren't "protecting" the client. They're projecting. They are pre-declining care on behalf of someone who hasn't even been offered the chance to care yet. It's medical gaslighting, but aimed at yourself.

We have turned assumptions into policy. We have turned doubt into standard operating procedure. We have mistaken pessimism for client advocacy.

"People here won't pay for that."

Bullshit. Show me your data. Show me your compliance dashboards. Show me the actual numbers, not your gut emotion at 4:30 p.m. when you're tired and frustrated and three clients in a row made you feel like you're negotiating for their attention instead of their pet's life.

I once visited a small-town practice in eastern Oregon—logging community, dusty trucks everywhere, two diners, one grocery store, and a blinking red light instead of a traffic signal. Median household income? About 40 grand. The kind of place outsiders would point at and say, "Oh, people there only want bare-bones care. They can't afford real medicine."

Except this hospital crushed that stereotype into powder.

Four doctors. Every single one of them grossing north of $800K a year. Not because they were upselling. Not because they were aggressive. Because they believed—unapologetically—that every pet deserved gold-standard medicine whether the postal code screamed "wealth" or not. They didn't play small. They didn't "treat based on perceived affordability." They didn't water down care because of assumptions.

They ran full-service everything. Comprehensive dentistry—not "cleanings when it smells bad," but proper periodontal protocol. Internal medicine that looked like a specialty department in a metro area. Preventive care dialed in like religion: heartworm, flea/tick, lab work, and weight management. Client education is so consistent the community could probably teach CE courses themselves.

And here's where it gets beautiful—they put their money where their mouth was. They invested $2,500 per tech, per year, in CE and travel to conferences. Not just "when the budget allows." Not "when the schedule is slow." Every. Single. Year. They treated growth like oxygen, not a reward.

When I asked the owner why they were so committed to this level of care and development, he said something I will never forget: "I refuse to teach my team we live in a 'poor town.' That's not a diagnosis. It's a mindset. We show our community what's possible—and they meet us there."

Boom.

He told me about a rancher who once came in with a 12-year-old Cattle Dog. Full dental disease. Pain. Infection. Liver values creeping. This rancher walked in with oil-stained hands and boots older than some of the techs. In most hospitals, someone would've prejudged immediately—*He's not going to go for diagnostics. Just give antibiotics and pray.*

Not here. They presented full care. Diagnostics. Dentistry. Pain control. Follow-ups. Full plan. Educated, not assumed. The rancher listened, nodded, then said, "Do whatever she needs. She's worked beside me her whole life. She deserves it." $2,200 invoice. Paid in full. No blink. No resentment. No drama.

Most clients don't say no to care. They say no to feeling judged, rushed, or underestimated. They say no when they don't understand the why. They say no when nobody bothered to believe they might say yes.

This town, this so-called "economically limited" community, didn't need pity. They needed leadership. They needed someone to raise the standard first, not wait for the standard to magically rise.

And here's what else they were seeing:
Staff turnover? Nearly nonexistent.
Client loyalty? Unreal.
Profitability? Through the roof.
Reputation? Legendary in the region.

Not because the town was rich ... *but because the practice's mind-set was.*

They didn't wait for the population to earn more money. They didn't look at census data and decide what medicine to offer. They decided who they were first—and then built a community around that standard.

They didn't say, "People here won't do it." They said, "Our job is to advocate. Their job is to decide."

Once you run your hospital through that lens? Everything changes. The ceiling blows off. The care elevates. The community rises to meet you. And suddenly, you realize scarcity was never financial—it was cultural.

Meanwhile, I've seen more practices in wealthy suburbs than I can count acting broke because their mindset was broke.

The problem isn't ZIP codes. It's headspace. Our job is to be advocates, not accountants in exam rooms. The moment your brain decides, *"They can't afford it,"* you've stopped being a doctor or credentialed tech or trained CSR and started being a cashier with a stethoscope. You're practicing wallet medicine, not veterinary medicine.

And look, I get it. You've got emotional scar tissue. Everyone in vet med does. You offered care once, twice, a hundred times, and you got burned with a "Let me think about it," or a blank stare, or a lecture about "just a dog." So now you play small. You pre-edit. You shrink your recommendations like you're apologizing for caring too much.

But shrinking never saved a life. Playing small never built trust. And low expectations never built great medicine.

So, let me rip the Band-Aid off:

Assumptions kill patients faster than disease sometimes.

When you assume someone "can't" or "won't," you steal their chance to say yes. You rob them of informed consent. You rob the pet of health. You rob your team of pride. And then you sit around wondering why burnout is up and morale is down.

Burnout isn't always about workload—sometimes, it's about the heartbreak of not living up to the medicine you swore you'd practice.

Every time you don't offer dentistry, periodontal disease wins. Every time you skip diagnostics, pathology keeps growing. Every time you soften your language to avoid discomfort, disease progresses quietly.

And here's the kicker—your team feels that. They *know* when they're not advocating at their best. They *feel* when they've lowered the bar. Which means slowly, painfully, their professional identity erodes.

You think it's "being nice" or "being realistic." They feel it as "we aren't the hospital I thought we were." That's culture rot. And it starts inside someone's skull long before it shows up on your P&L or your Google reviews.

Beliefs shape recommendations. Recommendations shape outcomes. Outcomes shape trust and lifetime value. And lifetime value shapes legacy.

So, no—culture isn't established by throwing pizza parties. **Culture is established when leaders establish and reinforce healthy belief systems that your team carries into every appointment**.

So, stop deciding what clients will or won't do. Instead, start educating them so they can tell you what they truly value.

Stop letting fear set the ceiling. Instead, start letting conviction set the floor.

Never let your team forget: your team's job is not to *offer services*. It's to **lead people to the best possible health outcomes for the beings they love**.

If you believe you're in the business of transactions, you've already lost. You're in the business of trust. You're in the business of influence. You're in the business of extending the good years and minimizing the suffering ones.

You don't sell diagnostics; you sell clarity.
You don't sell dentistry; you sell dignity and comfort.
You don't sell prevention; you sell more time together: extra Christmas mornings, more snoring at the foot of the bed, more walks, more stupid tennis balls, and more family memories. That is the product. Everything else is just a delivery mechanism.

Beliefs aren't soft; they are the steering wheel of your entire hospital. If you don't set them intentionally, they will default to insecurity, exhaustion, and scarcity—and that's how great practices become average and average practices become ghost towns.

Let's get tactical about this. I strongly hold that every high-performing practice has preferred care pathways: wellness, dermatology, senior care, chronic pain, obesity, GI upset, dentistry, cardiology, and behavioral support—not scripts, pathways. Clear starting points. Clear policies. Clear language. Clear expectations.

Weak cultures will tell a coughing dog owner, "Let's try antibiotics first." Strong cultures explain, "Coughing can mean everything from allergies to heart disease. The fastest way to give your pet comfort and protect them is imaging and bloodwork—let's take a look together."

One is guessing. The other is guiding.
One is fear. The other is leadership.

You can't scale a business on doubt. You scale on conviction, clarity, and courage to recommend what pets *actually* need.

Raise your belief ceiling.
Raise your care.
Raise your outcomes.
Raise your legacy.

That's culture. That's leadership. That's medicine that wins.

Why So Many Practice Owners Get Stuck

Let's talk about the traps that quietly choke practices—not because owners don't care, but because they care so damn much they smother the business instead of scaling it. If you see yourself in any of these, good. Awareness is the starting line. Denial is the prison.

Superhero Syndrome: The "If I Don't Touch It, It Will Break" Lie

You know this person. Or let's be real, maybe you are this person. The owner who claims it's about "quality control," but really, they can't stand handing anything off. The "if I don't personally intervene, everything breaks" leader. The one who runs the business like it's being powered by their adrenaline, caffeine, and existential dread instead of systems and people. They don't delegate—they hoard control and call it excellence. But it isn't excellence; it's exhaustion dressed up as heroism. Let me slap a truth bomb down on the table:

If your hospital only runs well when you're physically present, you haven't built a business—you've built a hostage situation. And the hostage is you.

You checking every invoice isn't quality. You approving every treatment plan isn't high standards. You micromanaging every client interaction isn't excellence.

It's fear, dressed up as leadership.

You don't trust your systems, because you don't have any. You don't trust your team, because you never empowered them. You don't trust outcomes, because everything lives inside your brain.

You're not being a hero—you're being the single point of failure.

Systems don't make you less necessary—they make your legacy possible.

You want consistent care? Standardize it.
You want team autonomy? Train for it.
You want freedom? Let go of the wheel and build the car so it drives straight.

Every practice that scales knows this truth: if the medicine drops when you leave the building, that's not a doctor problem—that's a leadership problem.

Conflict Avoidance Disguised as Kindness

Veterinary medicine has a PhD in people-pleasing. We're wired to soothe, support, comfort, and protect. And that's beautiful ... until it becomes the reason your standards collapse. Telling yourself "I don't want to hurt their feelings" is just a cute way of saying "I don't have the guts to lead."

Avoiding direct conversations doesn't protect your team. It traps them in mediocrity. It suffocates their growth. It breeds resentment in high performers. It signals to your best people that excellence is optional and excellence is the only reason they came.

You think you're being nice, but you're actually being selfish.

You don't want *your* discomfort. You don't want *their* reaction. You don't want to feel like "the bad guy." But leadership is not for the comfort-addicted. In truth, radical candor isn't cruelty; it's respect. And silence isn't kindness; it's abandonment.

In other words: your team deserves clarity, not vibes.

Fear of Losing Staff: The Culture Cancer

Nothing destroys culture faster than saying: "We can't lose them."

Yes. You can. In fact, sometimes you must. Because the minute you protect the wrong person, you sacrifice the right ones. Every great practice I've studied had a moment where leadership said: "I will not negotiate my standards to keep someone comfortable." And every struggling practice had a moment where leadership whispered: *"Let's just put up with it … we can't afford to lose them."*

Guess what? The day you said that, you already lost something bigger than that employee: you lost psychological safety. You lost accountability. You lost the moral authority to coach. You lost the respect of your best performers. You lost your standards, the heartbeat of your culture.

People don't quit jobs. They quit tolerance. They quit inconsistency. They quit environments where excellence is optional and chaos is rewarded with job security.

If someone holds your culture hostage, they're not an asset. They're a liability disguised as talent. And your A-players are watching. Your future leaders are watching. Your reputation is watching.

You don't lose people by holding standards. You lose them by not holding them.

Culture Is Your Operating System

Most people still think "culture" is about vibes—smiles, morale, a Top Golf outing, some branded hoodies, a pizza party, and a hope that everyone magically buys in. Let me be blunt: **culture is not a vibe. Culture is the operating system of your hospital**. You can remodel your lobby, install new software, hire more techs, and squeeze more appointments—but if your operating system is broken, everything else is lipstick on a cracked foundation.

Every hospital runs on one of two systems: intentional culture or accidental culture. One produces excellence. The other quietly sabotages everything you're trying to build. Most leaders keep trying to fix chaos with tactics—better scheduling, more meetings, and new protocols—while ignoring the underlying code. That's why giants like United Airlines and even the Cleveland Clinic stumbled: they tried to fix outcomes without fixing culture.

Culture starts long before the first patient of the day. It shapes who you hire, how you onboard, and whether you're building confident professionals or overwhelmed staff terrified of making a mistake. It dictates how your team communicates when things are busy, when a patient crashes, when a client is upset, or when exhaustion sets in. It determines whether team members boldly educate clients—or freeze up because they're unsure, unsupported, or afraid of being wrong.

Culture is the difference between consistent, proactive medicine and reactive, "just survive the day" medicine. It's the difference between a transactional appointment and a transformational healthcare experience that clients rave about. It becomes the lens for every decision, the language for every interaction, and the heartbeat behind every patient moment. Until a leader sees culture this way, they will always be fighting fires instead of preventing them.

There are only two cultural realities: Toxic/Accidental or Healthy/Intentional. Mediocre cultures drift until they rot.

Toxic/Accidental Culture

Toxic culture isn't always loud; often, it's quiet, hidden, and creeping. It shows up as reactive medicine—late diagnoses, missed preventive opportunities, and constant firefighting. It sounds like "everyone does it differently," because there is no shared philosophy or consistent playbook. It feels like churned-out appointments rather than relationship-driven healthcare.

In toxic cultures, client education becomes inconsistent or non-existent. Team members hesitate to speak up. Doctors cut corners because they're exhausted or don't believe the team can support best practices. Fear and defensiveness shape behavior. People avoid problems, distrust each other, and operate with a survival mindset. And revenue leaks everywhere—**not** because clients are cheap, but because belief barriers suffocate your team's ability to advocate.

Healthy/Intentional Culture

Healthy culture feels completely different. It creates preferred pathways to health, not just reactions to whatever walks in. It aligns every team member behind a unified care philosophy and a shared language. Appointments become empathetic, educational, and empowering experiences. Clients feel guided, understood, and cared for.

As the Veterinary Trust Flywheel shows, when culture is healthy, team consistency fuels client trust. Trust fuels compliance. Compliance fuels better outcomes. Better outcomes drive revenue as a natural byproduct—not as the primary goal. Healthy culture is built on shared identity, standards, and accountability. When it's in place, people grow, contribute, stay, and refer. The hospital evolves into the kind of place clients and professionals fight to be part of.

You Don't Sell Medicine ... You Sell Meaning

Clients don't come to you for rabies shots, X-rays, or dental cleanings. They come for peace of mind, for clarity, for guidance, for dignity, for partnership—and ultimately, for more time with the heartbeat sleeping at their feet.

Nike sells shoes. Chipotle sells burritos. You sell maximizing vitality and minimizing suffering for their pet.

When you forget that, culture slides into "treating cases" instead of serving lives.

And here's the truth: poor culture always shows up in medical decisions. Always.
It shows up in "try antibiotics first" medicine.
It shows up when CSRs send clients to Costco for meds because "it's cheaper."
It shows up in inconsistent recommendations, weak advocacy, and exhausted teams doing the bare minimum to get through the day.

Culture and Valuation: The Hard Financial Truth

My time working in veterinary acquisitions has taught me additional lessons about the value and importance of healthy culture: weak culture leaks into compliance rates, client loyalty, turnover, reviews—and eventually, your practice valuation. When you go to sell your practice (if you choose to someday), buyers don't just buy your profit. They buy your culture engine—or they discount your lack of one. Two practices with identical profit can differ in sale price by over a million dollars because one has trust, systems, stability, and empowered staff—and the other has dependency, dysfunction, and chaos.

Investors don't pay for what you did. They pay for what they believe your hospital will consistently do without you holding it together by sheer willpower.

A culture of trust and clarity? Worth multiples more. A culture where no one speaks up and the owner makes every decision? Sympathy offers.

The marketplace pays for predictability, trust, accountability, leadership depth, consistent medicine, and systems that scale. Not stress. Not intensity. Not martyrdom.

What a Culture-driven Hospital Actually Looks Like

A culture-driven practice doesn't happen by accident. It looks like:

- Leaders who know their values and repeat them until they become muscle memory.
- Teams are empowered to make decisions because trust is earned and reinforced.
- Leaders who catch people doing things right 10 times more often than catching mistakes.
- The courage to remove toxic high-producers because culture outranks volume.
- Client communication training is treated with the same seriousness as surgical training.
- Onboarding that indoctrinates behavior, not just "how to use the software."
- Exam rooms where team members confidently explain: *"Here's what's going on. Here's what we recommend. Here's why it matters. And here's how we'll partner with you to give your pet the longest, healthiest life possible."*

And yes, data matters. Not for judgment, for growth. Tracking diagnostics, dentistry, rechecks, prevention, and follow-ups isn't about numbers. It's about truth. Culture isn't "everyone gets along." **Culture is alignment + accountability in service of higher standards and better outcomes**.

Culture Isn't Dessert. It's the Ingredients

The biggest mistake leaders make is treating culture as a perk or a luxury—something to work on after the next fire is put out. That's backward.

Culture isn't what you fix last. Culture is what you build first.

When you take culture seriously—build it intentionally, reinforce it relentlessly, protect it fiercely—you stop reacting and start architecting. You prevent fires instead of fighting them. You stop being the bottleneck and start being the catalyst. You stop hoping your hospital improves and start designing a hospital that stays excellent.

Culture is your operating system.
Culture is your competitive advantage.
Culture is your trust engine.
Build it right, and the Veterinary Trust Flywheel doesn't just spin—it catches fire.

Teams don't burn out from hard work. They burn out from meaningless work, inconsistent leadership, low trust, and standards that slip without consequence. Your job is to build a place where excellence feels normal, advocacy is expected, kindness is practiced, and accountability is respected.

Do this, and you won't just have a profitable practice. You'll have a legacy.

A culture people talk about. A place people fight to work. A client base that evangelizes your name. A business that prints trust, loyalty, fulfillment—and yes, profit.

Great medicine matters. But great culture makes great medicine inevitable.

Example 1: The Dental Turnaround

A hospital on the East Coast had three doctors, all with wildly different philosophies on dentistry. One recommended full-mouth rads every time, one only recommended them when "needed," and one hated dentistry entirely.

After building clarity, alignment, and psychological safety, the team committed to a unified standard:

Every dental is a full-mouth rad dental. Period.

They trained, built scripts, fixed bottlenecks, and aligned the entire hospital.

Result?

- Dental compliance increased 42%
- Average dental revenue doubled
- Post-op calls dropped in half because pain scoring and anesthesia protocols were optimized
- Patients had better outcomes
- Clients raved
- The team felt proud because their care had consistency

That increased revenue?
It funded:

- heated surgical tables
- new monitoring equipment
- advanced training for two technicians
- a raise for the CSR supervisor

Better medicine → better business → better culture → better medicine.

That's the Flywheel.

Example 2: The Recheck Revolution

A hospital in the Midwest struggled with rechecks.
Nobody knew whose job it was.
CSRs didn't schedule them.
Doctors assumed techs would.
Techs assumed CSRs would.
Clients left without clarity.

The team invested in client experience standards and scripting, not just medical training. And it worked.

They built psychological safety around speaking up:

- CSRs started asking for rechecks confidently
- Techs reinforced value
- Doctors explained "why" instead of just "what"

Outcome?

- Recheck compliance increased 37%
- Chronic diseases were caught earlier
- Patients stabilized faster
- The emotional burden on doctors decreased
- Clients trusted the team more
- Revenue increased *without adding appointments*
- That additional revenue paid for an extra technician, reducing burnout

That's the power of culture.

The secret to veterinary success is embarrassingly simple: do the common things uncommonly well, with clarity, heart, and zero compromise on your standards and identity.

That's how you win.
That's how you lead.
That's how you change this profession from the inside out.
And that's how you build a practice—and a life—you're damn proud of.

Suggested Readings

Collins, Jim. *Good to Great: Why Some Companies Make the Leap... and Others Don't.* HarperBusiness, 2001.

DeBowes, Richard M. *Turning Profit into Long-Term Value.* Presentation, Washington State University, 2025.

Edmondson, Amy C. *The Fearless Organization: Creating Psychological Safety in the Workplace for Learning, Innovation, and Growth.* Wiley, 2019.

Goleman, Daniel. *Primal Leadership: Unleashing the Power of Emotional Intelligence*. Harvard Business School Press, 2002.

Heath, Chip, and Dan Heath. *Decisive: How to Make Better Choices in Life and Work*. Crown Business, 2013.

Kahneman, Daniel. *Thinking, Fast and Slow*. Farrar, Straus and Giroux, 2011.

Kotter, John P. *Leading Change*. Harvard Business School Press, 1996.

Lencioni, Patrick. *The Five Dysfunctions of a Team: A Leadership Fable*. Jossey-Bass, 2002.

Maslow, Abraham H. "A Theory of Human Motivation." *Psychological Review*, vol. 50, no. 4, 1943, pp. 370–396.

O'Reilly, Charles A., Jennifer A. Chatman, and David F. Caldwell. "People and Organizational Culture: A Profile Comparison Approach to Assessing Person–Organization Fit." *Academy of Management Journal*, vol. 34, no. 3, 1991, pp. 487–516.

Pfeffer, Jeffrey. *The Human Equation: Building Profits by Putting People First*. Harvard Business School Press, 1998.

Schein, Edgar H. *Organizational Culture and Leadership*. 5th ed., Wiley, 2016.

Sinek, Simon. *Leaders Eat Last: Why Some Teams Pull Together and Others Don't*. Portfolio, 2014.

Thaler, Richard H., and Cass R. Sunstein. *Nudge: Improving Decisions About Health, Wealth, and Happiness*. Yale University Press, 2008.

Chapter 7

Embrace a Servant Leadership Style

Opening Story: Dr. Halloran's Hospital

Before we get into servant leadership, let me tell you a story I've seen play out in a dozen different ZIP codes.

Let's call him Dr. Halloran—brilliant clinician, beloved by clients, and absolute force of nature in a 1,200-sq-ft building with too many patients and not enough oxygen.

He didn't mean to monopolize the hospital.
He didn't *try* to be the sun everyone orbited.
He just ... became it.

Because when something mattered, he stepped in.
When something broke, he fixed it.
When someone hesitated, he took over.
When a decision needed to be made, he made it before the question even left someone's mouth.

And in the beginning? It **worked**. He kept the hospital alive on caffeine, adrenaline, and sheer willpower. Clients adored him.

Team members bragged about "working with a legend." Every problem funneled to him, and he took pride in being the guy who could handle it all.

But slowly—almost invisibly—his hospital stopped being a hospital and became a museum of one man's competence. The techs stopped making decisions because "Dr. H will want it done his way." The Client Service Representatives (CSRs) stopped de-escalating upset clients because "Dr. H is better at handling those people." The associates stopped taking initiative because every time they tried, Dr. H corrected, re-explained, or just said, "Here, I'll do it."

So, the team learned.
Not medicine.
Not confidence.
Not leadership.
They learned one rule: "Let Dr. Halloran handle it."

And because he loved the hospital, he did.

Until one Tuesday afternoon—the kind where the lobby is an airport terminal, the phones won't stop ringing, and everyone's cortisol levels are double their heart rates—something snapped.

A tech asked him a basic question she'd been trained on three times. A CSR interrupted him with a client complaint he'd coached her through literally last week.
An associate hovered behind him in surgery, waiting to ask whether she should call a radiologist for a case she'd handled a dozen times.

And Dr. Halloran, exhausted and stretched thin, looked up and said the quiet part out loud: "Why am I the only one here who can do anything without a checklist?"

Silence.
Everyone froze.
But the truth? He wasn't wrong.

Because he'd spent 10 years answering every question, he had accidentally trained his entire team to *never* answer anything themselves. By being the hero for so long, he'd built a hospital entirely dependent on him—and now he resented the very dependency he created.

That night, after the last appointment left and the lights were shut off, he sat in his car and realized something brutal:

His team wasn't incompetent.
They were underdeveloped.
Under-trusted.
Under-empowered.
Undergrown.

And all of that traced back to one root cause: he led like the hero, not the builder of heroes. He wore every hat. Held every answer. Carried every burden. Owned every fire. He thought that's what leadership required.

But all it did was turn his hospital into a place where *nobody else ever learned to lead.*

And here's the kicker: the more he tightened his grip, the smaller the hospital stayed.

This story matters. Why? Because a lot of hospitals out there have their own version of Dr. Halloran.
Some are louder.
Some are quieter.
Some hide it under perfectionism.
Some hide it under "I just want things done right."
Some hide it under "It's faster if I just do it myself."

But the pattern is the same:
The leader becomes the bottleneck.
The team becomes dependent.
The culture becomes fragile.
The owner becomes exhausted.

It's so important to me to hit home on this as we broach the topic of servant leadership. Because contrary to popular misconceptions, servant leadership isn't soft. It's not "being nice." It's not stepping back. It's the opposite: it's building systems, trust, and capability around you so the hospital doesn't rest on one person's shoulders—especially yours.

If you lead like Dr. Halloran, there's only one possible ending: a brilliant doctor trapped inside a hospital that cannot function without them.

And that's not leadership. That's captivity.

Most Veterinary Leaders Feel Alone

If you want to understand leadership in veterinary medicine, start here: **there are only two kinds of leaders in this industry: leaders who see themselves as the hero and leaders who exist to build heroes around them**.

Most hospitals—no matter their size, profit, equipment, or resume—are held back by leaders stuck in the first category. Not because they're bad people. Not because they don't care. But because they were never taught that leadership isn't about direction—it's about service.

The problem is that too many leaders in this profession honestly believe that controlling every decision, owning every answer, and tightening their grip is what keeps the hospital strong. In reality, it's what keeps the hospital small.

Most practice owners, medical directors, and hospital leaders I've met—and maybe this is you—know a version of loneliness most people will never understand. It's not quiet. It's not gentle. It's loud, relentless pressure. It's the feeling that you are the emotional shock absorber for every damn thing that goes wrong—staffing issues, client meltdowns, surprise call-outs, personality collisions, the tech who's crying, the doctor who's frustrated, the CSR who's burned out, the client threatening a horrible review because "you don't care about animals," and the team staring at you like, *So ... what's the plan?*

You are the container for everyone else's stress. But where's your container? Exactly.

You go home wiped, not because you just worked a full day, but because you spent the whole day being the emotional chiropractor for grown adults who "didn't want to say anything earlier"—so now you get a 4:30 p.m. parade of problems that could have been solved at 8:00 a.m. if people weren't terrified of having uncomfortable conversations.

Every decision feels like a referendum on whether you're a tyrant or too soft. Every boundary you set gets tested like a toddler pushing buttons to see what they can get away with. Every time you try to delegate, someone does it halfway, hands it back, and shrugs like, "Well, I tried." Then it's your problem again. Suddenly, you're not just leading a hospital; you're running a daycare with anesthesia machines.

Leadership means holding the line when nobody else will. Leadership means carrying the emotional rubble when others crumble. Leadership means having your name on the door when the internet mob decides to weaponize a one-star review. Leadership means making payroll decisions while losing sleep at 2 a.m. wondering if the people you fought for even know how hard you fight.

And the brutal truth? Nobody prepared you for this. This is the part nobody tells you when you step into a leadership role thinking leadership means "help guide a team." Not one class in school. Not one professor saying, "By the way, you're going to spend half your career managing human emotion, conflict, and belief systems." No one said, "Hey, one day you'll sit in your car before walking into your own building, psyching yourself up like an athlete for a place you literally created."

Leaders burn out not because they don't care—but because they care so much it hurts. They carry the mission. They carry the standard. They carry the silent parts—the fear of losing good people, the guilt when someone quits, and the frustration of constantly motivating adults who say they want excellence but act like excellence is optional when they're tired.

And here's the dagger: when you don't build culture intentionally, you become the culture by default. That means every value lives inside your chest instead of inside your systems. Everything depends on you showing up perfect every day—emotionally bulletproof, infinitely patient, endlessly inspiring, always rational, never tired, never discouraged, and never needing help.

That's not leadership. That's martyrdom dressed up as management. And martyrdom is not noble—it's unsustainable.

Burnout at the leadership level rarely comes from lack of love for the medicine. It comes from lack of shared ownership in the mission. It comes from trying to carry an army on your back instead of building an army that marches beside you. It comes from being the only one who sees the big picture, the only one prioritizing purpose over comfort, and the only one eating stress so everyone else can feel safe.

Nothing will break you faster than leading a team that expects you to solve everything while they "give input." Nothing will suffocate you faster than being surrounded by people who want the benefits of a great workplace but aren't brave enough to build one with you.

You don't need more grit; you clearly have enough grit to power a city. You need distributed ownership. You need shared standards. You need a culture that can hold itself up—so you don't have to hold it alone.

Because there's a fine line between being the leader and being the only adult in the building. One of those is empowerment ... The other is collapse waiting for a time stamp.

This chapter is blunt because it needs to be: if you want to build a hospital that grows, retains, inspires, and delivers medicine at scale, servant leadership is the only leadership model that works long-term.

Let's break down what servant leadership is not, what it is, and how to become the kind of leader people run toward—not run from.

What Non-servant Leaders Do (Even If They Don't Realize It)

You know these leaders. You've worked for them. Some days, you've probably been them.

1. **They choose control over empowerment**.

   These leaders grip the wheel so hard the steering column bends. They need approval on everything, they want to be the final word, they hoard information, and they become the bottleneck that slows the entire practice down. Their identity is tied to being "needed."

   But when you build a hospital where everything must run through you, you're not leading—you're shackling.

2. **They focus on tasks over people**.

   They obsess over KPIs, throughput, production, and efficiency—but never ask,

   "What will it feel like for my team to actually carry this out?"

   If you ignore the human experience behind your operational demands, you won't raise performance. You'll raise burnout.

3. **They elevate their image over their team's growth**.

   These leaders want to look good to the medical director, the owner, the regional manager, the clients—anyone who can validate them. They protect their reputation even when their team is drowning. They take credit instead of giving it. They lean on their team when it benefits them and disappear when their team needs something back.

This is how you lose good people.

4. **They pick short-term efficiency over long-term trust**.

They push for today's output at the expense of tomorrow's stability. They cut corners.
They rush exams. They sacrifice training. And they justify it by saying, "We just don't have time."

Short-term wins become long-term losses.

5. **They want compliance instead of commitment**.

Their mindset is "Do it because I said so," not "Do it because you believe in why it matters." But teams don't give discretionary effort to leaders they fear; they give it to leaders they trust.

6. **They avoid hard conversations**.

These leaders delay accountability like it's a tax bill. They tolerate toxic behavior because "we can't afford to lose them." They let issues simmer until they explode.

But avoidance is not kindness. It's cowardice dressed up as compassion.

7. **They want to be the hero instead of building heroes**.

They jump in to solve everything themselves. They hoard answers. They love being the fixer because it feeds their ego.

But here's the truth: If everything depends on you, you're not leading. You're babysitting. And that babysitting is costing your hospital trust, retention, clarity, revenue, and your sanity.

What Servant Leaders Actually Do

You can call it whatever you want—culture-first leadership, human-centered leadership, or trust-based leadership—but servant leadership is one of the strongest, most powerful ways you can lead, because it flips the script: instead of your team existing to serve you, you exist to serve your team. But let's get something straight. Servant leadership isn't soft. It's not weak. It's not "letting people walk all over you." It's the exact opposite.

That means your title—hospital manager, medical director, and owner—doesn't make you "the boss." It makes you responsible. Responsible for clearing roadblocks. Responsible for giving your team what they need to succeed. Responsible for taking the punches first, so they don't always have to. Responsible for giving credit rather than taking it for yourself.

In practice? A huge part of servant leadership is transparency. It's saying, "Here's where we're struggling. Here's what's working. Here's what I don't know yet." It's owning mistakes. It's telling your CSR, "You're right, I should have supported you better with that client. That one's on me." It's vulnerability. It's the courage to say, "I'm learning too."

And most importantly, it's action. Servant leadership requires rolling up your sleeves to *do the work* your people need from you, so they can do the work pets and clients need from them.

As mentioned in the summary of the Flywheel and as we'll dig deeper into, in Chapter 8, psychological safety empowers your team to think, speak, act, and grow without fear. And servant leaders build it intentionally, every single day.

Servant leadership is how the hospital's clear mission, vision, values, and standards are maintained and modeled in the hospital every day. With a servant leader at the helm, these ideas and standards don't just live on a poster collecting dust on your hospital's wall; they become ingrained in the everyday practices, norms, decisions, and behaviors.

Here's how servant leaders succeed:

1. **They create clarity, not chaos**.

   Nothing destroys psychological safety faster than confusion. When people don't understand expectations, standards, or priorities, they don't feel safe—they feel exposed. Servant leaders eliminate guesswork by making mission, vision, values, and expectations painfully clear and repeating them until they become second nature. In other words, once the hospital's mission, vision, and values are established and clear behavior norms are established to ensure a culture rooted in clear standards, a servant leader ensures that those standards and hospital's identity are never compromised. A servant leader, in other words, ensures that this clarity—of mission, vision, purpose, standards, etc.—is unapologetically maintained and defended.

   Why? Because clarity reduces anxiety. Clarity builds confidence. Clarity creates safety.

2. **They build trust before they demand performance**.

   People don't perform at their highest level because a leader demands it—they perform because they trust the person asking.

   In veterinary medicine especially, nobody is taking clinical, operational, or interpersonal risks if they don't feel safe with their leader. Risk requires vulnerability, and vulnerability only happens when people believe, *"My leader is steady. My leader is fair. My leader is predictable. My leader has my back."*

   Servant leaders understand this. They don't sprint straight to performance expectations. They invest first in trust—emotional consistency, honesty without volatility, accountability without humiliation, and clarity without condescension. They show up the same way on their worst days as they do on their best days. Their team never has to wonder, *"Which version of my boss am I getting today?"* That emotional predictability is not soft; it's the structural beam that holds psychological safety in place.

And when people feel psychologically safe, they stop operating from survival mode. They stop overthinking every move. They stop hiding mistakes or withholding ideas. Instead, they start stepping up, stretching, and contributing—exactly the behaviors high-performance hospitals depend on. When a team trusts its leader, initiative spikes. Collaboration deepens. Learning accelerates. Doctors and techs speak up earlier, ask more questions, and make fewer assumptions. That's not a coincidence. That's trust doing its job.

Trust is psychological safety in action.
Trust is what turns direction into alignment.
Trust is what makes standards feel achievable instead of threatening.
Trust is what transforms accountability from punishment into partnership.

Without trust, you get compliance at best and burnout at worst. With trust, performance becomes the natural byproduct of people feeling safe, supported, and seen.

Servant leaders know this: you build trust first, and performance follows automatically. Demanding performance without trust is like demanding loyalty from strangers. But when trust is strong, performance isn't forced; it's unleashed.

3. **They grow people to grow outcomes**.

Psychological safety doesn't appear because you hung a poster in the break room. It blooms when people actually feel themselves getting better—not performing for approval, not walking on eggshells, not trying to avoid being the next public example of what went wrong.

Servant leaders understand a truth most hospitals ignore: you don't get better medicine without better people. And you don't get better people without better leadership.

This is where psychological safety stops being a "feel-good" concept and becomes an economic engine. It's the understanding that: Growth Drives Confidence. Confidence Drives Courage. Courage Drives Performance.

Think about this way, the real sequence hospitals live and die by: *Skill → Confidence → Courage → High Performance → Retention.*

Every arrow in that chain rests on one core environment: psychological safety.
People don't build skill if they're terrified of making mistakes.
They don't gain confidence if they only get feedback when something's on fire.
They don't build courage if every question is treated like an inconvenience.
And they definitely don't stay if their growth feels optional, unsupported, or punished.

Research across multiple industries (including healthcare) shows that people don't leave workplaces—they leave stagnation:

- Employees who feel they are developing are 2.9 times more likely to be engaged in their work.
- Employees who receive weekly coaching instead of annual reviews show up to 46% higher performance over time.
- In healthcare environments specifically, hospitals with strong learning cultures see 25–30% higher retention, better patient adherence, and significantly improved clinical accuracy.
- Teams with high psychological safety outperform low-safety teams by up to 60% on complex tasks (Edmondson, 2019).

These aren't soft numbers. These are operational outcomes.

Servant leaders turn growth into a system. In other words, the best leaders in vet med don't "hope" their people grow. They design for it: they coach instead of correct. They ask instead of accuse. They debrief instead of blame. They teach openly instead of hoarding expertise like intellectual property. They normalize feedback instead of weaponizing it.

They treat growth like rounds at a teaching hospital: deliberate, accountable, and safe. Because here's the uncomfortable truth: If people only get feedback when they screw up, they will spend their entire career trying not to screw up. And teams built on fear never innovate, never stretch, and never hit peak performance.

For us humans, growth is not a perk. It's a psychological need. Humans stay where they believe their future is getting brighter.

In one national workforce study, the top three reasons people stayed long-term were:

1. *"I am growing."*
2. *"I feel supported."*
3. *"I trust my leadership."*

Not salary. Not PTO. Not "pizza party Fridays." Growth, support, trust—exactly what servant leaders cultivate.

When you invest in people, you don't just produce better teammates. You produce better medicine, better outcomes, better client trust, and better hospital longevity.

Grow people → grow courage → grow outcomes → grow the hospital.

4. **They remove obstacles instead of creating them**.

You can't feel safe if your leader leaves roadblocks in your way. Servant leaders hunt for friction points—broken workflows, unclear protocols, equipment that's been "acting weird for months," and miscommunication between departments—and they fix them. And here's the key: they don't see any of it as "beneath them."

They don't say, "That's the techs' job," or "That's inventory's problem," or "Someone else should handle that." They don't float above the details like they're too important to care. Servant leaders know that small problems become big culture killers. They understand that when a scale never works, when a stapler is always missing, when the bandage cart is always empty, and when exam rooms don't reset consistently—those "tiny" annoyances compound into resentment, stress, and fear.

A servant leader never says, "I don't have time for that." They say, "If it matters to my team, it matters to me."

When work is predictable and processes are clean, psychological safety skyrockets. When systems are clunky and leaders look away, people stop trusting the environment—and stop trusting the leader. Chaos creates fear. Bottlenecks create self-doubt. But streamlined systems? They create calm. And calm is where people think clearly, speak honestly, advocate confidently, and grow.

Servant leaders fix the small things because they know the small things are what shape how safe and supported their team actually feels.

5. They model the standards.

Nothing destroys psychological safety like hypocrisy. If leaders say one thing and do another, people stop speaking up. Servant leaders embody the standards they expect from others. Their behavior is the most stable thing in the building.

When people see the leader owning mistakes, asking questions, being vulnerable, and seeking feedback, they feel safe doing the same.

6. They confront issues early and consistently.

Psychological safety does not mean an absence of conflict. It's the absence of *fear* around conflict.

Servant leaders don't avoid hard conversations. They don't sugarcoat issues until they rot. They don't wait until the fourth time someone blows up, melts down, or drops the ball before they say something. They don't weaponize politeness.

They go early. They go respectfully. They go consistently.

They know that problems don't disappear when you ignore them; they metastasize. And in veterinary medicine, small interpersonal cracks can turn into full-blown culture earthquakes: miscommunications in surgery, passive-aggressive shift handoffs, gossip loops that poison the hospital from the inside out, or a CSR who's afraid to speak up about a safety concern because "last time it didn't go well."

Research across healthcare, aviation, and high-reliability industries shows the same pattern:

- Teams that avoid conflict experience higher error rates, lower collaboration, and faster burnout.
- Environments where issues are not addressed quickly create a "psychological tax"—people spend mental energy tiptoeing instead of performing.
- Employees in low-feedback environments are three times more likely to disengage within a year.

Avoidance creates an invisible tension that everyone feels but nobody names. People start assuming, guessing, or resenting instead of communicating. And you know who ends up carrying all of that weight? The leader. Because every problem avoided eventually boomerangs back.

On the other side of the spectrum, blunt-force leadership doesn't create clarity—it creates trauma. A leader who brings a flamethrower to every conversation may get momentary compliance, but never long-term trust. Health care studies show:

- Harsh correction increases error rates by up to 43% in the following 24 hours because it spikes cortisol and narrows cognitive bandwidth.
- Teams exposed to demeaning feedback show drops in problem-solving accuracy and communication quality (Cohen et al., 2014).

So, aggression might feel efficient in the moment. But it destroys psychological safety—the very thing high-performance teams depend on.

Servant leadership is about holding two things at the same time:

1. **Truth:** "This behavior isn't aligned with our values," "This pattern can't continue," and "We need a higher standard."
2. **Respect:** "I'm with you in fixing this," "We'll work through it together," and "Your growth matters to me."

This combination is rocket fuel. It tells your team, "You matter too much for me to let you fail quietly." It creates accountability without shame, boundaries without brutality, and standards without fear.

Clean feedback strengthens trust, even when it stings. Studies show people actually prefer direct, constructive feedback over vague positivity—as long as it's delivered with fairness and dignity. In fact:

- 72% of employees say they wish their leaders gave more honest, straightforward guidance.
- Teams that receive timely feedback report 30% higher trust in their leadership.
- In healthcare settings, "respectful assertiveness" is associated with safer handoffs, better surgical outcomes, and lower turnover.

Which means confronting issues isn't just a culture move. It's a clinical and financial one. When you set boundaries early and consistently, you eliminate ambiguity—the #1 driver of workplace anxiety.

Boundaries do three things:

1. They protect the team: Everyone knows what behavior is acceptable, what's not, and what happens next.
2. They reduce emotional volatility: Expectations become predictable instead of explosive.
3. They increase team confidence: People feel safer when they know the leader will intervene before things get toxic.

Servant leaders become the emotional thermostat of the hospital. They keep the temperature steady. They prevent boiling points long before they happen. They don't let issues simmer. They don't let resentment ferment. They don't collect emotional debt hoping it magically disappears. They address issues with speed, clarity, respect, and consistency.

Not to punish.
Not to dominate.
But to protect the team, the culture, and the mission.

Because psychological safety isn't built in the easy moments; it's built in the hard ones, handled well.

7. **They build systems that outlive them**.

A psychologically safe environment is one where people aren't scared the whole place will fall apart if the leader steps away. Servant leaders create systems, pathways, scripts, standards, and communication frameworks so the hospital can perform without panic—even when they're not present.

When people know the system will hold them—even when the leader isn't there—psychological safety becomes structural, not situational.

Servant Leadership Practices for Navigating Animal Hospital Change

I've covered the key tenants of servant leadership in general, but look: leading a team through culture change is particularly messy. It's uncomfortable. It's emotional. But shifting your culture and priorities toward a focus on earning client trust, and embracing the Veterinary Trust Flywheel, is MANDATORY if you want to build a hospital where people love to work, clients feel cared for and trusting, and pets get the best shot at healthier, longer lives.

When you talk about shifting a team's focus toward prioritizing trust-building client experience (CX), you're not just tweaking a script or updating a policy manual. You're not hopping straight to tactics like Cleveland Clinic mistakenly did. You're asking people to think differently. To care differently. To show up differently. That doesn't happen because you told them to. It happens because you *led* them there. You made a case for *why*. And the only leadership style that works in the veterinary space—which needs a pretty dramatic overhaul to recognize itself as a service industry and which needs to better value client trust, service, and hospitality—is servant leadership.

Leading Culture Change with Transparency

When you're steering a culture shift, you don't get to keep secrets. Teams can sniff out bullshit faster than clients can smell fear in an exam room. If you're trying to "spin" the truth, they'll know.

So, be transparent. Talk about the Google reviews that sting. Talk about the client complaints that shook you. Talk about the financial challenges, or the opportunity to expand, or the dream of being the go-to hospital in your town. When your team feels like you're leveling with them, they'll lean in. When they feel like you're sugarcoating or hiding, they'll disengage and question whether to trust you.

Transparency builds trust, and trust is oxygen in a cultural change. Without it, your team will suffocate.

Owning Mistakes as a Leadership Superpower

Your team doesn't expect perfection. They expect honesty. They expect consistency. They expect you to own it when you drop the ball.

If a scheduling change created chaos, own it. If a price conversation with a client went sideways because you didn't prepare the team, own it. If you promised to fix something and didn't follow through, own it.

Owning mistakes isn't weakness. It's leadership. It shows your team that accountability isn't a weapon to be feared; it's a standard we all hold ourselves to. And when you model it, they'll follow suit.

Recognizing Vulnerability as the Unlock

Here's the uncomfortable truth: your team doesn't just need your authority. They need your humanity. Vulnerability is the unlock.

When you admit, "I don't have all the answers, but I believe in us," it does something powerful. It creates space for others to step up. It shows your team that they don't have to be perfect either—they just have to keep trying.

I've seen managers cry in front of their teams when talking about burnout or lost pets. And you know what? That team didn't lose respect. The team leaned in closer. Vulnerability connects people. And connection drives cultural change.

Serving Your Team to Serve Clients Better

At the end of the day, this whole shift toward CX isn't about buzzwords. It's about pets getting the care they need, clients feeling like they can trust you, and teams having the energy and pride to deliver on that.

But that chain starts with you serving your team. If your techs don't feel supported, how are they going to support Mrs. Johnson when she's crying about her cat's diagnosis? If your CSRs feel invisible, how are they going to make the nervous new puppy owner feel seen?

Your job as a servant leader is to serve the people who serve the clients. Period.

Quick Guide: Modeling Servant Leadership Through Change

Here's your cheat sheet. Print this out. Tape it to your office wall. Live it.

- Lead with transparency. Share the good, the bad, and the ugly. Don't spin. Don't hide.
- Own your mistakes. Say "That's on me" out loud. Model accountability.
- Be vulnerable. Share the real stuff—your fears, your hopes, your struggles. It connects.
- Clear roadblocks. Ask your team what's getting in their way, then fix it. That's leadership.
- Celebrate progress. Call out wins, big or small. Energy compounds.
- Put the team first. Make decisions through the lens of "Does this help my team succeed?"
- Reinforce the why. Remind them: this isn't about numbers; it's about pets, clients, and people.
- Serve relentlessly. Never forget: The leader's job is to serve. Serve your team, so they can serve pets and clients.

Bottom line: culture change doesn't come from mandates or slogans. It comes from leaders willing to serve first. You don't have to be perfect. You just have to be real, transparent, and committed. That's how you win trust. That's how you shift culture. That's how you build a hospital people love, inside and out.

Case Example: How One Manager Flipped the Script with Servant Leadership

Let me tell you about a hospital manager I worked with, whom we'll call *Rachel*. When I first met Rachel, her hospital was in rough shape. Staff morale was tanking. Clients were leaving frustrated. Google reviews were slipping fast. The vibe in the building was heavy; you could literally feel the burnout when you walked in.

I dug deeper to learn what was happening, and not surprisingly, most of the issues started with leadership and strategy. I saw a lack of transparency, lack of perceived fairness, lack of clarity of direction, very little training and feedback, and rampant miscommunication— just complete mismanagement. To compensate, Linda and the hospital owner had increased prices four times in the past year, 7% each time. And the team was poorly compensated.

I remember the conversation I had with Rachel when I saw what was going on. It wasn't easy and it wasn't pretty. It's not easy to deliver tough love, but she needed it. I was really real with her about what direction her hospital was heading in (down) and what would soon happen as a result: closed hospital doors. I said bluntly, "Until you step up as a leader, you're going to keep bleeding talent, trust, and money. This isn't mismanagement anymore; it's leadership malpractice. And if you don't fix it now, the only thing you'll be managing is the wreckage."

Rachel could have gone the "command-and-control" route. She could've cracked down, pointed fingers, and demanded better numbers. Instead, she chose servant leadership. And everything changed.

Here's what she did:

1. She owned her part. At the next staff meeting, Rachel stood up and said, "I know I haven't supported you the way I should. That's on me. I've been more focused on the bottom line than

on you, and it shows. I want to rebuild trust, and I'm asking for your help." Vulnerability. Right there in the open.

2. She got transparent. Instead of hiding the ugly data, she printed it. She put the reviews and client complaints on the wall. She showed the financials. She didn't spin it. She said, "This is where we're at. This is what our clients are saying. This is what's at stake." That honesty turned what felt like a blame game into a shared mission.

3. She asked the team what was broken. Rachel planned and led a "Moments That Matter" session. The team called out some truly painful pain points. Some of them focused on a lack of leadership. Instead of defending, Rachel wrote it all down. And she said, "Thank you. Keep going."

4. She cleared roadblocks. When her CSRs told her the phones were a nightmare—constantly ringing, unrealistic client hold times, and angry clients—Rachel didn't just say, "Do your best." She pulled call data, proved the volume was too high for one person, and fought to bring in a part-time floater to help at peak hours. The pressure lifted: her front desk team finally had breathing room to actually talk to clients instead of just surviving call after call. That one change gave her team confidence and gave clients a calmer, more human experience from the first ring. Simple. Immediate. Effective.

5. She celebrated the wins. Within three months, with Rachel relentlessly supporting people who were owning the goals the team had set in the workshop, things were turning around. Financials and Google review scores were recovering. The time was actually smiling again. One client said that she "finally felt heard." Instead of pocketing that progress, Rachel brought cupcakes to a staff meeting and read the reviews out loud. "This is you," she told her team. "You made this happen."

When I asked Rachel what flipped the switch, she didn't talk about the new part-time floater or the cupcakes. She said: "I stopped trying to be 'the boss' and started being their partner. Once they saw I was in it for them, everything else followed."

That's servant leadership in action. It's not complicated. It's not about titles. It's about humility, courage, and action.

Summary

Servant leadership isn't weakness. It's not "being nice" or letting people walk all over you. It's the strongest, boldest way to lead, because it means you're willing to go first. You're willing to be transparent when the numbers suck. You're willing to admit when you screwed up. You're willing to clear the roadblocks that crush your team's energy. You're willing to take the punches so they don't have to. That's not soft; that's steel.

In practice, servant leadership is strength aimed in the right direction: it's discipline married to empathy. It's clarity delivered with compassion. It's truth delivered with respect. It's power used to elevate others instead of yourself. It's the hardest, strongest, and most courageous way to lead.

Culture change doesn't happen because you bark orders, hand out scripts, or paste motivational posters on the wall. It happens because you *serve first*. Period.

And the payoff? Massive. Teams stop checking out. Clients start leaning in. Pets get better care because the people delivering it feel supported, valued, and proud. Trust flows both ways. The flywheel spins.

Rachel's turnaround proved it. She didn't claw her way back by doubling down on control or hiding the ugly truths. She flipped the script. She served her people. And once they trusted her again, everything changed: reviews, revenue, morale, and medicine. That's not luck. That's leadership.

So, here's your takeaway: your title doesn't make you the boss. It makes you responsible. Responsible to serve, to model vulnerability, to celebrate wins, and to put your people in a position to win. That's the only way to lead real change.

And if you're brave enough to lead this way? You won't just change your hospital. You'll change lives—your team's, your clients', and every single pet that walks through your hospital's doors. Servant leadership is the leadership that lasts. It is the leadership that multiplies. It is the leadership that transforms veterinary hospitals from stressful, reactive workplaces into aligned, resilient, high-performance teams.

Build *this* level of safety, and your hospital stops depending on you—and starts thriving because of you.

That's servant leadership. That's culture leadership. That's the leadership that wins.

In the Appendix, I outlined some of the core behaviors that servant leaders should model to support healthy culture, create emotional safety, and put the Veterinary Trust Flywheel in motion. I hope these are helpful to you.

Suggested Readings

Brown, Brené. *Dare to Lead: Brave Work. Tough Conversations. Whole Hearts.* Random House, 2018.

Cohen, Geoffrey L. and David K. Sherman. The Psychology of Change: Self-Affirmation and Social Psychological Intervention. *Annual Review of Psychology*, vol. 65, 2014, pp. 333–371.

Deci, Edward L., and Richard M. Ryan. *Intrinsic Motivation and Self-determination in Human Behavior.* Plenum Press, 1985.

Edmondson, Amy C. *The Fearless Organization: Creating Psychological Safety in the Workplace for Learning, Innovation, and Growth.* Wiley, 2019.

Gallup, Inc. *State of the Global Workplace 2022 Report.* Gallup, 2022, www.gallup.com/workplace

Goleman, Daniel. *Primal Leadership: Unleashing the Power of Emotional Intelligence*. Harvard Business School Press, 2002.

Greenleaf, Robert K. *Servant Leadership: A Journey into the Nature of Legitimate Power and Greatness*. Paulist Press, 1977.

Kahneman, Daniel. *Thinking, Fast and Slow*. Farrar, Straus and Giroux, 2011.

Lencioni, Patrick. *The Five Dysfunctions of a Team: A Leadership Fable*. Jossey-Bass, 2002.

Maslach, Christina, and Michael P. Leiter. *The Truth About Burnout: How Organizations Cause Personal Stress and What to Do About It*. Jossey-Bass, 1997.

Schein, Edgar H. *Organizational Culture and Leadership*. 5th ed., Wiley, 2016.

Sinek, Simon. *Leaders Eat Last: Why Some Teams Pull Together and Others Don't*. Portfolio, 2014.

Thaler, Richard H., and Cass R. Sunstein. *Nudge: Improving Decisions About Health, Wealth, and Happiness*. Yale University Press, 2008.

Zenger, Jack, and Joseph Folkman. *The Extraordinary Leader: Turning Good Managers into Great Leaders*. McGraw-Hill, 2019.

Chapter 8
A Case Study in Veterinary Client Experience—Part 2

Linda's False Start

In Chapter 3, I discussed the well-intentioned but misguided approach that Linda, the Regional Operations leader, took trying to instill client experience (CX) as a priority in her region.

I'm excited to report that Linda turned things around, but before I discuss how she did that, let's rewind and recap. Because the way she started is exactly how so many well-intentioned leaders blow up their own CX strategy.

Linda wanted her region to be the best in the company. She looked at survey data and saw clients didn't feel welcomed, and her hospitals weren't pulling in enough positive reviews online. So, she built a "premium, high-touch service" initiative, and it sounded pretty damn good on paper.

So, she rolled out strict guidelines: greet every client within 20 seconds, offer water and treats, say "We're so happy you're here," use the client's and pet's name twice, and ask for reviews at checkout. She trained the hell out of it, made guidebooks and videos, hired secret shoppers, and even dangled pizza parties as rewards.

And technically, it worked. Teams followed the rules. Secret shoppers gave them high marks. But clients? Thcy hated it.

The experience felt scripted. Robotic. At times, downright awkward. Client Service Representatives (CSRs) chased clients into the parking lot yelling their names just to check a box. Frustrated clients were still being asked for Yelp reviews on their way out the door. Doctors checked their watches while reciting scripted lines like "We're so happy you're here."

The reviews came in brutal: *"They're trying too hard." "It's all for the reviews." "I'd rather they explained my dog's bloodwork than asked me three times if I wanted water."*

Linda's team hated it too. They felt like puppets on strings. Words like "robotic," "superficial," and "tone-deaf" came up again and again. Morale dropped, and even some long-tenured staff left.

Bottom line: Linda's original approach was all tactics, no culture. All scripts, no heart. And it backfired—hard.

Linda's Turnaround: From Checklists to Momentum

Linda genuinely cared about CX. She wanted her 16 hospitals to lead the company in satisfaction scores, yes, but she also wanted to help pet owners. At first, she made the classic mistake of leading with tactics instead of vision—just like Cleveland Clinic.

After rolling out her "premium, high-touch service" strategy, Linda had the guts to admit it wasn't working. And instead of doubling down on control, she pivoted. She embraced the Veterinary Trust Flywheel and started over.

Instead of lists and mandates, Linda started with *why*. During her next regional meeting for all of her Hospital Managers, she opened by saying:

> *"I need to be honest with you. Our clients are telling us something we can't ignore: they don't feel seen. That hits me hard, because I know how much every single one of you cares. It means that somewhere along the way, our clients aren't feeling the heart that I know this team has. And that's not who we are.*
>
> *Here's the vision I want us to chase together: every client walking out of our hospitals should feel welcomed, heard, and absolutely certain they made the right choice by trusting us with their pet. When we earn that kind of trust, everything changes. Clients stay with us for years, they bring us more of their pets' care, they tell their friends about us. And that trust doesn't just help clients and pets. It helps you. It keeps our hospitals strong, stable, and resourced so you can do your best work and actually enjoy this job again. I know that, right now, very few of you do.*
>
> *We're starting over. I misstepped in throwing a bunch of lists and rules at you. So this isn't about scores or secret shoppers anymore. This is about us being who we say we are. This is about rebuilding trust with our clients, with our pets, and honestly, with each other."*

The difference was night and day. When Linda led with lists and secret shoppers, the team felt policed. They felt like pawns in a game. Their creativity, their judgment, their compassion—all the things that made them good at this work—got buried under scripts and rules.

But when Linda stood up, admitted mistakes, and spoke from the heart, everything shifted. Vulnerability cracked the door open. The team didn't hear a corporate directive. Instead, they heard a leader who trusted them, believed in them, and cared enough to take accountability and own the truth.

That's why it resonated. People don't rally behind rules; they rally behind purpose. They don't get inspired by "say the client's name twice." They get inspired when they're reminded of the *why*: that their work matters, that their compassion changes lives, and that trust is the real scoreboard.

Linda's heartfelt approach gave her team back what they were missing: dignity, ownership, and the freedom to be authentic. And that's the fuel that actually drives momentum.

Her teams didn't need more rules. They needed a reason.

Linda swapped scripts for culture. She gave teams freedom to connect authentically. Instead of demanding "Say every name twice," she said, *"Make every client feel known."* Instead of "Ask every client for a review," she said, *"When someone leaves smiling, that's your moment to invite them to share their story."*

Together, she and her team came up with a renewed vision and mission for their group of hospitals. Linda then asked them really direct questions: What was burning their teams out? What was getting in the way of connecting with clients? She heard some brutal truths—like lack of support and a constant pressure to hit metrics—but Linda kept her cool and used the intel to drive the conversation toward brainstorming solutions.

Linda then walked her leaders through the Veterinary Flywheel Workshop and six-step process to equip them to run the exercises in their own hospitals, equipping them to lead innovative culture change. This was an immense step that showed her managers that she trusted them. They felt empowered, excited, and motivated.

Over the next three months, all of her Hospital Managers led their own workshops, and Linda was present to help each one. Each hospital came up with their own gameplan for improvement.

But even better, the hospital leaders started sharing their teams' ideas with each other. Momentum spread hospital to hospital, powered by results and peer inspiration, not mandates. The region established a culture of creative problem-solving and shared inno- vation. Several hospitals adopted new strategies after being inspired by other hospitals' ideas. They felt they had each other's backs and were now excited about their shared goal to strengthen their collec- tive reputation and lead the company—not only in scores (although they did take pride in trying to out-compete!), but also in develop- ing a reputation for innovation and a healthy culture.

Many of them made major changes. Improved scheduling. Hired relief help. Created space in the day for staff to breathe. Suddenly, they had more emotional bandwidth to be present with clients.

Predictably, hospital teams felt empowered by having been involved in the creative innovation process. They expressed feeling more appreciated, valued, and involved. Suddenly, the staff had more emotional bandwidth to be present with clients. Those who raised their hands to lead the implementation and measurement of spe- cific ideas were excited by the opportunity to grow their skills and establish themselves as leaders within the team. For many of them, it was their first opportunity to lead and own their own projects and initiatives, and they loved the responsibility.

Six months later, the cringe-worthy moments were gone.

- No more CSRs chasing clients into the parking lot yelling their names. Instead: *"Liz, thanks for coming in. I hope Buddy feels better. If you need anything, we're here."*
- No more robotic review requests to frustrated clients. Instead: "I can see today was tough. Thank you for sticking with us. If you ever want to share feedback, we'd love to learn from it."
- No more doctors rushing through scripted lines. Instead: eye contact, pets being acknowledged, and conversations instead of interrogations.

CX improved because team experience improved. That's the Veterinary Trust Flywheel in action. Staff retention rates improved across the board, and CX scores—both in client surveys and in online reviews—steadily increased over the next six months. Within eight months, Linda's region had gone from near the worse in the company to #1. That year, Linda was invited to speak at her company's annual meeting.

Bottom Line: Linda's Lesson

Linda stopped obsessing over secret shopper compliance. Instead, she tracked real signals of loyalty: retention, referrals, and survey comments that used words like *trust, listened,* and *cared for.*

Those metrics told the truth. And over time, they improved—steadily, authentically, sustainably.

By shifting to the Veterinary Trust Flywheel, Linda went from "corporate and disconnected" to a leader who inspired her region. Staff retention improved. Client complaints dropped. Positive reviews started to pour in—not only because people were asked, but because they were moved.

Linda's story proves the point: checklists don't create connection. Culture does. Purpose does. Trust does.

Summary

Linda's story is the perfect reminder of what happens when you get CX wrong—and what happens when you finally get it right. At first, she went all-in on rules, scripts, and secret shoppers. And it flopped. Clients felt patronized. Staff felt like robots. Morale tanked. Trust eroded.

But here's where she earned respect: she admitted it. She owned the failure. And then she flipped the script. Instead of chasing compliance, she started chasing connection. Instead of handing down lists, she gave her managers ownership, purpose, and the tools to lead change themselves. And once the culture shifted, everything shifted.

The turnaround was night and day. Staff leaned in, clients leaned back in, and the flywheel spun harder than ever. Retention improved. Reviews skyrocketed. Linda didn't just climb out of the hole. She turned her region into the #1 performer in the company.

And the lesson is another reminder: checklists don't build trust. Culture does. Rules don't create loyalty. Purpose does. When you lead with authenticity, vulnerability, and vision, you stop managing tactics and start building momentum.

That's how you move from cringe-worthy scripts to genuine connection. That's how you turn "trying too hard" into "I'll never take my pet anywhere else." That's the Veterinary Trust Flywheel in action.

Chapter 9

Psychological Safety Builds Trust Within Your Team

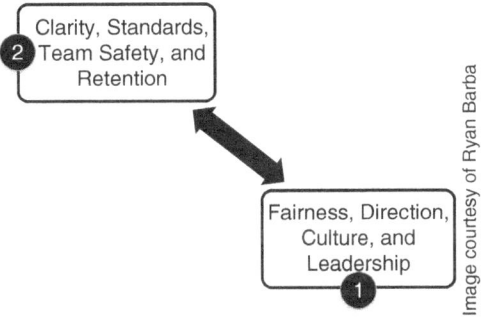

Image courtesy of Ryan Barba

Trust Within Your Team Will Never Exist Without Psychological Safety

When your culture is strong, standards are nonnegotiable, and your Mission, Vision, and Values are crystal clear—not corporate jargon, but daily behavior standards—something powerful happens inside a veterinary team.

People stop guessing.

They stop asking, "What does leadership really want from me?"
They stop wondering, "Am I going to get punished for trying something?"
They stop tiptoeing around decisions.

Culture, direction, and clarity create a sense of certainty and comfort. Fear and hesitation die. And when fear and hesitation die, psychological safety—that is, the freedom for your team to speak, try, and be vulnerable without fear of harm—emerges.

You can't have psychological safety without clarity. You can't have empowered teams operating in a fog. You can't expect people to speak up, take initiative, and challenge ideas if they don't understand the mission they're protecting.

Without a sense of psychological safety, your team will clam up and armor up. They don't feel safe to ask for help. They don't feel safe to make a mistake. They don't feel safe to say, "I'm overwhelmed," "I'm confused," or "I don't understand—can you walk me through that again?" They perform instead of connect. They shut down instead of speak up. They nod politely, then quietly panic. And every time that happens, trust evaporates drop by drop.

But when a hospital is clear on who it is, what it stands for, and when clear standards and values are defined so that your team understands clearly what "right" looks like, employees stop playing defense. They start creating. They start owning. They start innovating instead of waiting for permission like it's a rationed resource.

When the team understands the destination and the rules of the road, they don't white-knuckle the wheel. They drive. They accelerate. They explore. They raise their hand and say, "I have an idea," instead of, "Please don't shoot the messenger."

Mission gives direction.
Values give guardrails.
Vision gives energy and purpose.
Culture, supported by servant leadership, brings it all to life.

And psychological safety? That's what your team feels when these things are all in place.

That's when the quiet assistant starts asking brilliant medical questions.
That's when the Client Service Representative (CSR) suggests a better way to handle check-ins.
That's when the new grad doctor stops internalizing stress and starts collaborating.
That's when you stop losing people because of silence, shame, and uncertainty.

When your team feels safe—they communicate early, not after mistakes compound. They solve problems instead of hiding them. They learn faster. They take pride instead of taking cover. They move from "I hope I don't get in trouble" to "I'm going to help us win."

This is the evolution. "Culture + Clarity" isn't the goal—it's the soil. You planted values. You planted expectations. Psychological safety is the sunlight and water that helps people grow into their potential instead of shrinking into roles.

Welcome to the part of the journey where your leadership equips people to step into their highest contribution. This is where the foundation has been established, and the Flywheel begins to spin.

In veterinary medicine, people don't get burned out because they don't love animals.
They get burned out because they don't feel safe.

The psychological truth is that **safety is the emotional space that creates trust.**

Safety is a feeling. Trust is a belief.

When your brain feels safe, you learn faster, you communicate honestly, you take initiative, and you advocate for what's right. In contrast, when your brain feels unsafe, you protect, defend, hide, and survive. You clam up and stop thinking creatively.

That's neuroscience. That's human behavior. And that's the game we're playing—inside every lobby, every exam room, and every break room.

So, you don't build trust by saying "trust me." You build trust by making people feel safe at every touchpoint—every shift, every phone call, every tough medical conversation, every "Can you show me again?," and every "Hey, I disagree."

If your team doesn't feel safe emotionally, they cannot trust fully. If they don't trust fully, they won't communicate fully. And if they don't communicate fully, mistakes, conflict, fear, and turnover walk right in.

That's why this matters. This isn't kumbaya fluff. This is how you build a hospital people stay in, believe in, and rave about.

Safety Is Built over Time—And It's a Ladder

Most hospitals treat trust like a binary: you either have it in place or you don't. And many hospital leaders think that trust is this one-time thing you just "get" by default. You're the vet, you care about animals, and you got the degree—boom, trust, right?

Wrong. Dead wrong. Trust isn't automatic. And it's not a one-time thing that's magically earned. Trust results from establishing a sense of safety within the team, rooted in a strong and healthy culture, consistent and nonnegotiable standards, and a clarity of what the hospital stands for and where it's going.

Safety is a ladder, and people climb it one rung at a time. Everyone on your team climbs it step by step—your techs, your CSRs, and your doctors—or they don't climb at all.

This idea that safety is built in phases isn't something I invented in a coffee shop. The *Four Stages of Psychological Safety* come from Dr. Timothy R. Clark, a global expert in workplace culture and leadership. His research breaks down how humans build trust and safety in any environment—step-by-step, no shortcuts, and no corporate buzzwords.

And here's why it's powerful: for years, "psychological safety" was treated like this fuzzy, feelings-based idea. But Clark quantified it, structured it, and made it *trainable*. He showed that safety grows in four predictable stages, and people don't graduate to the next one until the environment earns it. Let's dig deeper into his research findings.

People move through trust the same way every time:

1. **Inclusion Safety**—First, they check to see if they're welcome. They ask themselves, "Do I belong here? Do I feel wanted and valued here?"
2. **Learned Safety**—Then, they check to see if they're in a space where it's safe to ask questions and experiment. They ask themselves, "Is it okay for me to ask questions or admit when I don't know something without feeling embarrassed or being judged?"
3. **Contributor Safety**—Then, they check to see whether it's safe to push the envelope—to contribute their ideas and insights. They ask themselves, "Do I feel safe to share my ideas here?"
4. **Challenger Safety**—Finally, they check to see if they can challenge without fear. They ask themselves, "Is it safe for me to question established norms and decisions without fear of retaliation or risking my career?"

That's the ladder. Your team members climb this ladder over time. If they don't, and if they feel stuck at any one point, safety dies and everything suffers.

Morale drops.
Communication gets tight and weird.
Clients get defensive.
Leaders get frustrated.
People start whispering.
Clients start price-shopping.
Eventually, turnover and negative reviews start showing up as symptoms.

But imagine the benefits when your team members actually *mature* through these four stages. I'm not talking about a cute poster on the breakroom wall. I mean your people *living* this. Breathing it. Trusting it. They feel safe to be human. Safe to ask for help. Safe to speak the truth. Safe to innovate. Safe to *own* outcomes without fear of humiliation or punishment. When that happens, everything changes.

Instead of techs whispering in the back hallway about what went wrong, they raise their hand and say, "Hey, we missed something. Let's fix it together." Instead of a receptionist quietly drowning because they're afraid to ask the doctor for clarity, they ask. Instead of a new assistant being terrified to say they don't understand a procedure, they *learn it faster*, become competent sooner, and stick around longer because they feel supported instead of judged.

And here's the kicker: when people feel included, when they feel safe to learn, when they feel safe to contribute, when they feel safe to challenge the status quo, you don't just get better medicine. You get momentum. Fear disappears. And once fear exits the building, possibility walks in.

Turnover drops. Drama dies. Gossip becomes obsolete because people talk *to* each other, not *about* each other. New hires join the team and feel seen and supported instead of tossed into survival mode. Your senior staff don't feel threatened by new energy— they *mentor it*. Doctors stop being traffic controllers and become coaches. CSRs stop apologizing and start communicating with confidence and clarity. Techs stop waiting for instructions and start taking initiative.

This isn't soft fluff. This is a hard advantage. This is business armor.

When people operate in Stage 4—where they feel safe to challenge, to improve, to innovate—you start compounding ideas, not just hours worked. You unlock efficiency, creativity, and pride. Not the fake "family" talk. Real community. Real ownership. Real loyalty. Real growth.

This is how the best practices get better. This is how you stop playing catch-up and start leading. This is how you become *the hospital* people whisper about in recruitment groups, the place people would move zip codes for. The place where careers are made, not burned out. The place where pets and people win together.

Your Team's Psychological Safety Launches the Flywheel

You want retention? Start here.
You want standards? Start here.
You want innovation? Start here.
You want referrals, loyalty, trust, margins, and long-term enterprise value? Start here.

So, psychological safety isn't "nice." It's a strategy. It's a competitive edge. It's the foundation of a Veterinary Trust Flywheel.

A hospital where people feel psychologically safe isn't just nicer: it's more resilient, more profitable, more attractive to talent, and more trusted by pet owners.

Psychological safety has the potential to turn a group of tired veterinary professionals into a mission-driven, high-performing, retention-proof, and recruitment-magnet of a team. When a veterinary hospital builds psychological safety, everything changes—*and it changes fast.*

Let's get real: people don't leave veterinary medicine because of hard work. They leave because of toxic work environments where speaking up feels risky, being honest feels dangerous, and being human feels like a liability.

But in a psychologically safe hospital? The air is different. The energy is different. The way people walk through the door is different. They don't brace themselves for impact—they exhale. They settle in. They contribute.

Here's what this looks like, and here's how the psychological safety of your team starts to initiate the magic that is the Veterinary Trust Flywheel:

Daily Experience Skyrockets

When people feel safe, they stop wasting emotional energy worrying, or trying to survive the day, and instead start investing that energy into being excellent. Techs speak up before problems escalate, CSRs ask clarifying questions without shame, and doctors collaborate instead of operating in silos. Suddenly, the building runs more smoothly—not because the workload changed, but because the *fear* was removed. And when fear leaves, creativity, initiative, and ownership show up.

Belonging Becomes the Default

Psychological safety tells your people, "You fit here. Your voice matters. You are part of this." And when people feel like they belong, they don't clock in—they *commit.* They show up with heart. They advocate for patients more boldly. They support each other more naturally. They celebrate wins louder and recover from losses faster. Belonging is the emotional glue that keeps great teams together.

Internal Trust Becomes the Default Setting

When psychological safety takes root, something profound happens inside a veterinary hospital: trust stops being earned drop-by-drop and starts flowing like oxygen. Teams don't just like each other more—they *trust* each other more. They believe they've got each other's backs. And that trust completely changes the way a hospital operates.

In a psychologically safe environment, team members learn—through repetition, through clarity, through consistent leadership—people stop policing each other. They stop walking on eggshells.

They stop hovering over tasks being conducted by teammates like anxious helicopter coworkers. They trust that if someone says something is done, it's done. They trust that if someone needs help, they'll speak up. They trust that nobody is hiding mistakes or cutting corners out of fear.

This is the magic: psychological safety turns "I hope they got it" into "I know they've got it."

Technicians stop double-checking each other's work because they know their partner is focused, supported, and confident—not rushed, overwhelmed, or scared of making a mistake. CSRs don't feel the need to reconfirm every detail of an estimate because they know the team is aligned on standards and messaging. Doctors stop rewriting each other's treatment plans because they trust the consistency of the care philosophy they built together.

Teams begin to operate like a well-trained flight crew: clear roles, shared language, predictable behaviors, and mutual respect. Trust becomes muscle memory.

And here's the beautiful thing—once trust becomes the norm, speed goes up, friction goes down, and emotional load drops by half. People waste significantly less mental energy asking:

- "Did they do it?"
- "Should I check again?"
- "Do they know what's expected?"
- "Do I need to remind them?"
- "Are they going to get upset if I correct this?"

All that noise disappears. Instead, people operate in a rhythm—a confident, reliable, almost seamless flow where hands are metaphorically and literally passed from one team member to another without hesitation.

Trust transforms a group into a unit. Trust turns coordination into choreography. Trust turns "your job vs. my job" into "our patients, our clients, our hospital."

And when trust becomes the foundation, teams take smarter risks. They speak up faster. They collaborate more naturally. They problem-solve in real time. They protect each other—not from clients, but from burnout, overwhelm, and isolation.

In psychologically *unsafe* environments, everyone is checking on everyone because they're scared. In psychologically *safe* environments, everyone is supporting everyone because they're aligned.

And when a veterinary team moves with this kind of trust—this unshakable belief that "I can count on you and you can count on me"—medicine improves, morale skyrockets, and the entire culture becomes self-sustaining.

Trust isn't a perk.
Trust isn't a feeling.
Trust is a collective superpower created by psychological safety—and it's one of the most transformational shifts a veterinary hospital can experience.

Retention Goes Through the Roof

Veterinary medicine is competitive as hell right now. Everyone is hiring. Everyone is recruiting. Everyone is offering "signing bonuses" like candy. But here's the secret: people don't leave psychologically safe environments. They don't walk away from teams where they feel respected, protected, and valued. You can't poach someone who feels seen where they are. Safety is retention. Safety is glue.

Why? Because happy teams don't leave. This is what makes **retention** finally stick. Not gimmicks. Not signing bonuses. Not fear. Safety. Clarity. Culture. Leadership. Retention is not a mystery. It's not random. It's not luck. Retention is the direct result of a team that feels safe, connected, valued, and united under a shared mission, a clear set of standards, and leadership that actually walks the talk.

Engaged teams show 59% less turnover. According to North American Veterinary Community (NAVC) and Veterinary Hospital

Managers Association (VHMA), in vet med bad culture drives 70% of people out the door.

When psychological safety is strong, you unlock trust.
When leadership is strong, you unlock direction.
When culture is strong, you unlock belonging.

And when people trust each other, have direction, and feel like they belong? They stay. They grow. They give their best. They protect the hospital. They become ambassadors. They become evangelists. They become your competitive advantage.

That is the real win. That's the future. That's how you build the kind of veterinary hospital that outlasts trends, outperforms competitors, and becomes the place where the best people in the industry want to work.

If you want retention that actually sticks—retention you can build a future on—you need to understand that people don't leave hospitals; they leave environments. They leave toxic or absent cultures. They leave inconsistency. They leave poor leadership. They leave places where they don't feel psychologically safe.

Veterinary medicine isn't just physically exhausting; it's emotionally loaded. Every single day your team is navigating grief, fear, money stress, emergencies, euthanasia, compassion fatigue, client expectations, and their own internal pressure to "be perfect." When you place human beings inside that environment without psychological safety, you are essentially asking them to sprint a marathon while carrying sandbags.

Psychological safety is the removal of those sandbags.
It's the permission to be human.
It's the permission to not know everything.
It's the permission to make mistakes and learn.
It's the permission to raise a hand and say, "I need help."
It's the permission to speak honestly without fearing retaliation, humiliation, or punishment.

Without that, people burn out: not from the work, but from the emotional isolation.

Retention also builds momentum. When people stick, things click: communication flows, efficiency skyrockets, and trust deepens.

Here's why: when a team's been together for a while, they build rhythm. They communicate better. They're more efficient. They know each other's strengths. They know how everyone reacts under stress. They know how to support each other when shit gets tough.

This trust, momentum, communication, and efficiency within the team build over time. Every tough case, every emotional moment— the team battles through it together. The bonds get tighter. The trust gets stronger.

That's why a tenured team will deliver better outcomes, even in the hardest cases.
Why? Momentum. Communication. Trust within the team.

When turnover drops, something else happens: trust grows not just within the team, but between the team and leadership. People start to realize: "Wow, my hospital leaders built an environment where people actually want to stay."

This is when momentum kicks in. Less change (from turnover) means more comfort. And teams that work together over time better understand their role within that specific team. Everyone sees where they fit, how their strengths matter, and how they plug into the team. And if they have questions, they know they can ask their leaders. Morale skyrockets. Culture thrives.

When you put all of this together, the pattern becomes unmistakable: when leaders choose to bet on their people instead of cutting corners—when they invest intentionally in fairness, clarity, culture, and servant leadership—the team feels that, and, trust deepens. And when trust deepens, the team feels safer, more supported, and more empowered. Then, they reciprocate with loyalty and effort. So, a high-trust environment doesn't just create a happy team; it creates a team that stays.

And when a team stays, everything compounds. Communication gets sharper. Efficiency increases. Internal trust grows more and more over time—both within the team and between the team and its leadership—eventually becoming second nature. Morale rises because people aren't operating from survival mode—they're operating from confidence, connection, and rhythm. And culture goes from "aspirational" to "undeniable."

High-trust culture isn't fluff. It's not a bonus. It's the retention engine—the most powerful compounding asset your hospital will ever have.

Recruiting Gets Stupidly Easier

Psychologically safe teams basically recruit for you. When a team feels safe, respected, supported, and proud of where they work, they don't shut up about it. They talk about it at lunch with techs from other clinics. They talk about it in Facebook Vet Tech groups (which have hundreds of thousands of members). They talk about it at state Veterinary Medical Association (VMA) meetings, CE weekends, and over drinks with former coworkers. And research shows this isn't anecdotal—it's predictable.

A 2023 McKinsey study found that employees in high-trust, psychologically safe environments are three times more likely to recommend their workplace to friends. That's not fluff; that's recruitment firepower. A 2022 Workhuman report showed that when employees feel respected and psychologically safe, referral likelihood jumps by 56%. And across industries, referral hires consistently outperform every other recruitment method, with Harvard Business Review noting they have 25% higher retention and up to 70% faster time-to-fill.

You know what that means in veterinary medicine—where everyone is starving for credentialed techs, solid CSRs, and doctors who aren't burned to dust? **Psychological safety becomes a recruiting strategy. One of the most powerful ones.**

When your culture is strong and your team feels safe, you don't rely on desperate job ads or shotgun Indeed postings that attract burnt-out applicants who are just trying to escape something. Instead, you get pre-vetted humans sent by people who already thrive in your system. In vet med—where identity, mission, and belonging matter—that's massive.

Referrals start flowing.
Not the "warm bodies" you get from job boards.
The good ones.
The ones who give a damn.
The ones who stay.

Research backs that up too: LinkedIn's 2023 Global Recruiting Report found that referrals are four times more likely to be high-performing hires. And in fast-paced, emotionally heavy fields like healthcare, a 2020 Society for Human Resources Management (SHRM) study showed referral hires have 45% lower turnover in the first year compared to traditional recruits. Translation? Your culture literally selects for people who reinforce your culture. Flywheel economics.

In psychologically safe hospitals, referrals don't just "happen." They pile up. Because people who feel supported want to protect that environment. They don't bring you toxic coworkers. They bring you people who match the energy. They refer teammates who align with your standards, your medicine, your mission, and your pace.

High-trust teams recruit people who think like them, communicate like them, and care like them.

Low-trust teams? They recruit from desperation and patch holes with the first résumé that shows up.

When your hospital becomes known as a place where people stay, grow, and feel safe being themselves, you don't need recruitment gimmicks. You have walking, talking billboards wearing scrubs telling everyone, "You should come work with us."

That's the advantage. That's the compounding effect. That's culture doing your recruiting for you.

Individual Performance Explodes

Here's another really cool benefit of establishing psychological safety for your team: it literally makes people smarter—not IQ-smart, but impact-smart. When people feel safe, they don't waste mental bandwidth protecting themselves, tiptoeing around egos, or worrying about getting embarrassed. That freed-up cognitive space gets reinvested into doing the work BETTER: asking sharper questions, taking initiative, troubleshooting faster, collaborating without politics, innovating without fear, and acting like owners instead of passengers. And it's not just inspirational talk—the research backs this up in a big way.

A 2024 study of 580 employees across high-tech companies found that psychological safety directly boosts "employee innovative performance." When teams feel safe to share information, challenge ideas, and experiment without punishment, they generate better ideas, improve workflows, and solve problems faster. Another 2023 study showed that psychological safety drives stronger team learning behavior, higher team confidence, and better productivity. In plain English: safe teams learn faster, trust deeper, and execute better.

It gets even stronger. A massive meta-analysis covering 19,180 employees found that psychological safety has a significant positive correlation with both individual innovation and team-level innovation. Not a small link—a real, measurable jump. That's the difference between a team that just "does the job" and one that creates new ways of doing it. Other research in healthcare environments—a lot closer to veterinary medicine—shows that psychological safety reduces burnout, increases error reporting and early problem detection, and strengthens communication in high-pressure environments. Sound familiar?

Harvard's original work on psychological safety showed that teams who feel safe take more interpersonal risks—they speak up when something's off, ask questions, admit mistakes early, and communicate directly without fear. That's the foundation of innovation. You can't innovate while bracing for impact. And multiple recent studies confirm the same pattern: when people don't fear humiliation, they collaborate better, think clearer, and correct problems before they snowball.

And in a field like veterinary medicine—emotionally intense, medically complex, constantly changing—those gains aren't optional. They're competitive advantage. Psychological safety improves problem-solving, strengthens collaboration across roles, increases the quality of medical discussions, and reduces the cognitive load that burnout creates. When people stay longer, learn together longer, and trust each other longer, your hospital benefits from stronger institutional memory and more consistent patient care.

So yeah, psychological safety makes people smarter. Because it stops the brain drain caused by fear. It lets people use their full mental horsepower instead of keeping one foot on the brake. It multiplies the impact of fairness, good pay, strong leadership, and clear expectations. And when you combine all of that? You get a team that doesn't just show up—they show out. You get initiative, ownership, innovation, and excellence. Not because you demanded it, but because you created the conditions where it can actually exist.

That's the truth every elite workplace understands and every mediocre workplace avoids: psychological safety isn't soft. It's strategic. It's measurable. It's rocket fuel for performance.

Clients Feel It Too

And here's how it starts to power the Veterinary Trust Flywheel: a psychologically safe team exudes confidence and unity. Clients don't know the term for it, but they feel the difference instantly. They trust you faster. They follow medical recommendations more consistently. They stop doctor-shopping. They become loyal because your hospital feels steady, supportive, and aligned. Safety inside the building becomes trust outside the building. (We're going there next.)

So, in summary: psychological safety isn't soft. It isn't optional. It is the competitive advantage of the modern veterinary hospital.

It's how you build a team that not only performs, but stays.
Not only stays, but thrives.
Not only thrives, but recruits the next generation of people who turn your hospital into a powerhouse.

Psychological safety is the result of clarity and vision, of intentionally developed and supported culture that champions standards and clarity, and of passionate, intentional servant leadership. And once your team feels it, it changes everything.

We'll get into that in Chapter 11.

Suggested Readings

Clark, Timothy R. *The 4 Stages of Psychological Safety: Defining the Path to Inclusion and Innovation.* Berrett-Koehler, 2020.

Deci, Edward L., and Richard M. Ryan. *Intrinsic Motivation and Self-determination in Human Behavior.* Plenum Press, 1985.

Edmondson, Amy C. "Psychological Safety and Learning Behavior in Work Teams." *Administrative Science Quarterly*, vol. 44, no. 2, 1999, pp. 350–383.

Edmondson, Amy C. *The Fearless Organization: Creating Psychological Safety in the Workplace for Learning, Innovation, and Growth.* Wiley, 2019.

Gallup, Inc. *State of the Global Workplace 2022 Report.* Gallup, 2022, www.gallup.com/workplace.

Harvard Business Review. "What Google Learned from Its Quest to Build the Perfect Team." *Harvard Business Review*, 2016.

Kahn, William A. "Psychological Conditions of Personal Engagement and Disengagement at Work." *Academy of Management Journal*, vol. 33, no. 4, 1990, pp. 692–724.

Maslach, Christina, and Michael P. Leiter. *The Truth About Burnout: How Organizations Cause Personal Stress and What to Do About It*. Jossey-Bass, 1997.

McKinsey & Company. *Psychological Safety and the Critical Role of Leadership in the New World of Work*. McKinsey, 2023.

NAVC and Veterinary Hospital Managers Association. *Veterinary Team Retention & Engagement Survey Report*. NAVC–VHMA, 2022.

O'Reilly, Charles A., Jennifer A. Chatman, and David F. Caldwell. "People and Organizational Culture: A Profile Comparison Approach to Assessing Person–Organization Fit." *Academy of Management Journal*, vol. 34, no. 3, 1991, pp. 487–516.

Society for Human Resource Management. *Employee Job Referral Programs & Turnover Outcomes*. SHRM, 2020.

Workhuman. *The Global Human Workplace Index*. Workhuman, 2022.

Zenger, Jack, and Joseph Folkman. *The Extraordinary Leader: Turning Good Managers into Great Leaders*. McGraw-Hill, 2019.

Chapter 10

Case Study—The Day a "Successful" Veterinary Hospital Finally Faced the Truth

Before burnout ever showed up, before turnover spiked, before the eye rolls in the break room and the whispered "does anyone actually know how we do this?" moments ... Riverside Veterinary Care looked "fine."

Not broken. Not failing. Just ... unclear.

But "unclear" is the silent killer of veterinary hospitals.

Everyone at Riverside cared deeply. Everyone hustled. Everyone wanted to do great medicine—and on the good days, they did. But the inside of the building felt like running a marathon on gravel: lots of motion, no real smoothness. The medicine was solid, the hearts were enormous, and the effort was ridiculous. But the entire team carried a low-grade, constant anxiety—the "every day is a pop quiz" energy. You know the one.

No one said it out loud, but everyone felt it: "We're working hard ... but not always together."

Ask five people how to manage a vomiting recheck? Five different answers.

Ask three doctors when to recommend full-mouth radiographs? Three different philosophies, three different conversations, and three different client experiences.

Ask a Client Service Representative (CSR) how to explain the estimate? Depends on who trained them, what mood they're in, and how busy the lobby is.

This wasn't incompetence. It wasn't laziness. It was the real enemy: **inconsistent standards**.

The team wasn't failing. They were guessing. And in veterinary medicine, guessing is emotionally expensive.

The Day Everything Shifted

The turning point didn't happen during a crisis, or after a resignation, or in response to a bad review. It happened in a Tuesday staff meeting—one of those "everyone is tired but trying" mornings—when a quiet technician finally said the thing every person had been swallowing for months: *I want to feel like we all do things the same way. Right now it feels like every day is a pop quiz.*

Silence. But then, a collective exhale: the sound teams make when honesty becomes oxygen.

No drama. No anger. Just truth.

And in that moment, leadership finally understood: The team didn't need more effort. The team needed **psychological safety**: clarity, consistency, and leadership that didn't hide behind titles or fear conflict.

That single sentence cracked the door open. And from it eventually came the most powerful element any hospital can have: **Identity**.

Building Identity—Not Rules, but Purpose

Riverside's leadership didn't fix this by dropping a laminated HR binder from Mount Olympus. They fixed it by sitting down—doctors, CSRs, techs, assistants, and everyone—and asking three servant-leadership questions:

1. What kind of hospital do we want to be?
2. Why does this place exist?
3. How do we treat each other and our clients when we're at our best?

The answers weren't corporate. They weren't fluffy. They were *raw*:

- "We want to be known for kindness and competence."
- "We want clients to trust every doctor, not just their favorite one."
- "We want new people to feel supported, not tested."
- "We want to practice medicine we're proud of."

The mission became simple and powerful: *to protect the bond between pets, clients, and veterinary professionals through trust, empathy, and excellence.*

The vision: *a hospital where every team member practices with confidence because expectations are shared, not assumed.*

The values weren't posters—they were behaviors:

- We communicate directly and kindly.
- We back each other up before we blame each other.
- We close loops: with clients and with each other.
- We do the right thing even when it's slower.
- We leave egos outside and bring curiosity inside.

- We speak up without fear, and we listen without defensiveness.
- We fix small problems because small problems become big culture killers.

This was the first act of servant leadership—the act of giving the team a voice, a role, and a shared purpose. It wasn't a policy. It was psychological safety becoming real.

No fluff.
No corporate jargon.
Just a team deciding who the hell they were going to be, together.

The Transformation You Could Feel in the Hallway

Culture doesn't change overnight. But it does change through consistency: servant leadership showing up in small, daily behaviors that compound.

And here's what began to happen at Riverside:

1. **CSRs stopped asking "Let me check with the doctor."**

   Because they finally had clarity.
   They knew the hospital's standard pathways, and they felt supported in using them.

   This is psychological safety: the freedom to act confidently without fearing they'll be corrected, contradicted, or embarrassed.

2. **Technicians shifted from waiting to anticipating**.

   With clear standards, techs weren't guessing the plan; they were preparing for it. Servant leadership had removed the friction that once made every shift exhausting.

3. **Doctors stopped practicing alone in silos**.

   Shared medical pathways meant shared philosophy.
   Shared philosophy meant shared identity.
   Shared identity meant collaboration instead of comparison.

4. **New hires weren't "tested by fire."**

They were onboarded into consistency, not chaos.
Servant leaders didn't expect them to "figure it out."
They expected them to grow—and protected that growth.

5. **Morning huddles actually mattered**.

Updates had purpose.
Communication had alignment.
People felt seen, heard, and grounded.

6. **Rechecks were intentional, not reactive**.

No more "just come back and we'll see."
There were standards.
There was a shared plan.
There was trust.

7. **Debriefs became safe spaces, not blame-fests**.

When something went wrong, the question shifted from "Who messed up?" to:
"What system failed and how do we fix it together?"

That is servant leadership in action.

8. **Clients stopped saying "I only want to see Dr. ___."**

Instead, they said: "Your team is incredible." Because the TEAM finally *was* incredible: aligned, confident, and empowered.

Not coworkers. Not shift-mates. Not exhausted firefighters in matching scrubs. A team.

The Quiet Victory That Changed Everything

Six months later, Riverside saw the moment every hospital should be chasing.

A new grad—barely one year in—walked into a complex senior-care follow-up. She took the case from start to finish with a level of confidence and clarity far beyond her experience. She educated the client without faltering. She built trust. She delivered medicine like someone who belonged.

The tech assisting her smiled. The CSR overheard and nodded. A seasoned doctor peeked in and, instead of feeling threatened, felt *proud*.

After the appointment, the new grad walked into treatment and said the four words that prove culture change is real:

"I felt supported today."

Not "I knew everything." Not "I nailed it." Not "I did it alone."

"I felt supported."

That sentence is the sound of psychological safety.
That sentence is the sound of servant leadership.
That sentence is the sound of a hospital with an identity.

The Real Lesson

Riverside didn't change because of rules or memos or management buzzwords. It changed because leadership stopped trying to be important—and started trying to be useful.

This hospital shifted when leaders:

- listened instead of defended
- clarified instead of assumed
- fixed instead of ignored
- empowered instead of controlled
- set standards instead of letting preference rule
- protected psychological safety instead of protecting their ego

- removed obstacles instead of pretending they were "someone else's job"
- modeled vulnerability instead of faking invincibility

When a veterinary team knows:

- Why we exist
- Where we're going
- How we behave
- What great looks like here
- That speaking up won't get them punished or embarrassed
- That small issues matter because small issues create big stress
- That their leader is in the details with them, not above them

Everything improves:

Medicine.
Communication.
Confidence.
Client trust.
Morale.
Retention.
Revenue.
Pride.
Stability.
Trajectory.

Clarity doesn't box people in. Clarity frees people.

Psychological safety doesn't soften expectations. It strengthens them.

Servant leadership doesn't make leaders small. It makes teams limitless.

Riverside didn't become robotic. They became dangerously capable humans operating with alignment, purpose, and pride.

They stopped guessing. They started owning. And for the first time, their hospital wasn't surviving on effort—it was thriving on culture.

Chapter 11

How Your Team's Psychological Safety Translates Directly to Client Experience

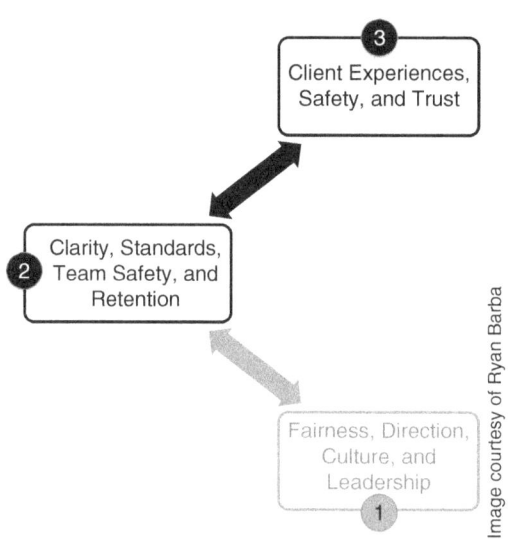

Image courtesy of Ryan Barba

Once you've built a culture with real clarity—where everyone knows what the hospital stands for, what good medicine looks like, how to communicate, and how to support one another—you create psychological safety for your team. And when your team feels safe to speak, question, think, and advocate without fear, everything about their communication shifts. They narrate. They empathize. They slow down instead of rushing. They show up as their best selves. And clients feel it instantly.

Clarity and safety turn your staff from a group of individuals into a unified force. The hospital becomes predictable in the best possible way—steady, organized, and aligned. Clients walk in and feel the energy: *these people know what they're doing. These people actually like working with each other.* That emotional stability is the first spark of trust.

Then retention enters the picture: when clients see the same faces month after month, year after year, trust becomes effortless. Familiarity becomes emotional safety. Continuity becomes reassurance. Clients no longer brace for inconsistency because they know the team knows them, their pet, and their story. And your long-tenured team communicates with efficiency, coordination, and competence that only time can build. Clients notice. They feel the smoothness, the cohesion, and the "these people have their shit together" vibe. They don't have to repeat themselves. They're not re-explaining history. They're not wondering whether the new doctor will contradict the last one. The whole experience just feels better.

That's competent support. That's how you build massive trust.

And yes, the data backs it up: Deloitte found that employee engagement directly drives customer satisfaction. In veterinary medicine, clients who feel your staff is warm, consistent, and invested are two to three times more likely to return.

But here's what makes this part of the flywheel so powerful: the relationship goes both ways.

Clients can tell when they're dealing with a trusted, appreciated, and empowered team. They can feel when the culture is healthy and the people enjoy working together. And when clients trust the team, they show up differently: they give grace instead of suspicion, patience instead of pressure, and kindness instead of blame. Their trust becomes validation. Their gratitude becomes fuel. Their loyalty becomes emotional reinforcement. It strengthens the team's sense of purpose, deepens psychological safety, and increases retention even further.

This is why the arrow between "Team Experience, Efficiency, and Retention" and "Client Experience (CX) & Client Trust" points both directions. It's a feedback loop.

When trust is missing, you feel the opposite instantly. Stress skyrockets. Clients start questioning everything—your methods, your intentions, and your prices. They second-guess every move. Their worry comes out sideways as criticism, defensiveness, or hostility. And that emotional friction wears teams down. Staff feel attacked, scrutinized, and micromanaged by clients. Their confidence dips. Their morale cracks. Their desire to stay slips away.

But with clients who trust the hospital? It's night and day. They assume good intent. They collaborate instead of confront. They listen instead of challenge. They take guidance instead of fighting it. And they say *thank you* more. They remind the team why the work matters. They bring meaning back into the building.

I've said it before and I'll say it again here: You cannot—*cannot*—build a CX that consistently earns client trust if your team isn't standing on solid psychological ground. You can duct-tape the cracks with scripts, slogans, mission statements on the wall, and Pinterest-pretty handouts—but none of that moves the needle if your people are scared, second-guessing themselves, or bracing for the next internal landmine.

But when your team feels psychologically safe? The CX doesn't just "improve." It **transforms**. It evolves. It compounds. It becomes something clients *feel*—not because you taught them a new greeting or passed out a "smile more" memo, but because your people show up real. Confident. Aligned. Calm. Human. Supported by a culture and leadership team that actually earns the word *trust*.

A team that feels safe doesn't fake it at the front desk and then fall apart in the treatment room. They don't freeze when a client questions a care plan. They don't get defensive when something goes sideways. They breathe. They collaborate. They think. They absorb pressure instead of transmitting it. They stop *performing* customer service and start *being* it.

And as we've discussed: clients don't trust scripts. They trust **energy**. They trust consistency. They trust a team that clearly knows its standards, knows its medicine, and knows each other.

This is what psychological safety creates.

At the core, it's simple: distrust breeds conflict; trust builds partnership. And in a profession already loaded with emotional weight, that difference is everything.

Trusted teams create trust with clients. Trusted clients reinforce trust with teams. And that cycle boosts morale, confidence, and retention in ways no bonus, no policy, and no incentive can touch.

This is the flywheel. This is the compounding effect of culture done right. This is how trust multiplies between your team and your clients and transforms your hospital from the inside out.

Safety Unlocks Personality. And Personality Builds Trust

Fear suppresses personality. Safety unleashes it.

A psychologically safe team doesn't operate from "don't mess up." They operate from "I belong here, I matter here, and what I say carries weight." When fear isn't running the show, you start to see:

The Client Service Representative (CSR) who radiates warmth not because it's part of the job, but because she finally feels valued enough to show up fully.
The tech who kneels to greet a nervous dog without rushing— because he's not terrified of falling behind or being judged.
The doctor who explains medicine in clean, human language— because she doesn't need jargon to protect her ego.

Authenticity is not fluff. Authenticity is **operational advantage**.

Because when clients feel that authenticity, *they* feel safe. And when they feel safe, they stop holding back. They tell you the whole story. They ask questions. They express concerns. They approve treatment. They stop Googling in the parking lot. They stop needing to "think about it." They start trusting you.

Authenticity + Safety = Trust
Trust = Treatment Acceptance
Treatment Acceptance = Healthier Pets
Healthier Pets = A Hospital That Wins Long Term

This isn't emotional fluff. It's operational math. It's the Flywheel in action.

Safe Teams Communicate Clearly, Consistently, and Confidently

Psychologically safe teams communicate differently. They speak with clarity, not hesitation. They don't waffle. They don't contradict each other or interrupt each other. They don't give clients five versions of the same recommendation—or different recommendations for the same type of case—depending on who's in the room.

When a team feels safe:

They Portray Confidence

They know their role. They know the hospital's standards. They know they're valued. That confidence bleeds into every client interaction, and clients instinctively translate confidence into competence.

They Feel Comfortable Validating Information

A safe team asks for help when they're unsure. They double-check facts instead of guessing because they're ashamed to need help or afraid of looking "dumb" to their team or leaders. They confirm dosing, protocols, and plans without shame, which leads to cleaner, safer medicine and messaging.

They Feel Valued and Empowered

When your team feels genuinely valued—not performatively, not "pizza party for morale" valued, but *my-leader-trusts-me-with-real-decisions* valued—everything changes.

This is where empowerment stops being a buzzword and becomes a behavior.

A team member who knows their voice matters doesn't walk into an exam room as "the assistant" or "the CSR." They walk in as an advocate. A translator. A guide. A partner in the pet's care. They don't wait for permission to help. They don't silently defer and hope the doctor fills every gap. They step up, they explain, they anticipate, and they own the CX like it's theirs.

And clients feel that energy instantly.

People can tell when someone is genuinely confident and supported versus when they're nervous and trying not to get in trouble. Clients may not know veterinary medicine, but they know humanity. They know when someone is speaking from empowerment instead of obligation.

That is trust-building gold.

It's the difference between a client thinking, *"They were nice,"* and a client thinking,

"These people know me, they know my pet, and I know we're in good hands."

They Communicate Clearly, Which Clients Interpret as Competence

Clarity is one of the most underrated superpowers in veterinary medicine. When your team feels psychologically safe on the inside, they stop second-guessing themselves, stop tiptoeing, stop hunting for the "right" phrasing, and start communicating with confidence. And here's the magic: clients read confidence as competence. Every. Single. Time.

Clients don't need the Latin root of the disease.
They don't need a five-minute dissertation on pathophysiology.
They don't even need all the details you think are impressive.

They need plain language spoken by a team that sounds aligned, calm, and clear.

"Here's what's going on."
"Here's what we recommend."
"Here's why it matters."
"Here's what happens next."

When your team communicates like that—consistently, across doctors, across techs, across CSRs—and when they stop trying to prove themselves and their worth by showing off every bit of detail they know, clients stop feeling overwhelmed and start feeling supported. They stop Googling during the appointment because your explanation actually lands. They stop shopping around because you didn't confuse them or bury them, you guided them.

Aligned Teams Create Aligned Messaging

Here's the truth nobody wants to admit: most client confusion isn't a "client problem." It's an alignment problem inside the hospital.

When your team trusts each other—when the culture is safe, consistent, and collaborative—they stop sending clients mixed signals. The doctor isn't saying one thing while the tech says another. The CSR isn't promising something the medical team can't deliver. Nobody is accidentally undermining anyone else's recommendations.

Instead, the whole team starts speaking with one voice.

The doctor, tech, and CSR aren't three separate touchpoints anymore; they're one unified experience. They're all playing the same game, running the same playbook, and reinforcing the same standard of care in different ways, through different roles, but with the exact same message.

And clients feel that alignment instantly.

A unified team creates this powerful sense of, *"Wow, these people know what they're doing."*
Clients stop wondering who to believe.
They stop worrying about missing information.
They stop feeling like they're driving the appointment.
They relax, because everyone they interact with is saying the same thing, in the same style, with the same confidence and clarity.

In other words: alignment kills doubt. Alignment kills hesitation. Alignment kills mistrust.

When clients sense that everyone on your team is on the same page—same philosophy, same priorities, and same communication style—they naturally assume the care is stronger, the medicine is better, and the hospital is more competent.

And they're right.

Aligned teams *are* more competent, because aligned teams are the byproduct of intentional leadership and psychologically safe culture. Without that? Mixed messages, inconsistent communication, and clients who walk out the door feeling unsure—even when the care was good.

But with alignment?

Your hospital feels coordinated.
Clients feel confident.
And trust becomes the default, not the exception.

Calm Teams Create Calm Clients

Clients don't walk into your hospital as blank slates. They walk in with adrenaline already in their bloodstream. Their dog's limping. Their cat hasn't eaten. Their new puppy is coughing. Their credit card balance is top of mind. Fear is sitting in the passenger seat long before they pull into your parking lot.

And humans—all humans—read emotional tone before they process information. That's neuroscience. Our brains are wired to scan our surroundings for safety before logic. So, when a client walks through your doors, the very first thing they're evaluating isn't your credentials, your equipment, or your medical brilliance.

They're evaluating:
"Do I belong and feel safe here?"
"Does this team feel like they've got me?"
"Do I need to be on guard?"

This is where a psychologically safe team becomes your hospital's secret weapon.

A team that feels safe internally brings a different presence into the room: things like steady posture, relaxed tone, unhurried explanations, and grounded eye contact. The client feels that calm before the first word is even spoken. It's contagious. It spreads. It immediately downshifts the entire emotional environment.

Suddenly, the client isn't bracing.
They're breathing.
They're receiving.
They're listening.

And here's the multiplier: when your people feel safe, they don't leak micro-stress.
No clipped sentences.
No rushed body language.
No side-glances.
No tension in their voice.
No "I don't have time for this" energy.

Clients pick up on micro-stress more than any clinical detail. If your team looks panicked or overwhelmed, clients assume the situation is worse than it is. If your team looks irritated or rushed, clients assume they are being judged. If your team looks checked-out, clients assume you don't care.

But when your team is psychologically safe, those micro-stresses disappear. The team moves as one. They communicate fluidly. They regulate each other. Their calm becomes the backdrop of the appointment—something the client doesn't consciously notice but deeply feels.

And because the client feels calm, they show up differently:

They ask clearer questions.
They express concerns earlier.
They stay open instead of defensive.
They follow recommendations instead of shutting down.
They make better decisions for their pet because they aren't in fight-or-flight.

Calm is not the absence of chaos; it's mastery in chaos. Calm is not passive; it's powerful. Calm is leadership. And you cannot fake calm. You cannot script calm. You cannot "train" calm in a seminar.

Calm is the natural output of a team that feels safe, supported, respected, and connected. If you build a hospital where your team can breathe, your clients will too. And when clients breathe, they trust. And when they trust, you win—medically, emotionally, and financially.

Trust Erases the "Weak Link" Effect

Every hospital knows the "weak link effect," even if they've never named it.

It's that one moment, that one person, and that one interaction that tanks the entire appointment—even when everyone else did their job perfectly. The CSR with the flat tone. The tech who seems rushed. The doctor who communicates brilliantly but is followed by a checkout process that feels cold or chaotic. Or worse, the doctor who's incredible ... but the tech is terrified to speak up, so information gets lost, and the whole visit collapses in confusion.

In an unsafe hospital, this happens constantly. Why? Because the organization relies on a few high performers to carry all of the emotional weight while everyone else operates in fear, inconsistency, or silence.

And here's the psychological truth: clients judge the whole hospital based on the weakest moment. So, your CX is only as strong as its weakest point. Broken links define the brand more than polished ones.

One insecure explanation. One dismissive tone. One breakdown in handoff. Boom—trust gone.

But in a psychologically safe hospital, the weak link effect disappears.

Why? Because every role is empowered. Every voice is respected. Every team member feels confident stepping into their part of the CX with clarity, consistency, and ownership.

The CSR isn't "just the front desk." The assistant isn't "just helping." The tech isn't "just grabbing vitals." Everyone becomes a co-owner of the experience.

That means the doctor doesn't have to compensate for a shaky handoff. The tech doesn't have to guess what the doctor wants. The CSR doesn't have to apologize for something she didn't understand. Everyone plays the same game, on the same team, with the same mission.

When trust flows internally—horizontally across peers and vertically between leaders and staff—it creates a hospital where nobody freezes, nobody hides, nobody undermines, and nobody drops the baton in the relay.

And because the culture lifts everyone, not just the "stars," the entire client journey becomes stable, predictable, and strong at every single touchpoint.

A safe hospital doesn't rely on heroes. It relies on systems and psychological safety that make *every person* a strong link.

And when every link is strong? The chain never breaks.

Purpose Beats Fear Every Damn Time

Fear-based performance is the fastest way to make your hospital feel cold, scripted, and transactional. When your team is scared—of being wrong, of being snapped at, of being judged, and of being thrown under the bus—they stop being human and start acting like robots. They say the "right lines" but with zero heart. They follow the checklist but avoid real connection. They focus on *not messing up* instead of *showing up*. They stop showing initiative and creativity.

And clients can smell that fear a mile away. They don't have to be trained in veterinary medicine to feel when someone is tense, guarded, or performing instead of caring.

But when your team is rooted in purpose, not fear, you unlock something completely different. People communicate with warmth. They advocate with conviction. They guide with confidence. They stop hiding behind scripts and start speaking from their gut. They stop worrying about punishment and start focusing on the pet and the person in front of them.

Purpose makes your team magnetic. Clients feel safer. They trust deeper. They let their guard down because the energy in the room tells them, *"These people care about my pet, not about covering their ass."*

Fear manufactures compliance. Purpose builds connection.

And connection is what drives trust, adherence, loyalty, and every damn metric that matters.

When your culture runs on fear, your team survives the day. When your culture runs on purpose, your team transforms the experience.

Clients know the difference instantly, because energy doesn't lie.

Safe Teams Innovate in the Moment

Here's what leaders forget: innovation in a veterinary hospital doesn't always come from a whiteboard session. It comes from the hallway. The exam room. In the moment.

A psychologically safe team doesn't sit around waiting for permission or instructions. They don't think, *"Is this my job?"* They think, *"What does this pet, this client, this moment need?"* And then they just do it.

Real-time innovation looks small from the outside, but it's enormous to the client.

It's the assistant who notices the shaking hands of a grieving pet owner and quietly grabs a glass of water without disrupting the exam.

It's the tech who steps in to hold the fractious cat before the doctor even asks, because she's tuned into the room and unafraid to act.

It's the CSR who prints a handout, sketches a diagram, or pulls up a visual because the client's eyebrows just did that "I'm smiling but I'm lost" thing.

It's the nurse who texts a nervous puppy parent later that day: "Hey, just checking in."

None of that is in an SOP. None of that is "policy approved." But all of it builds loyalty like crazy.

Because clients don't remember the medical code or the exact phrasing you used. They remember how cared for they felt. They remember the initiative. They remember the effort they didn't have to ask for.

And here's the key: that kind of initiative only shows up in a culture that says:
"We trust you."
"We value you."
"We see you."

Psychologically safe teams don't innovate because they're trying to impress. They innovate because they're not afraid of being wrong. They're not worried about being reprimanded. They're not stuck in the paralysis of "What if I make a mistake?"

When your team feels safe, they act human. When your team acts human, they act creatively. And when they act creatively, clients feel seen, supported, and emotionally carried through the experience.

That's innovation. That's trust. That's what turns a veterinary hospital from "good" into unforgettable.

Safe Teams Handle Hard Moments with Grace

Let's get real: veterinary medicine is emotionally heavy in a way most industries will never understand. You've got puppy joy, blunt-force emergencies, frantic "Do something!" energy, financial stress, moral stress, fear, guilt, grief, and uncertainty—sometimes all in the same hour. The building hums with emotion every single day.

A scared team collapses under that weight. A safe team rises to meet it.

When a team doesn't feel safe—psychologically or emotionally— hard moments hit like a tidal wave. They rush. They snap. They shut down. They avoid eye contact. They default to defensiveness. They say things that sound clinical instead of compassionate. Everything tightens.

But a psychologically safe team? They show up differently. When the stakes are high, they slow down instead of spiraling. They get curious—"Help me understand what you're feeling"—instead of defensive. They make clients feel seen, not judged or dismissed. They hold the emotional weight of the moment with presence, not panic.

They can talk to the euthanasia client without their own anxiety leaking into the room. They can guide the panicked pet parent without sounding irritated or overwhelmed. They can de-escalate financial tension because they're grounded enough to hear the fear underneath the anger. They can give a CPR update, a cancer diagnosis, or bad news with honesty and humanity because they're not fighting their own internal stress while doing it.

That kind of emotional steadiness isn't talent. It's culture.

You can't deliver calm to a client if your team doesn't have calm within themselves. You can't create safety for a family in crisis if your staff feels unsafe in their own workplace.

This is the hidden engine behind emotional intelligence in veterinary care: not scripting empathy. Not forcing "be kind" as a mandate. It's giving your team psychological safety so real empathy can actually flourish.

A safe team has the bandwidth to care. A safe team has the composure to hold space. A safe team has the emotional reserves to show up for people who are falling apart.

That's grace. That's leadership. And that's what turns hard moments into healing ones—for pets, clients, and your own people.

Confident Recommendations Build Compliance

Confidence is the engine behind every "yes" in veterinary medicine. You can have the perfect treatment plan, the most ethical recommendation, and the cleanest medical reasoning. But if your team presents it with hesitancy, the client feels that wobble and mirrors it right back.

A team that feels safe—truly safe—doesn't tiptoe around recommendations. They don't apologize for good medicine. They don't shrink their voice when clients look confused or overwhelmed. They don't hedge every sentence with "maybe," "possibly," or "it's up to you."

They speak like professionals who know their craft and know the value of what they're offering.

"Here's what's going on."
"Here's what your pet needs."
"Here's why it matters."
"Here's the plan."

And the client's nervous system responds to that clarity. Certainty is contagious. When your team shows up grounded, steady, and confident, the client borrows that emotional stability. Most pet owners are scared in the exam room—scared of the cost, scared of the diagnosis, scared of being judged, and scared of losing their pet. They're not looking for options; they're looking for *leadership.*

When the team believes in the recommendation, the client believes in the recommendation.

This is psychology, not sales.

We follow people who sound like they know where they're going. We trust people who speak with conviction. We say yes when someone confidently walks us through the why, the what, and the next step.

Confident communication is built in a culture of psychological safety. When your staff isn't worried about being ridiculed, corrected in front of clients, or punished for misspeaking, they show up bolder, clearer, and more human.

Clients don't comply because you pressure them. They comply because your team communicates with the kind of calm, grounded certainty that says: "We know what your pet needs, and we've got you."

That's what builds trust. That's what drives adherence. That's what elevates medical outcomes across the board.

High-retention Teams Build High-trust Clients

Psychological safety doesn't just make teams *happier*—it makes them *stay.* And in veterinary medicine, team retention isn't a "nice perk." It's one of your biggest competitive advantages. Because when a team feels safe to speak up, safe to ask questions, safe to make mistakes, safe to grow, and safe to be human at work ... they don't leave.

They're not burned out. They're not looking over the fence. They're not daydreaming about jumping ship to the clinic down the road.

Safe culture creates sticky culture. Sticky culture creates long-term teams. Long-term teams create long-term trust.

And here's the part most hospital owners forget: client trust skyrockets when staff retention is high.

Clients notice everything. They notice when the CSR who checked them in last year is still there this year. They notice when the tech who helped with their new kitten is now helping with their adult cat. They notice when the doctor who walked them through a terrifying diagnosis also gets to see the recovery.

Consistency feels like safety. Familiarity feels like competence. Seeing the same faces over time feels like, *"Okay, this place is stable. This place is healthy. I trust these people."*

High retention tells clients:

- "This hospital treats its people well."
- "The team must work well together."
- "If the staff is this loyal, the care must be good."
- "My pet's health is in consistent hands."

Clients don't consciously say that, but they *feel* it ... instantly.

Staff turnover, on the other hand, destroys psychological safety for clients. Constantly changing faces makes clients wonder:

- "Why can't this place keep people?"
- "Is something wrong here?"
- "Are the team members even trained?"
- "Does the doctor even know my pet's history?"
- "Am I going to have to re-explain everything every time?"

When turnover is high, client anxiety goes up, even if the medicine is great. When retention is high, client anxiety drops, even before the appointment starts.

And here's the kicker: long-term staff become long-term storytellers. They know the pets. They know the families. They remember the details, the quirks, the histories, and the emotions. They can say things like:

- "How's Max's arthritis since winter hit?"
- "I remember his last dental; he bounced right back."
- "You switched foods last year and his weight stabilized. Let's revisit that."

That familiarity hits clients *deep*. It signals continuity, competence, and care.

You can't fake that. You can't teach that in onboarding. You can't create that with scripts. It only comes from time, and time only happens when your team stays.

A psychologically safe team gives you consistency. Consistency gives clients confidence. Confidence gives clients trust. And trust is the currency of loyalty—the thing that keeps your hospital thriving, growing, and emotionally grounded year after year.

So, retention isn't an HR metric. It's a trust strategy. It's a clinical strategy. It's a business strategy. And it all starts with psychological safety.

Clients Move Through the Four Stages Too, and It Changes Everything

Carter's model of the Four Stages of Psychological Safety is often used to describe dynamics within teams. And yes—that's foundational. But here's the unlock most practices miss: clients go through the same four stages.

It's not just the technicians and CSRs learning to speak up. It's the pet owners learning to trust, ask questions, advocate, listen, accept guidance, and partner in care.

A client doesn't walk in day one feeling confident, understood, and part of the decision-making process. They *learn* that comfort the same way a new CSR or assistant does.

And elite hospitals—the ones clients rave about and return to year after year—*design for this progression.*

Let's walk their journey.

Stage 1: Inclusion Safety—"Am I Welcome Here? Do They See Me and My Pet?"

For clients, psychological safety starts the second they walk through your door (or land on your website, honestly).

Seeking to understand whether they belong in your hospital, a client is silently asking themselves:

- Do they look up when I walk in, or do they keep typing?
- Do they talk *to* me or talk *at* me?
- Did they use my pet's name?
- Do I feel judged ... or included?

Inclusion Safety for clients means *I feel like I belong here as a pet parent. I don't feel rushed. I don't feel like a transaction.*

When you nail this stage, the client's defense system lowers. They stop preparing rebuttals and start preparing to trust.

This is the emotional on-ramp.

Stage 2: Learner Safety—"Can I Ask Questions Without Feeling Stupid?"

Once a client feels welcome, they test the next boundary: "Am I allowed to not know things here?"

This is huge.

If they feel dumb for asking about vaccines ...
If they feel embarrassed about misinterpreting symptoms ...
If they feel inferior when they say "my baby" instead of "my dog" ...

They shut down. They nod along. They pretend they understand. They leave confused. They go home and Google symptoms instead of trusting you.

Learner Safety means a client feels safe to say:

- "I don't understand that—can you explain it again?"
- "What are my options?"
- "I'm nervous."
- "I've never had a pet with this condition before."

A psychologically safe veterinary environment celebrates client questions, not tolerates them.

Because curious clients become informed clients.
Informed clients become committed clients.
And committed clients follow the care plan.

Stage 3: Contributor Safety—"Can I Actively Participate in My Pet's Care?"

This is where the magic starts happening, when the client transitions from spectator to participant.

They:

- Share concerns honestly
- Ask for clarity instead of guessing
- Tell you when something isn't working

And they start trusting you enough to collaborate—not challenge, not hide, and not fight for control.

Contributor Safety is the moment a client says, **"We're in this together."**

That's when treatment adherence jumps.
That's when recheck rates climb.
That's when clients feel emotionally bonded—not just serviced.

Stage 4: Challenger Safety—"Can I Express a Concern or Idea Without Being Dismissed?"

This is the highest level of trust a pet owner can give you. It's when a client feels safe enough to say:

- "I'm worried about finances. Can we talk options?"
- "I'm nervous about anesthesia. Can you walk me through it?"
- "Last time, Fluffy seemed stressed. How can we make this easier?"
- "Can I show you a video of what I saw at home?"

They're not questioning your competence. They're partnering in care.

That's the highest form of trust.

And when clients reach this stage? They're yours. Forever.

They refer. They advocate. They defend your prices. They send cookies at the holidays. They mourn with you when their pet passes.

And when they get a new pet? There's no shopping around. They already know where they belong.

Establishing Psychological Safety for Clients with Past Veterinary Trauma

This section is about how to treat the visit you can't see.

INTRO: The Wound You Can't See Hurts the Most

Every day, veterinary teams walk into exam rooms assuming they're starting from zero.

But clients walk in carrying stories—some silent, some buried, and some still bleeding.

A dog who crashed during anesthesia.
A cat who deteriorated suddenly after a missed diagnosis.
A hospital that dismissed their fear.
A doctor who talked over them.
A bill they didn't understand.
A euthanasia that shattered them.
A miscommunication that spiraled out of control online.
A tech who made them feel stupid.
A receptionist who made them feel judged.

And the heaviest trauma of all: the feeling that they failed their pet.

You will never see these experiences unless you ask. Clients almost never volunteer them. And because they don't speak it, teams unknowingly step right on the bruise.

The client becomes tense. Then the team becomes defensive. And the appointment derails. And everyone walks away feeling attacked or misunderstood.

This is the unseen battle happening inside exam rooms every day.

Not because clients are difficult. But because their nervous systems are still holding onto the last experience they survived.

So, let's talk about how to recognize that trauma, how to respond to it with emotional intelligence, and how to create psychological safety so powerful it rewires the entire relationship.

This isn't soft. This is strategy. Because psychological safety isn't only for your team. It's for your clients, especially the ones who've been hurt.

What Client Trauma Looks Like (Even When They Hide It)

Clients with veterinary trauma rarely look "traumatized."

They look:

- Hypervigilant
- Distrustful
- Question-heavy
- Emotionally reactive
- Quick to assume the worst
- Prone to catastrophizing
- Sensitive to tone
- Easily triggered by small delays or small missteps

Or the opposite:

- Polite but distant
- Quiet
- Numb
- Afraid to ask questions
- Agreeing to everything but visibly anxious

This is fear of wearing socially acceptable clothing.

Trauma doesn't show up as tears. It shows up as tension. And if you interpret that tension as "difficult client behavior" instead of "someone who's been hurt," you lose the entire visit.

Reinforce this important point with your team: clients with trauma are not trying to be challenging. They're trying to protect themselves.

Why Veterinary Trauma Hits Harder than Other Types of Trauma

There are three unique factors that make veterinary trauma especially intense:

1. **It involves a loved one who cannot speak**.

   This guilt is enormous. Clients think: "If I miss something, they suffer silently." The emotional stakes are massive.

2. **It involves money + uncertainty**.

People feel guilty spending, guilty not spending, and guilty guessing wrong.

Money + fear = emotional combustion.

3. **They often blame themselves**.

"I should've known."
"I should've brought them in sooner."
"I should've asked more questions."
"I should've trusted my gut."

Self-blame amplifies trauma more than anything else. This is why a normal medical recommendation—bloodwork, hospitalization, imaging—can feel like a threat to clients with past trauma. They are not reacting to *your* hospital. They are reacting to *their memory of another one.*

The Trauma-informed Veterinary Care Framework

Here is the operationally tight, emotionally intelligent framework for supporting clients who may be carrying past trauma.

1. **The Emotional Check-in**

This should happen during the first 90 seconds of the visit.

Here's an example script: "Before we dive in, how are you feeling about today's visit? Anything on your mind from past experiences that you want us to be aware of so we can make this easier for you?"

This question is a master key. It unlocks everything.

It tells clients:

- You see them
- You care about their emotional experience
- You're not rushing

- You're not judging
- You're willing to partner, not dictate

Most clients answer with relief:
"Yes, actually ..."
"We had a rough experience last time ..."
"I'm nervous because ..."

And once they say it aloud, the fear loses its power.

2. The Normalization Technique

When clients express fear, normalize it.

Try saying something like, "A lot of pet parents feel this way after what you went through. It makes complete sense you're feeling cautious today."

Normalization removes shame. Shame is what makes clients defensive.

3. The Reassurance Loop

Clients with trauma need more touchpoints, not fewer. A reassurance loop includes:

- Time expectations
- Step-by-step narration
- Frequent updates
- Explicit confirmation that their pet is safe

For example: "We're going to run X-rays now. It should take about 10 minutes. If we're running longer than that, I'll come update you. If anything changes, you'll know right away."

Clients don't need perfection. They need predictability. Predictability *is* safety.

4. The Transparency Protocol

Trauma hates ambiguity, and ambiguity fuels fear.

Be extra clear about:

- Why you're recommending something
- What it costs
- What happens next
- What choices they have

For example:

"I want to walk you through every option so you feel fully in control.
Here's path A …
Here's path B …
Here's what I recommend and why …
But you get to decide what feels right for you and Shadow."

This restores agency—something trauma steals.

5. Permission-based Medicine

Never push. Invite.

"Would you like to talk through what the next steps might look like?"
"Would it help to see images or diagrams?"
"Do you want a moment to think this over?"

Permission conveys respect. And respect rebuilds trust.

6. Soft Transitions Between Moments

Transitions are dangerous for anxious clients:

- Going "to the back"
- Leaving the pet
- Waiting alone
- Moving from exam to treatment
- Getting bad news
- Signing estimates

Each transition needs narration.

"We're going to move to the next step, and here's exactly what that looks like …"

This simple phrase prevents emotional spirals.

7. **Affirm the Relationship**

Clients with trauma don't trust they're doing "a good job."

Affirm them (as you might remember, that's one of the key things clients want to feel). Tell them: "Thank you for being so thoughtful about your Shadow's care. You're doing right by him; he's so lucky to have you."

This lands deeper than you think.

A Real Case Example—And the Transformation

Let's call the client Melissa.

Melissa had previously lost a cat during a dental procedure because of a communication breakdown at another hospital. She walked into your ER with her new cat, Harper, for vomiting.

She looked calm at first glance—but the moment you mentioned bloodwork, she stiffened.

Your tech said, "We'll take her to the back now," and Melissa said, "Why? What are you doing back there?"
Her voice shook.
Her body language changed.
She became hyper-alert.

In a traditional hospital, this becomes conflict.
"Ma'am, this is standard procedure."
"You have to trust us."
"We do this with every pet."

But a trauma-informed team sees the real story.

Doctor: "Hey Melissa, I want to check in. It seems like this moment feels stressful. Did something happen in the past that makes this part hard?"

Melissa breaks. "Yes. My last cat—during a procedure—no one told me what was happening …" And suddenly, the entire emotional world changes.

Doctor: "Thank you for sharing that with me. Given what you went through, this fear makes complete sense. Here's what we'll do instead: we'll bring the equipment in here so Harper can stay with you. And I'll narrate every step. You won't be out of the loop for a second."

Two things happen immediately: Melissa relaxes. Harper relaxes.

The bloodwork goes smoothly.
Melissa thanks the entire team.
She becomes a loyal, lifelong client.

Not because of the medicine. But because of the emotional skill. This is how trauma-informed care changes everything.

Summary

When clients feel psychologically safe:

- They ask honest questions
- They follow through with care
- They approve diagnostics
- They trust your recommendations
- They come back sooner
- They refer more
- They leave positive reviews
- They spend more confidently
- They become lifetime clients

And as we've covered, all of this improves patient outcomes, team morale, and hospital financials, which increases the hospital's ability to invest in better equipment, invest in a better team experience, hire and retain better staff, reduce burnout, and reduce errors.

Which raises client trust ... And the flywheel accelerates again.

Next, to summarize, here are my "Trauma-Informed Veterinary Care Principles":

1. Ask how the client is feeling.
2. Normalize their emotions.
3. Narrate every step.
4. Provide predictable timelines.
5. Offer choices.
6. Use permission-based language.
7. Emphasize relationship and partnership.
8. Confirm understanding before moving forward.

Remember: clients aren't difficult. They're scared. Your job is not to fix the trauma; it's to create a safe space where new trust can grow. You are not just healing pets. You're healing everything that happened before the client walked in your door.

Suggested Readings

Clark, Timothy R. *The 4 Stages of Psychological Safety: Defining the Path to Inclusion and Innovation*. Berrett-Koehler, 2020.

Deloitte. *The Employee Experience Imperative: How Engagement Drives Customer Satisfaction*. Deloitte Insights, 2017, www2.deloitte.com

Edmondson, Amy C. "Psychological Safety and Learning Behavior in Work Teams." *Administrative Science Quarterly*, vol. 44, no. 2, 1999, pp. 350–383.

Edmondson, Amy C. *The Fearless Organization: Creating Psychological Safety in the Workplace for Learning, Innovation, and Growth*. Wiley, 2019.

Harvard Business Review. "What Google Learned from Its Quest to Build the Perfect Team." *Harvard Business Review*, 2016.

Kahn, William A. "Psychological Conditions of Personal Engagement and Disengagement at Work." *Academy of Management Journal*, vol. 33, no. 4, 1990, pp. 692–724.

Levy, Pamela, et al. "Trauma-Informed Care in Medical Settings: A Framework for Safety and Healing." *Journal of Behavioral Health Services & Research*, vol. 45, no. 4, 2018, pp. 626–638.

Maslach, Christina, and Michael P. Leiter. *The Truth About Burnout: How Organizations Cause Personal Stress and What to Do About It*. Jossey-Bass, 1997.

McKinsey & Company. *Psychological Safety and the Critical Role of Leadership in Performance and Innovation*. McKinsey, 2023.

Porges, Stephen W. *The Polyvagal Theory: Neurophysiological Foundations of Emotions, Attachment, Communication, and Self-Regulation*. W. W. Norton, 2011.

Rogers, Carl R. *On Becoming a Person: A Therapist's View of Psychotherapy*. Houghton Mifflin, 1961.

Workhuman. *The 2022 Global Human Workplace Index: Psychological Safety and Belonging at Work*. Workhuman, 2022.

Zenger, Jack, and Joseph Folkman. *The Extraordinary Leader: Turning Good Managers into Great Leaders*. McGraw-Hill, 2019.

Chapter 12
Client Trust Drives Pet Medical Outcomes

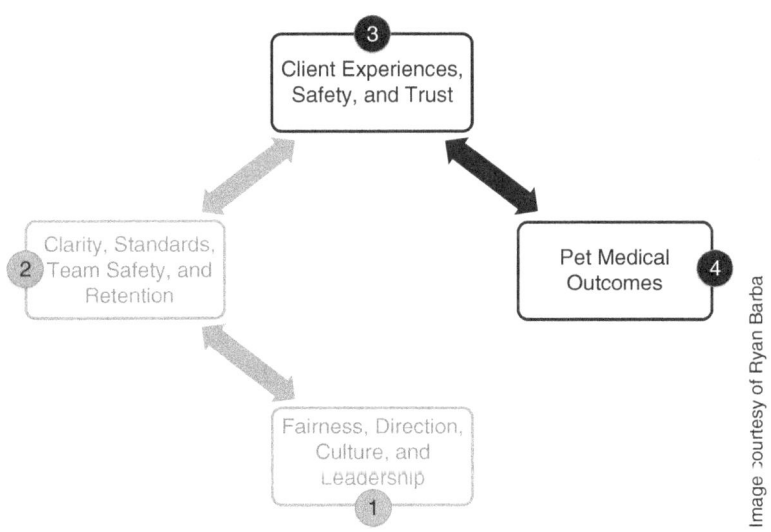

Image courtesy of Ryan Barba

Clients Who Trust You Take Your Medical Advice

By now you've seen how psychological safety transforms a veterinary team. You've seen how trust becomes the engine of communication, confidence, and daily flow inside the hospital. You've seen how it spreads outward—into exam rooms, into tone of voice, into how your team educates, advocates, and guides. And you've seen how it then creates psychological safety for clients.

Now it's time to talk about what happens next: momentum—real, compounding, or unstoppable momentum. The kind of momentum that turns a normal veterinary hospital into a magnetic, trusted, and high-performing machine. The kind of momentum that shows up in your compliance rates, your recheck adherence, your dentistry numbers, your online reviews, your retention, your recruiting pipeline, and your bottom line.

As we've discussed in detail, it all starts with psychological safety inside the team. That's the ignition. That's the spark. the catalyst that makes everything else possible. Because once your people feel safe—truly safe—the entire flywheel of your practice starts spinning in a way you cannot fake, cannot manufacture, and cannot shortcut. And that translates into psychological safety for clients who move through the same four phases of psychological safety your team does. And as that trust continues to build, clients increasingly trust you.

And this is where the Veterinary Trust Flywheel comes alive.

This part is simple. It's direct, and it's the heartbeat of veterinary outcomes: when clients feel safe enough to trust your recommendations, you get higher medical compliance.

This is THE GAME. Trust = compliance.

It is the greatest unlock in veterinary medicine: that compliance is not about persuasion. Compliance is about trust.

Higher Compliance Leads to Improved Medical Outcomes for Pets

Compliance lives or dies on trust. A Mars Veterinary Health study showed that strong client trust boosts compliance with recommended care by 30–40%. The American Veterinary Medical

Association (AVMA) confirms it: when trust is high, clients stick to treatment plans—vaccines, preventatives, and chronic care. National compliance rates are often below 40%. But in high-trust hospitals? Those rates can double.

Why? Because trust makes clients feel included. And inclusion—along with the other four feelings every client craves (affirmed, known, supported, and appreciated)—builds that trust. When I believe my pet's doctor is on my side, I listen. I don't push back. I don't doctor-shop. I don't wonder if the recommendation is about revenue. I move forward with the plan. I follow instructions at home.

The data is clear: when clients trust your team:

Diagnostics get approved.
Dentals get scheduled.
Rechecks get booked.
Preventives get purchased.
Prescriptions are filled and refilled.
Treatment plans get followed.

Of course, trusting clients will still ask questions. They'll want clarity. They may need to weigh options based on budget. That's normal. But they're not questioning intent. They're not doubting quality. They're not second-guessing qualifications.

Because in their minds:
The doctor is on *my* team.
She's on *Buddy's* team.
I know it. I trust it.
And because of that, I'll follow her lead.

For your team, compliance isn't about money. It's not about "selling services." It's about keeping pets alive longer and healthier. That is the core of veterinary medicine, the reason why your team joined this industry and ultimately comes to work every day. Period.

When clients trust your team, they say yes. When they say yes, medicine gets better.

Let's talk diagnostics, for starters. As we all know, diagnostics aren't really optional. They're not "extras." They're how medicine works. When clients say yes to bloodwork, radiographs, urine tests, fecal screens, and dental X-rays—the stuff we all know they *should* say yes to—your team gets a full picture instead of a blurry one.

With diagnostics, you don't guess. You don't assume. You don't treat symptoms blindly. You get information that actually tells you what's wrong, how bad it is, what's been missed, what's brewing under the surface, and what's coming next if you don't act. Compliance to diagnostic recommendations turns medicine from detective work into precision work.

When compliance improves and you're armed with real data as a result, you make real clinical decisions. Better information means:

- Catching kidney disease before it's stage four
- Finding heart disease before the cough starts
- Seeing arthritis progression before mobility collapses
- Spotting diabetes early enough to stabilize
- Identifying dental disease before infection spreads
- Detecting endocrine issues before they become expensive, painful crises

In other words, information is the difference between reactive medicine and preventive medicine. Reactive medicine is expensive, stressful, and often too late. Preventive medicine is predictable, stable, and dramatically more effective.

Pet owners *feel* that difference. And pets *live* that difference.

This is the whole point.

Higher compliance means better diagnostics. Better diagnostics mean better decisions. And better decisions lead to longer lifespans, better quality of life, fewer emergencies, fewer surprises, less suffering ... More years of tail wags, couch cuddles, and mornings with the pet that's their whole heart.

So, good medicine isn't magic; it's information obtained by earning your clients' trust. If you want healthier pets, you need clients who trust your team enough to say yes.

This is not complicated. This is not philosophical. This is the real-world chain reaction that every great hospital understands.

This is the point where the flywheel stops being conceptual and becomes tangible. You can measure this part. You can see it in your data. You can watch it happen in real time.

Quality Medicine Reinforces and Multiplies Client Trust

Trust helps clients say yes to better medicine. But also, the medicine you deliver is one of the most powerful trust-building tools you have. It's the *proof*. It's the receipts. It's the moment when a client realizes, "These people actually know what they're doing, and I'm not risking my pet's health by listening to them."

This is why the arrow between client trust and medical outcomes in the Flywheel is also bidirectional. Because trust isn't just emotional; it's experiential:

When a pet finally stops itching after months of misery, that's trust reinforced.
When a diagnosis is caught early because your doctor insisted on a blood panel, that's trust reinforced.
When a post-op call reveals a pet healing exactly the way your team said they would, that's trust reinforced.
When a technician explains a treatment plan in plain English and the pet improves exactly as predicted, that's trust reinforced.

Every accurate diagnosis, every clean surgery, every thoughtful pain protocol, and every well-executed treatment plan becomes a trust deposit in that client's emotional bank. You stack enough deposits, and loyalty becomes automatic. You don't have to "sell" anymore—clients start assuming you're right. They *expect* excellence. They stop questioning the estimate and start asking, "What's best for her?"

Clients trust what works. And when your medicine works consistently, visibly, and predictably, it cements you as *their* hospital—not a hospital, not the closest hospital, but **their** hospital. The one they recommend. The one they drive across town for. The one they defend in Facebook groups. The one they return to year after year.

This is the reverse engine of the Flywheel: **trust drives medicine → medicine drives trust.** It's a loop. A compounding asset.

Every time the medicine delivers, the client feels more confident approving the next recommendation.
Every time the medicine delivers, the team feels more confident giving the next recommendation.
Every time the medicine delivers, the hospital becomes more aligned, more credible, and more unstoppable.

Quality medicine doesn't just support trust—it *supercharges* it. It turns trust from a feeling into a fact. Into a story the client will tell their friends, their family, their coworkers, and their dog park crew. Into a reputation that no amount of marketing dollars can buy.

Because at the end of the day, you can talk all you want about client experience and brand voice and hospitality. But nothing builds trust faster than a pet who walks out healthier than they walked in. Great medicine makes already-established trust unshakeable. And unshakeable trust is the most valuable asset your hospital will ever own.

Suggested Readings

American Veterinary Medical Association. *AVMA Guidelines for Preventive Healthcare for Dogs and Cats*. AVMA, 2023, www.avma.org

American Veterinary Medical Association. *Economic State of the Veterinary Profession*. AVMA, 2022, www.avma.org

Christiansen, Sophie B., and Peter Sandøe. "Veterinary Clinician–client Communication and Shared Decision-making." *Veterinary Clinics of North America: Small Animal Practice*, vol. 48, no. 2, 2018, pp. 303–318.

Deloitte. *Experience Matters: Customer Trust and Business Performance*. Deloitte Insights, 2018, www2.deloitte.com

Edmondson, Amy C. *The Fearless Organization: Creating Psychological Safety in the Workplace for Learning, Innovation, and Growth*. Wiley, 2019.

Fogle, Bruce. *Caring for Your Aging Dog: From Puppy to Golden Years*. St. Martin's Press, 2012.

Kahn, William A. "Psychological Conditions of Personal Engagement and Disengagement at Work." *Academy of Management Journal*, vol. 33, no. 4, 1990, pp. 692–724.

Mars Veterinary Health. *The Role of Trust in Veterinary Care Compliance*. Mars Veterinary Health Institute, 2021.

National Academies of Sciences, Engineering, and Medicine. *Preventing Chronic Disease: The Role of Prevention and Early Detection*. National Academies Press, 2020.

Peterson, Mark E., and Steven E. Nichols. *Small Animal Endocrinology*. Elsevier, 2020.

Shaw, John R., Bonnie Adams, and Joy M. Bonnett. "What Can Veterinarians Learn from Studies of Physician–patient Communication about Veterinarian–Client–Patient Communication?" *Journal of the American Veterinary Medical Association*, vol. 232, no. 7, 2008, pp. 1000–1008.

Volk, Janice O., et al. *Executive Summary of the Bayer Veterinary Care Usage Study*. Bayer Animal Health, 2011.

World Health Organization. *Adherence to Long-Term Therapies: Evidence for Action*. WHO, 2003.

Chapter 13
Quality Medicine Becomes Cultural Proof and Builds Team Pride

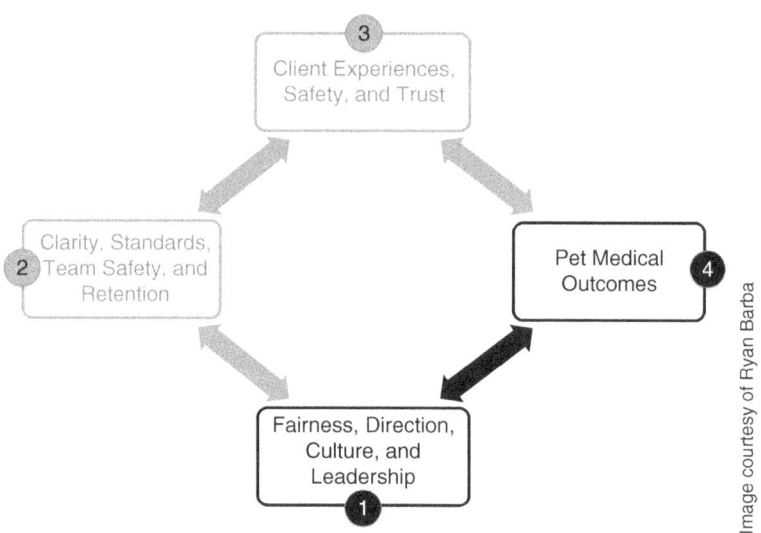

Image courtesy of Ryan Barba

Here's where we complete the Flywheel's circle, the moment where great medicine stops being "clinical" and becomes **cultural fuel**. Because when your hospital consistently delivers high-quality care, catches disease early, manages chronic conditions well, prevents avoidable suffering, and helps pets live longer, healthier lives, the impact doesn't stop at the patient. It ripples outward. It strengthens team identity. It reaffirms purpose. It reinforces your mission, vision, and values more powerfully than any speech, poster, or all-hands meeting ever could.

Nothing aligns a team faster than seeing their work *work*.

And the data backs that up. The American Animal Hospital Association (AAHA) found that hospitals with high adherence to clinical guidelines report **22–30% higher team morale scores** and **significantly lower turnover**, especially among technicians. Another study in the *Journal of Veterinary Internal Medicine* showed that hospitals with consistent preventive care protocols see **up to 40% earlier disease detection**, which directly correlates to better patient outcomes and, importantly, **higher clinician job satisfaction**—because nothing burns a team out faster than preventable suffering.

Every win matters.
Every early catch matters.
Every life saved matters.
Not just to the pet ... to the people who showed up that day and made it happen.

When a diagnosis is caught early because your team followed the protocol ...
When a dental patient returns pain-free and the owner says, "I had no idea he could act like a puppy again" ...
When chronic issues improve because the hospital finally communicated clearly and consistently ...
When a critical patient pulls through because your team was aligned, focused, and brave ...

Your people don't just feel proud. They feel **united**. They feel the mission in their bones. They feel the values coming alive in real time. They can point at the outcome and say, "We did that. Our standards did that. Our teamwork did that."

High-quality medicine builds team pride. When your doctors see outcomes improve, they get more confident. When your techs see that their catheter placement, their restraint technique, and their recheck notes actually changed the course of a patient's life, they feel ownership. Pride turns into engagement. Engagement turns into consistency. Consistency turns into a brand.

High-quality medicine becomes cultural proof.
It's the receipts.
It validates the standards you've set.
It makes the mission real instead of theoretical.

And here's the psychological kicker: when the team sees great outcomes happening because of the systems, protocols, and behaviors your hospital stands for, they become emotionally invested in repeating those behaviors. They believe in the work. They believe in the hospital. They believe in each other. And culture begins to compound.

Data from Gallup shows that employees who can *directly see* the impact of their work are **2.8 times more likely** to be engaged and **5 times more likely** to stay long-term. In human healthcare, research from the Agency for Healthcare Research and Quality found that high-reliability units—the ones with tight protocols and consistent outcomes—report **25–30% higher psychological safety** and **dramatically lower burnout**, because consistent success creates team stability. Veterinary teams are no different. When medicine is better, the environment calms. The chaos decreases. The team breathes again.

Better medical outcomes strengthen team confidence. The hospital starts to feel competent, capable, and cohesive. Doctors trust their techs. Techs trust their CSRs. Everyone trusts the system. The hospital becomes less reactive and more intentional. People communicate more clearly because they have conviction behind the care they're delivering.

Confidence isn't swagger—it's stability. It's a team quietly knowing, "We do good work here."

And the more great outcomes a hospital delivers, the more the team wants to repeat the behaviors that made them possible—listening, narrating, caring, slowing down, collaborating, protecting psychological safety, and supporting each other. For leadership, servant leadership stops being a philosophy and starts becoming instinct. Leaders embrace the idea of "we, not me," because they've seen what "we" can do. They've watched excellence unfold right in front of them, powered by the entire team.

Better medicine isn't just better medicine.
It's cultural oxygen.
It's mission fuel.
It's values reinforcement.
It's the spark that ignites servant leadership.
It's the confidence engine that powers the Trust Flywheel.

And that's how a hospital becomes unstoppable.

Case Study: How Better Medicine Transformed Riverbend Animal Hospital

To see how this plays out in the real world, let's look at a hospital I'll call Riverbend Animal Hospital—a mid-sized, three doctor practice in Illinois that had quietly slipped into "just okay" medicine. Nothing awful. Nothing dangerous. Just ... average. Vaccines? Sure. Sick visits? Yes. But preventive care compliance hovered around **28%**, dental compliance was under **20%**, and internal team morale surveys showed low confidence in medical consistency: "Every doctor does things differently," "We don't know what the standard is," "We feel rushed," "We don't have time to do it right."

Turnover followed.
Two techs left in six months.

The CSRs were drowning.
The doctors felt frustrated and isolated.
Clients felt the inconsistency.

Then the medical director made a simple decision that changed everything:
"We're going to build and follow real protocols. And we're going to track outcomes."

They started small:

- Preventive care guideline refresh
- A unified dental protocol
- Mandatory chronic disease recheck schedule
- Technicians empowered to initiate diagnostic conversations
- Weekly medical rounds celebrating wins (not just reviewing mistakes)

Within four months:

- Dental compliance jumped from 18 to 46%
- Preventive care bundle acceptance rose 31%
- Early-stage kidney disease diagnoses doubled (which meant earlier intervention and better long-term outcomes)
- Team morale scores increased 22%
- Technician retention stabilized completely. Not one tech left
- Client NPS rose 19 points

But the biggest shift wasn't on a spreadsheet. It was emotional.

A 12-year-old cat named Milo came in for routine bloodwork as part of the new senior protocol. His values showed early renal changes—subtle ones that would have been missed without the updated guidelines. The team acted fast, coordinated beautifully, and Milo improved within weeks because of early intervention.

The client came back for a recheck and said, with tears in her eyes, "Thank you for giving me more time with him. You caught what no one else did."

That moment went up on the breakroom wall.
The team stopped rolling their eyes at "new protocols."
They believed.
They trusted the system.
They trusted themselves.
They trusted each other.

And the Flywheel turned.

Riverbend ended the year with the highest retention in its history, the highest revenue in its history, and more importantly, the **highest morale and confidence** the team had ever felt.

This is the real power of quality medicine:
It doesn't just heal pets.
It heals teams.
It heals culture.
It builds pride that cannot be faked.

And it's available to *every* hospital willing to commit to doing the work.

Suggested Readings

Agency for Healthcare Research and Quality. *Patient Safety and High Reliability in Healthcare.* U.S. Department of Health and Human Services, 2022, www.ahrq.gov

American Animal Hospital Association. *AAHA Guidelines for Veterinary Preventive Care.* American Animal Hospital Association, 2022, www.aaha.org

American Animal Hospital Association. *Utilization and Capacity Study.* AAHA, 2023, www.aaha.org

Edmondson, Amy C. *The Fearless Organization: Creating Psychological Safety in the Workplace for Learning, Innovation, and Growth.* Wiley, 2019.

Gallup. *State of the Global Workplace Report.* Gallup, 2023, www.gallup.com

Kahn, William A. "Psychological Conditions of Personal Engagement and Disengagement at Work." *Academy of Management Journal*, vol. 33, no. 4, 1990, pp. 692–724.

Polzin, David J. "Evidence-Based Stepwise Approach to Managing Chronic Kidney Disease in Dogs and Cats." *Journal of Veterinary Internal Medicine*, vol. 27, no. 3, 2013, pp. 765–778.

Shaw, John R., et al. "The Role of the Veterinary Team in Preventive Care Delivery." *Journal of the American Veterinary Medical Association*, vol. 238, no. 3, 2011, pp. 305–312.

World Health Organization. *Burnout and Occupational Mental Health in Healthcare Workers*. WHO, 2021, www.who.int

Chapter 14
Trust and Medical Outcomes Drive Profitability (And Yes, That's a Good Thing)

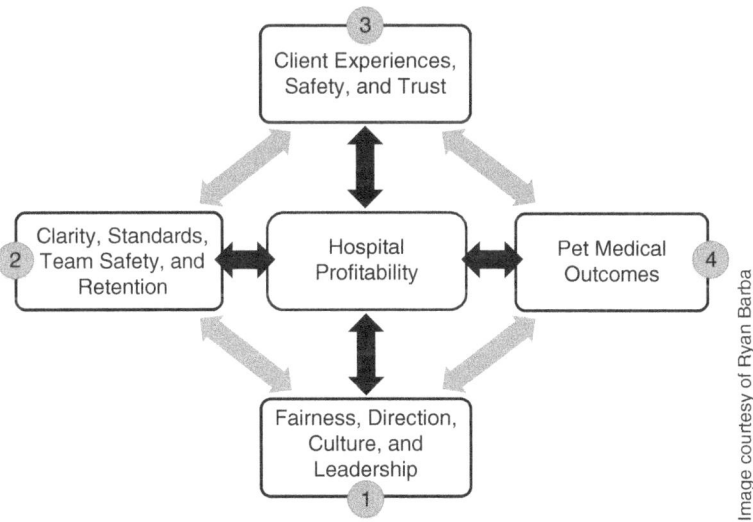

Image courtesy of Ryan Barba

Let's state what I hope is obvious by now: if you want a profitable hospital, stop obsessing over the next marketing gimmick, stop relying on price increases, stop skimping out on your team's comp and benefits, and start *obsessing* over trust, retention, and outcomes.

Better Medical Outcomes Drive Loyalty, Growth, and Reputation

When clients consistently feel safe and see great outcomes, several things are put into motion.

First, client trust increases even further. When clients trust your medical advice and thereby see consistent, quality medical care, they'll see that they (and their pet) have been rewarded for the trust they have in you. Result? Even more trust.

And with that comes ... loyalty: clients who genuinely believe, "These are my people. This is my hospital." That kind of loyalty cannot be bought. It can only be earned. And I'm talking lifetime loyalty: not one visit. Not one year. A lifetime. Ten, fifteen, twenty years of care. Generations of pets.

Second, loyalty, or client retention, is a straight-up money machine. Bain & Company found that across industries, a simple 5% bump in customer retention can raise profits by 25–95%. That's insane leverage. That's what the data shows. And it's why investing in client experience isn't a "nice-to-have." It's one of the highest-ROI decisions a veterinary hospital can make.

Third, your clients become your marketing engine. They become evangelists for your hospital. They tell friends. They tell coworkers. They tell neighbors. They post online. They defend your hospital on social media without you even asking. This is the most powerful growth channel in veterinary medicine—and it is free.

And fourth, your reputation stands on its own ... and even attracts talent. When your hospital is known as a place where teams thrive and clients trust, you stop chasing talent. Talent chases you. People want to work in places where the culture feels alive, healthy, supportive, and clear.

Net Promoter Score: What It Is and Why It Matters in Vet Med

One of the most widely used tools to measure client satisfaction across all industries is Net Promoter Score (NPS). If you've ever seen a survey asking, "How likely are you to recommend this hospital (or brand) to a friend or family member?"—that's NPS.

Clients answer on a 0–10 scale (0 = not at all likely, 10 = extremely likely):

- Promoters = 9 or 10
- Passives = 7 or 8
- Detractors = 0 to 6

The hospital's overall score is calculated from the percentage of Promoters minus the percentage of Detractors. But even before calculating that score, each client's answer tells you a lot about their likelihood to return, spend, and trust you.

Here's the truth: trust isn't just a warm, fuzzy feeling. It's an accelerant.

Across hundreds of hospitals, when veterinary clients rate their experience higher—measured through NPS—every key business metric lights up. But here's the wild part: the growth doesn't happen gradually. It **explodes** once you cross a certain threshold.

When NPS moves from "meh" territory into the eight-and-above range, everything starts to scale.

- Existing clients come back more often—in some hospitals, return rates jump by *30–50%*.
- New clients stick around, showing retention gains north of *25%*.

- Average visit spend climbs—often *10–20% higher* as trust deepens and clients say "yes" to recommendations more confidently.
- Product purchases rise steadily, because pet owners who trust your advice are far more likely to buy the food, meds, and preventives you recommend.

Add it up, and once you hit that NPS tipping point, you're looking at a compounding effect: loyalty, frequency, and spending all reinforcing each other.

It's not magic. It's momentum. When people *feel cared for*, they don't just return the favor—they return to *you*.

Higher NPS scores means stronger loyalty, higher client spend, and better patient outcomes. Trusting clients buy food, preventatives, medications, etc. They'll come back more often. They'll stick around longer. As such, I'm 100% convinced that earning and maintaining client trust is the single best strategy you've got to ensure long-term financial health.

NPS measures "likelihood to recommend." So, those who give you a high NPS score will tell their friends, their family, their coworkers—basically anyone who'll listen—to bring their pets to you. That's free marketing. And let me remind you—it's not only free, it's the most effective marketing on earth. That's how *reputation* gets built. You and I both know: you're 10 times more likely to try a new restaurant because your buddy raved about it than because you saw some random billboard or online pop-up ad. Same principle here.

Team Retention Drives Profitability, Too

Team retention is just as important. Because turnover is a silent killer.

Replacing one employee costs anywhere from 50 to 150% of their annual salary. For a vet tech, that usually means $25,000+ down the drain when you add up recruiting, training, and the productivity you lose. And in this industry, the hit is even worse because turnover disrupts clients, disrupts pets, and shreds morale.

On the flip side, when you keep your team intact, they get faster. They get sharper. They work more efficiently. That might mean shaving a few minutes off each appointment, which adds up to a couple extra patients a day. Or maybe they can handle a couple more walk-ins or drop-offs. Across the board, efficiency = cost savings + revenue gains.

And here's the long game: consistency + outcomes = reputation.

Pet Outcomes and Profitability

You want your hospital's name to be synonymous with "excellent medicine." Nobody wants to hand their pet over to a team they don't trust to keep them healthy. Over time, if your outcomes are strong, word spreads. Clients tell stories. Reviews pile up. Referrals increase. Reputation grows even more. And money pours in.

And nothing builds reputation faster than emotional proof. Picture this: a client breaks down in tears thanking your team after you save their dog's life. You think everyone else in that lobby just leveled up their trust in you? You better believe it.

Profitability Opens the Door for Reinvestment, and Increased Momentum

I think many in our industry (maybe a lot of industries) view "profit" as a dirty word. In reality, nothing could be further from the truth. Let's get this straight: profit isn't dirty. Profit is freedom. Profit is fuel. Profit is what allows you to reinvest in, and take care of, your people, your clients, and your patients.

On the Client Side

A financially strong hospital reinvests into better client facilities, better tech, and better communication tools—all of which improve the experience for clients. It can also mean more CE for the team, to improve team training on everything from communication to emotional intelligence to medical quality. Every one of those investments makes the experience smoother, more transparent, more valuable. Which equals, you guessed it: more trust.

And here's an underrated but really valuable part: a profitable hospital isn't under constant pressure to jack up prices. Clients hate feeling gouged. They'll trust you more if your pricing feels (and is) fair.

A client who is concerned about their ability to afford care for their pet is more likely to hold off on getting care "until things get worse," to delay getting their pet necessary vaccinations, or even to avoid getting their pet their care it needs altogether. But when prices are fair, clients are less likely to delay or avoid care. That means pets stay healthier. And that's literally the point of all of this.

We have a responsibility in our industry to price our services fairly, to make care accessible to as many clients and pets as possible.

Fair pricing = better trust + better pet outcomes.

On the Team Side

Profit means you can pay people better. Offer stronger benefits. Train them. Give them flexibility. Add wellness programs. Hell, upgrade the break room. Plan fun outings. All of that reduces burnout and makes people want to stick around.

Here's a bonus move: share your hospital's wins with the team. Show them how their work is actually driving success. Let them feel ownership in it. That pride builds culture like nothing else. That's the arrow from "Hospital Profitability and Investment" to "Two-way Trust between Teams and Leaders." Sharing your hospital's success gives the team even more ammunition to take pride in the work they're doing and the success that's driving, especially when you explain how this profitability will continue to make life better for them, clients, pets, and hospital overall. Don't keep your financial success a secret from your team.

On the Medical Side

Profit lets you buy better equipment. Pay for certifications. Fund training that makes your team sharper. That translates directly into stronger medical outcomes.

In summary: profit isn't greed. Profit is how you keep the cycle alive.

Without profit, you can't invest in your team, your clients, or better medicine. Profit lets you pay fairly, buy better gear, and price fairly. And fair pricing builds more trust, which drives outcomes, which drive reputation, which drives retention.

That's the loop. That's the Veterinary Trust Flywheel. Leaders who bet on people first? They're the ones who friggin win.

This Isn't Theory. This Is Reality

This isn't pie-in-the-sky philosophy. This isn't aspirational leadership fluff. This isn't a "maybe someday" ideal.

This is the lived reality inside elite veterinary hospitals—the ones that grow, retain, attract, and thrive.
The ones with waiting lists for appointments and waiting lists for job applicants.
The ones with doctors who stay 10 years, not 10 months.
The ones with clients who hand-write thank-you cards after euthanasias.
The ones with stable finances, even in volatile markets.
The ones where the phrase "we treat your pets like family" isn't a slogan. It's simply true.

They don't win because they hustle harder.
They don't win because they burn their teams out less slowly than competitors.
They don't win because they have shinier buildings or bigger budgets.

They win because they lead smarter.
Because they invest in psychological safety.
Because they understand the compounding force of trust—internally and externally.
Because they know that the Veterinary Trust Flywheel doesn't happen by accident.

It happens by design.
It happens through culture.
It happens through leadership.
It happens through intention.
It happens through consistency.

And once the flywheel spins, it becomes the most unstoppable force in your hospital.

The Flywheel in Action

Let me give you a real example to really drive this home for you.

I worked with a hospital that was completely stuck. They couldn't attract new clients, and they couldn't keep their team. When I dug into the books, I immediately saw why. The owner, whom we'll call Dr. Angela, and the hospital manager, whom we'll call Pam, had gone all-in on the strategies I warn people about:

1. Prices jacked up way above the local market.
2. Staff hired at below-market pay.
3. And to make it worse, they were constantly running short-staffed to "save money."

Here's what happened next. Predictably, the team figured it out. They realized they were making less than other local hospitals, or even local retail or fast-food jobs, and resentment spread like wildfire. Then they watched prices climb higher while their pay stayed low. The frustration became vocal:

> *"Why are we underpaid when we're now the most expensive hospital in town? Why are we always short-staffed while clients scream at us about prices?"*

And of course, the clients noticed. Negativity leaked, hospitality slipped, service dipped, and clients started asking the exact same thing:

> *"What am I even paying for here?"*

So they left. Many found other, more reputable hospitals nearby charging 30% less. Meanwhile, this place was stuck in the worst possible cycle: constant staff turnover, bleeding clients, zero momentum.

I told Dr. Angela to flip the script: cut prices back to market level, raise pay, and increase staffing hours.

She immediately pushed back: "That'll kill my margins."

She wasn't wrong: In the short term, it would. But I challenged her to bet on her people. Pay them fairly. Support them. Give them the tools to win. And then bet on herself as a leader who could rebuild culture from the ground up.

To their credit, Angela and Pam did it. At the next staff meeting, they laid it all out with total honesty:

> *"Team, our revenue dipped and we panicked. We raised prices and tried to save on labor costs while asking you to cover more. That was wrong. We're fixing it. Prices are coming down. Wages and hours are going up. We're betting on you—the team. Together, I know that we can turn this around. We trust you."*

Pam then led the staff through Veterinary Trust Flywheel exercises (you'll get those later in this chapter).

And here's the beauty: transparency worked. Trust started to rebuild. Margins dipped for a few months, sure, but the culture flipped. The team felt supported and trusted. They brought more energy. Clients noticed. Prices were fairer, so fewer clients left. Service improved. Referrals started to grow.

Here's the kicker: even after a 7% price increase, average client spend held steady because clients opted into more services. Within six months, the hospital had recouped the early losses. Turnover plummeted. Morale soared. Retention stuck. And positive reviews came pouring in.

One of the biggest reasons why the Veterinary Trust Flywheel works is because, as I often say, "A mindset of scarcity creates scarcity. A mindset of abundance creates abundance." By clinging to price increases to drive revenue, or by underpaying staff to save costs, Pam was embracing a scarcity mindset that suggests "we're just hanging on for dear life"—and that scarcity mindset was yielding scarcity within the hospital: a scarcity of joy, of trust, and frankly, of long-term team members and clients. But when Rachel flipped the script and embraced a mindset of abundance—that is, investing in her team and hospital with the faith that they'd drive growth and abundance once they were empowered—abundance followed. The Veterinary Trust Flywheel, at its core, is an abundance-assuming strategy. It challenges hospital leaders to give their teams the chance to succeed together, by assuming the best in their teams—that is, by assuming abundance—rather than embracing a mindset of scarcity—playing it safe to survive or to not fail.

An abundance mindset takes guts, no question. It can feel like a gamble, because your team will have to rise to the occasion. But in reality, you're embracing an abundance mindset in *yourself*—you're signaling to yourself that you trust your ability to lead your team toward change, successfully. And simply by thinking that way—having faith and confidence in your leadership and—by extension—your team, you're willing abundance into existence. I can't wait for you to see that fruit of that mindset.

The Veterinary Trust Flywheel, Summarized

The veterinary industry doesn't need more hacks, more shortcuts, or more shiny apps. It needs more trust: trust inside the team, trust between the team and clients, and trust between clients and the medicine you're recommending.

Most hospitals totally misunderstand client experience. They think CX is about being "nice," "making people smile," or slapping empty slogans on a wall. That's amateur hour. In veterinary medicine, client experience isn't a vibe—it's an ecosystem.

The Veterinary Flywheel shows that that ecosystem **starts with your team**. And in particular, must be built on a foundation of fairness. If your people feel underpaid, unclear, unsupported, or unsafe, you can forget CX, forget compliance, forget loyalty, and forget profitability. Nothing works when the foundation is cracked.

Then, champion clarity for your team. Give them a target. Remind them why they come to work every day. Set a vision WITH your team that they can be proud of. Set clear standards. Build a culture with a spine. Lead like a servant, not a dictator. When you do that, the magic happens: psychological safety rises, communication gets cleaner, trust forms, morale jumps, and—most importantly—your people stay. Retention becomes the engine that powers everything else.

And here's where the flywheel kicks in: strong teams that stick around create authentic experiences for clients, who then also stick around. Clients feel the clarity, the cohesion, the confidence. They walk in, recognize the same faces, trust the recommendations, and say "yes" to care. Trust skyrockets. And when clients trust you?

They give it back. They show gratitude, patience, and loyalty that refuels your team emotionally. That emotional validation deepens safety, strengthens culture, and drives even more retention. The arrow goes both ways—always.

That trust then fuels compliance. Compliance fuels outcomes. Outcomes fuel confidence. That confidence reinforces and refuels culture, motivating continued servant leadership and team retention. Retention fuels client trust. Client trust fuels revenue. Revenue fuels reinvestment. That's the Flywheel. That's how an entire hospital transforms from barely surviving to absolutely unstoppable.

This is the blueprint—not theory, not fluff, not corporate nonsense—for how veterinary hospitals actually win. You don't fix a hospital through marketing hacks or price hikes or "positive thinking." You fix it by betting on your people first and trusting the flywheel to do what it does: compound. Amplify. Accelerate.

Team wins.
Clients win.
Pets win.
The hospital wins.

That's the Flywheel. And once it's spinning? Good luck trying to stop it. The cycle continues—stronger every rotation. It's how great hospitals stay great—and how good hospitals become unstoppable.

If you invest in trust—anywhere in the cycle—the whole system lifts.

This isn't theory. This is physics. This is momentum. This is leadership.

So let's dig deeper now. I've explained the Flywheel in theory, and explained how it works. Let's get tangible now: if you're a hospital leader, how do you actually put this in place and do it? How do you establish a mission and culture? How do you build psychological safety for your team that translates to psychological safety for clients?

That's where we're headed next. Part 3 covers Steps 1 and 2 of Flywheel—ensuring fairness, providing direction, building culture, and embracing servant leadership to drive internal psychological safety, trust, and retention.

Suggested Readings

American Animal Hospital Association. *Utilization and Capacity Study*. AAHA, 2023, www.aaha.org

American Veterinary Medical Association. *U.S. Pet Ownership and Demographics Sourcebook*. AVMA, 2022, www.avma.org

Bain & Company. "The Value of Customer Loyalty." *Bain & Company Insights*, 2019, www.bain.com

Gallup. *State of the Global Workplace Report*. Gallup, 2023, www.gallup.com

Harvard Business Review. "The Economics of Customer Retention." *Harvard Business Review*, Jan. 2020, hbr.org

McKinsey & Company. "The Employee Experience: How Loyal Teams Drive Profitable Growth." McKinsey, 2022, www.mckinsey.com

Net Promoter Network. *Net Promoter Score (NPS) System Overview*. Satmetrix Systems, 2023, www.netpromotersystem.com

Society for Human Resource Management. *The High Cost of Employee Turnover*. SHRM, 2022, www.shrm.org

Weiss, Alexander, et al. "Client Trust and Adherence in Veterinary Medicine." *Journal of the American Veterinary Medical Association*, vol. 256, no. 9, 2020, pp. 1002–1010.

World Economic Forum. *Putting People at the Center of Rebuilding the Economy*. WEF, 2021, www.weforum.org

Part 3

Tangible Direction for Building Culture, Direction, Safety, and Trust

Up until this point of the book, I've been really tough on "tactics-first" strategies. I've shared disaster stories—the Cleveland Clinic story, Linda's failed rollout—because they prove a crucial point: you can't skip straight to scripts and start recommending behaviors without first establishing vision and purpose. Culture comes before tactics. The "why" has to be solid. Internal psychological safety needs to be firmly established. Leaders need to step into servant leadership behaviors that keep trust flowing between their team and clients.

One quick way to remember this is a (I'll admit, maybe a bit cheezy) line I've used when lecturing about this subject in the past: "Tactics Trail Target, Team and Trust." It's a quick way to remember: teaching your team client experience strategies (or "tactics") must come after you've established your hospital's "Target" (vision), nurtured a healthy environment and culture for your Team, and successfully established Trust.

That said, tactics aren't the enemy. Far from it. Once you and your team understand the why, adopting proven tactics—the specific, prescriptive practices that have been proven to build trust—is smart. And we'll get there. So, if you're already asking yourself, *"Okay, but how do we actually do this?"*—good. That's the right question.

So, let's get into specifics. In this part of the book, I want to share with you the valuable intel I've gained in leading client experience strategy for hospitals, regions, and entire veterinary companies.

I'll start by walking you through the exact, six-step approach I've used to lead teams through exercises to collaboratively define your hospital's mission, vision, and values—the clarity of direction they need to set the tone for hospital culture.

Then, we'll turn our attention to clients. For that part, I'll start by giving you a foundation of how clients truly want to *feel* when interacting with your team and hospital.

Then, in the next part of this book, I'll use this content as context to share some specific practices that data and my experience show have the best chance of equipping your team to truly connect with, build trust with, and improve the satisfaction needle with clients.

Let's go.

Chapter 15
The Six-step Process for Establishing Clarity

Alright—it's *how* time.

Up to this point, we've been talking mindset, principles, trust, retention, and culture. But none of that means a damn thing if you don't actually put it into action. The Veterinary Trust Flywheel isn't just theory. It requires execution. And execution starts with planning *and* then never taking your foot off the gas.

Here's the deal: the process I'm about to walk you through is going to ask a lot of you. It's not some quick, three-step checklist you half-ass in an afternoon and then let collect dust. This is a full-day workshop with your team. It's assigning ownership to key tasks. It's measuring and reporting. It's straight-up strategic planning. And yeah—if you've never done this before, it might feel a little uncomfortable. Good. That's where the growth happens.

I'm asking you to go full-throttle leader here. You're going to stand in front of your team, share a vision, and get them fired up about it. You're going to facilitate exercises that may push you outside your comfort zone. And you're going to have to get a little cozy with data: collecting it, reviewing it, and sharing results. If you've never thought of yourself as a "numbers person," this will stretch you. But trust me, you can do it.

And here's the thing: you don't have to be perfect. In fact, the worst thing you can do is pretend you're perfect. Your team doesn't want a flawless motivational speaker; they want a real human being who's willing to take risks and grow. Be straight with them:

"I'm trying something new here. It's outside my comfort zone. But I believe it's worth it—for you, for this hospital, for the pets we serve. Be patient with me, and let's figure this out together."

That's leadership. You go first. You embrace the discomfort before you ask your team to. That's how you earn their respect. That's how you model change. And you should feel proud for even *getting here*. If you've made it this far into this book, you're already in the top tier of leaders in this industry. You're committed. You're not looking for excuses; you're looking for execution.

And let me be crystal clear: there's no pressure to nail this flawlessly. The best leaders I know are not the polished, buttoned-up, "never make a mistake" types. They're the ones who are vulnerable, communicative, and humble. They say, "Here's what I'm trying. Here's what I'm learning. Here's how I messed up, and here's how I'm going to do better." That's what people connect with. That's what inspires loyalty.

Now, here's the best part: I've got you covered. In the pages that follow, I'll walk you step-by-step through the process. And in the Appendix, I've built out facilitator guides, complete with talking points, exercises, agendas, and material lists. You don't have to wing this. You've got the playbook.

So here's your only job right now: commit. Don't dabble. Don't dip your toe in. Commit to the workshop. Commit to the process. And most importantly, commit to never stopping. Because this isn't about one good meeting or one cool exercise—it's about building momentum you never let die.

Your hospital has the potential to be *that hospital*. The one clients rave about. The one other practices in town whisper about: *"How did they pull that off?"* The one where teams stick, clients trust, pets thrive, and the flywheel keeps spinning.

This is the moment you start building it.

Let's go.

The Six-step Process

Alright, welcome to the part of the book where we get even *more* tangible, and start digging even deeper into the "How." I have a six-step process for initiating and then actively growing momentum in your hospital. The first three steps? They happen during a live, full-day "Veterinary Hospital Identity Workshop" with your team. The other three? That's the follow-through: implementing, measuring, sharing results, revisiting, and adjusting goals as you go.

This is not theory. This is execution. And we're going to break it all down step by step.

The workshop is heavily focused on setting our sights on the future: who do we want to become and what do we want to be known for? As part of that, you're also going to ideate ideas to improve the client experience and deepen trust with clients, and then work as a team to prioritize where to focus.

What I cover here is the step-by-step overview of the process, which includes the full-day Veterinary Hospital Identity Workshop for your team. In the Appendix at the end of this book, you'll find more detailed facilitation guides, material lists, agendas, and even sample dialogues and examples that other hospitals generated through these activities.

Preparing for the Six-step Process

Here's the play. In the next few pages, I'm going to walk you through a six-step process to bring the Veterinary Trust Flywheel to life in your hospital.

But let's get into some logistics first about how you plan to hold your workshop.

Garner Team Commitment

Some hospitals literally close their doors for a day to make this happen. Others schedule it on a weekend or a day they're already closed. Either way, it takes planning. Your team needs advance notice. People will have to come in on a day they normally wouldn't. Some will need schedule adjustments. You may even have to pay some overtime, and that's okay. This is an *investment* in your culture. Don't look at it as lost revenue; look at it as planting seeds that will pay you back in trust, retention, and client loyalty.

And let's be real: make it mandatory. If you don't, you'll end up with half the team missing, and that kills the point. Will you get pushback? Absolutely. People will talk about their "me time," family commitments, or say it feels unfair. That's normal. But trust me that over time, they'll see the value. They'll realize you included them because their voice matters. They'll feel the benefits when the culture shifts. And at the end of the day, it's one day. They can handle it.

Here's a mistake leaders make: over-explaining. You don't need to hand your team a 10-page agenda weeks before. Keep it simple:

> *"We're doing full-team planning to make this hospital better ... for you, for our clients, and for the pets we care for. We need everyone there."*

That's it. The details come when they walk in the room.

Make It a Big Deal

Now, you've got to make the day *feel different*. Don't just drag them into a boring room with fluorescent lights and stale vibes. Make it a celebration. Stock the table with coffee, donuts, and pastries in the morning. Keep snacks and drinks flowing all day. Cater a solid lunch. Show your team you put thought into this, that you value their time, and that this isn't just another meeting. The food and vibe are symbolic; it says, "This matters."

Secure Space

You'll need a room that fits everyone comfortably, with wall space to hang posters, charts, and exercises. Some hospitals don't have that kind of room—and that's fine. Rent a conference room at a hotel or a community center. Yes, it costs money. But again: it's an investment. You're saying to your team, "This work is important enough that we're treating it seriously." That sends a message in itself.

Bottom line: this workshop is the launchpad. It's the day where everyone gets in the same room, puts their fingerprints on the hospital's future, and walks out feeling like they're part of something bigger. That's how you light the spark as a leader. I'm so excited to share how it works with you.

Step 1 (During the Workshop): Set the Tone

If there's one big takeaway from the Cleveland Clinic story and the "Linda the Regional Manager" case study, it's this: culture doesn't shift because you hand your team a checklist. You can't mandate trust. You can't force client experience. If you want your people to buy in, you've got to start by answering the question that every single human in your building is silently asking:

Why?

Why are we here? Why are we changing? Why should I care? Why should I trust you enough to come along on this ride?

Simon Sinek made this famous with his "Start With Why" TED talk, and it's not just a cute soundbite. It's a leadership law. People don't follow plans. They follow purpose.

So, when you kick off this workshop, this is where you lean in. Before you throw out exercises or posters or worksheets, you look your team in the eye and get real about what's happening and what's at stake.

An effective intro to the day is all about fire. There's no script that can do this for you. It has to come from you—your words, your energy, your truth. Don't overthink it. If you stand up there and sound like a corporate memo, you'll lose them in the first two minutes.

Instead, challenge yourself to be raw and emotional. Get excited. Let them feel the passion in your voice. Show them that you're not just "checking a box" today. You're lighting a fire.

Here are some ways you can do that (mix and match what feels authentic):

- Lay out the Veterinary Trust Flywheel in simple terms. Explain the vision of what happens when trust flows both ways—team to client, client to team—and how that changes everything.
- Talk about client trust. Spell out how clients want to feel when they interact with your hospital: valued, competently supported, known, included, affirmed.
- Be candid about your challenges. Maybe your Google reviews aren't where they should be. Maybe the team's stretched too thin. Maybe you see a big opportunity you've been missing. Own it.
- Get personal. Tell them why this place matters to you: why you wake up every morning to do this work, why you're betting on them to take it to the next level.
- Make it clear: everyone matters. Every single person in the room has a role—in the hospital, in this workshop, in what happens after. This isn't "management's project." This is ours.

At the end of the day, this moment is about hope. You're giving your team a reason to believe things can get better: not by magic, not by corporate mandates, but by their own hands.

Don't hide behind being polished or perfect. Be real. Be human. If you're nervous, say it. If you don't have all the answers, admit it. Vulnerability builds trust. And trust is the whole point.

Your job in this opening moment is simple: get your team leaning forward in their chairs. Get them excited about what's possible. Show them you're not here to waste their time. You're here to build something bigger, together.

Because once they feel that? The rest of the workshop—the exercises, the values, the planning—all of it lands 10 times harder.

Step 2 (During the Workshop): Vision and Values Setting

Here's the deal: if you want your hospital culture to be more than fluffy words on a poster, you've got to involve your team in building it. For it to work, it can't come from you, dictated from the top-down (in other words, "owner dictates and everyone else nods"). Instead, we'll run a collective, roll-up-your-sleeves activity to start our workshop where every voice gets a shot to contribute.

Every hospital, every business, needs three things locked down if they want to build something that lasts: mission, vision, and values. This isn't corporate jargon. This is the DNA of your hospital.

Without a mission, a vision and values, you're just winging it. You're just reacting every day, chasing problems instead of building momentum.

With them? You've got alignment. You've got culture you can actually enforce and celebrate. You're setting the foundation for how your hospital operates: how you treat patients, clients, and each other.

So let's break down Mission, Vision, and Values, and why each piece matters.

Mission: Why You Exist

Your mission is the "why we get out of bed every morning" statement. It's not a fancy marketing slogan; it's your core purpose. Present tense. Day-to-day. What do you actually *do* for pets and their families, and why do you exist at all?

For example, a veterinary hospital might say: "To provide compassionate, high-quality medical care to pets and peace of mind to their families."

That's the heartbeat. That's what anchors you today. If your team can't answer why your hospital exists in one sentence, you've got a problem.

Vision: Where You're Going

Now, the vision. This is about the future. It's not what you do today, it's what you're building toward: a long-term aspiration. Think 5, 10 years down the road. When people in your community talk about you, what do you want them to say? What do you want to be known for?

Something like: "To be the most trusted veterinary hospital in our community, known for innovation and exceptional client experiences."

This is your destination. It paints a picture. And here's the kicker: it should scare you a little. If it doesn't stretch you, it's too small.

Values: How You Behave

Values are the rules of the game. They're the principles that guide how you treat clients, patients, and each other, every single day. They're not just words on a page and they're not negotiable.

For a veterinary hospital, it might look like: Compassion. Integrity. Teamwork. Growth. Excellence.

But don't just write them down and pat yourself on the back. Values need to be lived. If "teamwork" is a value, that means nobody gets to say, "That's not my job." If "growth" is a value, then CE opportunities and mentoring can't be optional. This is the cultural playbook for your hospital, lived out every single day.

Putting it all together: mission grounds you, vision pulls you forward, and values guide how you behave.

Why This Works

Because it's not about you dictating values. It's about the team co-creating them. And when people help create the culture, they protect it. They defend it. They live it.

This workshop sets the stage for everything that comes next. Without vision and values, you're just running on fumes. With them, you've got direction, energy, and buy-in.

And trust me: the difference between a hospital with real, shared vision and values versus one without? Night and day. Hospitals that get this right stop playing defense. They stop just reacting to client complaints, turnover, and chaos. They play offense. They move with intention. And over time, that intention builds trust, culture, retention, and growth.

I've run these with hospitals all over the country, and when it's done right, the results are magic. Not only the output, but the feeling within the team: people leave feeling bought in. They leave with clarity. They leave knowing *why* they're here beyond "checking vitals" or "answering phones." And that's what builds momentum. So beyond actually defining your hospital's mission, vision, and values—which itself is super valuable—this activity LITERALLY builds buy-in and a foundation for building culture.

Step 3 (During the Workshop): Designing Your Future Team and Client Experience/Goal-setting

In the next section of the workshop, you get your whole team laser-focused on setting clear goals (1) to improve the team experience and (2) to deepen client trust.

This is deep "How" work: how do we actually take steps toward the Mission and Vision we just articulated? What are our strategic priorities? How are we going to better build trust as a team?

Defining the Team Experience

Team comes first. This is where you start putting petal to the metal and start crafting the future hospital environment, culture, and experience you and your team wants.

In case you need it, let's get real for a second and recap the value of this part: if your team hates coming to work every day, no amount of pizza parties, or even an awesome mission statement—is going to fix it. And I'm not even talking about pay or benefits here—we'll leave that in its own bucket. I'm talking about the *actual in-hospital experience* for your people. The day-to-day stuff. How they're onboarded. How they're trained. How they handle tough cases together. How they communicate. How it *feels* to work here. That's the stuff that makes or breaks culture, so that's what you'll focus on in this activity.

The activity is designed to take all that unspoken frustration—the rolled eyes, the under-the-breath comments, the "ugh, here we go again" moments—and turn it into actionable change. It's a workshop built for your team, by your team. And it works because instead of leadership dictating solutions from on high, you're creating space for the people in the trenches to say in a safe space, "Here's what sucks, here's what we think would fix it, and here's how we'll own it together." That's empowerment. That's culture.

I'm gonna keep it real with you: this exercise might sting. When your team starts unloading frustrations, it might feel like they're pointing the finger at you. You might get that defensive itch— like, "Wait, I'm not the problem here." Don't go there. That's ego talking.

This workshop isn't about blaming you, or making you prove your worth as a leader. It's about taking an honest look at what's broken today so you can start building the future tomorrow. Every hospital has blind spots. Every team has issues. That's not failure—that's fuel.

And here's the thing: by even running this workshop, you've already proved your value as a leader. Most people duck this. They avoid the hard conversations. You're stepping straight into it. That's leadership gold. That's you saying, "I care enough to hear the truth, even if it's uncomfortable, because I want us to win."

Your team's going to respect that more than you realize. They'll notice that you didn't shut down, didn't argue, didn't spin excuses. You just listened. That kind of openness? That's how trust gets built. And trust is the whole point of this.

So when the feedback comes in—and yeah, some of it might be brutal—don't flinch. Lean into it. Nod. Write it down. Thank them for being real. Because on the other side of that sting is growth, momentum, and a stronger team that actually believes you've got their back.

The activity will yield a list of high-priority initiatives you and your team agree to focus on to better the team experience. And you'll see: the energy at the end is just different. You can feel the optimism, the hope, the pride. You close by reminding everyone: this is how we shape the hospital we want to work in. This is how we stop just surviving and start building something that actually feels good. And the beauty is, it's repeatable. Do it quarterly. Stack small wins. Watch culture shift right in front of you.

Here are a few examples of team-focused priorities that I've seen result from this exercise in the past:

- Role Clarity: Within their first 30 days, 100% of new hires receive a written role description and checklist of core responsibilities and performance metrics.
- Cross-training: By the end of the year, 80% of team members are cross-trained to cover at least one additional role/responsibility.

- Anonymous Pulse Surveys: Run quarterly anonymous surveys to measure team morale, workload stress, and leadership trust.
- Culture Wins: Leadership shares at least three "small wins" from the team in every monthly staff meeting.

The best part? It's not theory. It's real. When your people feel like they had a hand in designing their own experience, they stop being passive employees and start becoming co-owners of the vibe. That's the type of energy clients feel the second they walk in the door. That's how you win.

Defining the Client Experience to Build Trust

Now we turn the attention toward your clients. You spend some time explaining how pet-owner clients want to feel, as we covered in Chapter 4. Then, you and your team get work setting clear, real-life goals for improvement.

The approach I lay out in the Facilitation Guide is a total game-changer if you're serious about elevating your client experience and building massive trust with clients. It's about 45 minutes of real talk and honest brainstorming with your team. The goal? Zero in on the exact moments in a client's journey where you either win their trust or lose it. These are the moments where clients either feel cared for or walk away frustrated. Think: that first phone call, the vibe in the lobby, how billing is explained, or whether anyone bothers to follow up after an appointment. These aren't small details. These are the moments that make or break trust.

Here's why this works: instead of leadership guessing what's broken or what could be better, you give every single person on your team a voice. They know the friction points better than anyone, because they live them daily with clients. Everyone gets their ideas out, you cluster them into themes, and then you prioritize ... together. No fluff, no "someday we'll fix this." You literally leave the session with your top three to five improvement ideas, owners assigned, and next steps locked down.

And the benefits? Massive. First, your team feels heard. They're not just cogs doing what leadership tells them; they're shaping the experience. That builds buy-in like crazy. Second, you're focusing your energy on the *right* stuff, the small shifts that clients actually feel. And third, you create a culture of momentum: you celebrate wins, track progress visibly, and revisit the process quarterly to keep leveling up.

This is how you stop spinning your wheels and start compounding wins. It's simple, it's practical, and it creates real change your clients notice. Don't overthink it—just get your people in a room, put the markers in their hands, and start fixing what actually matters.

Together, the two exercises of "Defining the Team Experience" and "Defining the Client Experience" give you a clear set of Strategic Priorities. These are what bring your Mission, Vision, and Values to life. They determine what you actually tackle first. Here's where most leaders get tripped up. Strategic priorities are not "everything we do." They're the handful of big bets you're making *right now* to move toward your vision while delivering on your mission.

Here are few examples of client-focused strategic priorities, complete with clear measures of success, that I've seen come out of past workshops:

- Transparency with estimates: Ensure 100% of clients receive and acknowledge a clear treatment plan/estimate before services are performed.
- Digital engagement: Increase use of text/email reminders to reduce missed appointments by 10% over the next six months.
- Treatment Plan Clarity: Ensure 100% of clients receive a written estimate and treatment plan *before* services are provided, with at least 90% confirming understanding in a follow-up question at checkout.
- Proactive Updates: For hospitalized or surgery patients, provide at least two proactive updates (call or text) per day. Target: 95% compliance tracked in logs.

- Follow-up Calls for Sick Visits: 100% of non-wellness visits get a personalized follow-up call within 24 hours. Target: 90%+ compliance.
- First-time Client Experience: Every new client receives a hand-written thank-you card (signed by at least two staff members) within five days of their first visit.

Notice what's not here? "Keep the lights on." "See patients." That's just daily business. Strategic priorities are the big rocks, the focus areas that get extra attention and resources because they move the needle.

Here's the hidden benefit there: these exercises aren't just about creating goals. They're about creating leaders. Each strategic priority goal is assigned a leader on your team to oversee and reinforce it. And every time you assign a goal, you're not just asking someone to "own a task." You're giving them a shot to step up, show what they're made of, and start flexing muscles they didn't even know they had.

For the less-tenured tech, the CSR who's been grinding quietly, or that assistant who wants to grow but doesn't know how—this is the golden ticket. Leading a goal is their chance to raise their hand and say, *I'm ready for more.* And when they do, you better invest back in them. Don't just hand them the keys and walk away. Sit down with them. Talk about the actual goal, yes, but also talk about leadership itself. Give them feedback. Show them what they're doing well, where they can push harder, how to navigate the challenges of getting people on board.

Because here's the truth: hospitals don't get better by accident. They get better because leaders, at every level, step up and grow. And leadership isn't just reserved for the doctor in the corner office or the manager with the title. Leadership is taught, built, and sharpened in the trenches, day by day, goal by goal.

If you're serious about building a hospital that thrives long term, you *have* to invest in your team's leadership potential. Every future superstar starts with small opportunities like this. You think you're just helping someone manage a goal around improving follow-up calls? Nope. You're training your next lead tech. You're shaping the future manager who will one day hold this hospital together when things get tough. You're building a leadership bench that makes your hospital unstoppable.

Ignore this, and what happens? You burn out your current leaders, and when someone leaves, you scramble. But when you pour into people now, when you treat these "small" leadership chances as training grounds, you're playing the long game. You're showing your team that growth is possible here, that they don't have to leave to find leadership opportunities. That's retention gold.

So don't sleep on this. Assign leaders. Coach them. Cheer them on. Critique them. That's how you build a team full of owners, not just employees. And when you've got a hospital full of owners? Clients feel it. The culture shifts. And the whole flywheel spins faster.

Remember that the Appendix has detailed materials for you to run this Veterinary Hospital Identity Workshop successfully: Facilitation guides, sample scripts, examples. They are designed for you to pick up and go, even if you've never run a workshop or managed a process like this before.

Step 4 (Post-workshop): Implement and Measure

Okay, so you've reached the end of your workshop, and are now equipped with a draft mission and vision, and your team has aligned on what they feel are your team's values. Your team has also brainstormed and prioritized what they feel are the most-impactful goals it can set to improve team experience and maximize client trust. You've assigned leaders to push the team forward toward those goals. What now?

You just pulled your team into a room and worked them hard for a full day. Don't let all that magic go to waste. Bring their ideas to life: implement. Measure.

Setting goals without tracking them is like joining a gym and never stepping on the scale, picking up a weight, or checking your progress. You might *feel* like you're moving forward, but you're really just running in place.

What gets measured gets managed. And in a hospital setting, whether it's improving client trust or creating a better team culture, you can't just throw goals out into the air and hope they land somehow. Hope isn't a strategy. If you don't measure, you don't know if the changes put in place are actually being implemented or actually working ... or worse, if you're sliding backward.

And listen, this isn't about creating some cold, corporate dashboard that nobody ever looks at. This is about giving your team *proof.* Proof that their effort is paying off. Proof that their ideas are making things better. Proof that clients are noticing, that wait times are shrinking, that follow-ups are happening, that trust is building. When people can actually see results, they get fired up. They buy in. They start believing in the vision because the numbers are showing it's real.

On the flip side, if you don't track? People lose faith. They'll say, "Yeah, leadership talks about change, but nothing actually happens." That's a culture killer, every time.

So here's the mindset shift: tracking is not micromanaging, it's storytelling. Every metric is a piece of the story you're writing as a leader. Client satisfaction scores? That's your story of trust. Staff turnover dropping? That's your story of culture. Wellness plan enrollments going up? That's your story of preventive care.

If you're not measuring, you're just guessing how you're doing. And if you're just guessing, you're gambling with your team's trust, your clients' loyalty, and your hospital's future. No bueno.

How you measure progress depends on the goals you set. Period. There's no cookie-cutter answer here. If your goal is to build client trust, then you've got to actually ask clients. Not once a year.

Not just when they leave a review. I'm talking surveys, quick check-ins, focus groups, even just real, informal conversations while they're standing in your lobby. Look them in the eye and ask, "How's your experience been? What can we do better?" That feedback is gold.

If your goal is financial health, then track the damn numbers. Look at return rates. Average client spend. Retention over time. Don't just assume things are going well because the lobby looks busy. Measure it.

If your goal is to improve how your team delivers, then document the actions. Did the tech actually call the client back after the sick visit? Did the CSR follow through with the follow-up? Put systems in place so those actions don't live in the land of "I think we did it." Make it trackable and visible.

You've got a ton of measurement tools at your disposal. Use them. Surveys. Dashboards. Whiteboards in the breakroom. Google reviews. Phone logs. It doesn't matter what you pick, what matters is that you're tracking consistently and showing the team the receipts. Because progress isn't about what you *hope* is happening. It's about what you can prove.

Step 5 (Post-workshop): Share Results and Celebrate Success

Then, once you have results to share, share them. And celebrate success and progress, even when it's small. As soon as you start celebrating that openly, you'll feel the shift.

People need to see proof that their work matters. You can talk vision and values until you're blue in the face, but when you actually show them the numbers, the reviews, the wins, they'll feel it in their gut. That's how you build pride. That's how you build momentum. That's how you create a flywheel that keeps spinning faster. And that's how you take your hospital from average to unforgettable.

And don't overcomplicate it. You don't need some fancy dashboard with a password nobody remembers. Whiteboard in the breakroom? Perfect. A quick slide at the monthly staff meeting? Awesome. A 30-second shoutout in morning rounds? Even better. The key is visibility and consistency.

Sharing results tells your team:

1. We're measuring what matters (not just production and dollars).
2. I see you. I notice your effort.
3. We're in this together. When the numbers go up, we all win.

This is culture. Not pizza parties. Not empty slogans. Culture is your people seeing their efforts play out in real time and feeling proud of their impact.

Step 6: (Post-workshop) The "3 Rs"—Reflect, Revisit, Raise the Bar

Hitting your goals isn't the finish line. It's the starting line for what comes next. Too many hospitals make the mistake of setting a goal, crushing it, and then ... moving on like nothing happened. Or worse, letting the energy fizzle out. That's how you murder momentum.

The great teams? They pause. They reflect. They ask, *What worked? What didn't? What did we learn?* They take a second to acknowledge the progress and celebrate wins because it builds pride and energy. But then they immediately pivot to, *"Okay, what's next?"*

Revisiting your goals has to be a recurring rhythm, not a once-a-year offsite. Your team should be looking at results regularly—perhaps monthly—and asking: "Are these still the right goals? Are they moving us closer to being the hospital we want to be? Do they still match what our clients and patients need from us?" The industry shifts. Client expectations shift. Your team evolves. If you're not reassessing, you're flying blind and falling behind.

And then comes the fun part: raising the bar. Once you've nailed something, don't just pat yourself on the back and coast. Build on the momentum. If your follow-up call rate went from 50 to 90%, awesome. Now make the calls *better*. Train the team to add more warmth, more empathy, more personalization. If you cut client wait times down by five minutes, celebrate it and then ask, *"How do we shave another five?"* This is where greatness comes from: stacking win on top of win.

Because here's the thing: momentum compounds. Clients feel it. Your team feels it. And when you keep reflecting, revisiting, and raising the bar, you're not just checking goals off a list. You're building a culture that's addicted to progress. A culture where "good enough" doesn't exist, and everyone is bought into the idea that tomorrow can—and will—be better than today.

That's how you separate your hospital from the one down the street. That's how you create a place clients rave about, a place your team is proud of, and a place where pets get the absolute best care possible.

Reflect. Revisit. Raise the bar. Repeat. That's the game.

Real Talk—For You, Leader

And for fuck's sake: don't forget to have fun with it. Watching these strategies actually *work*—seeing your hospital grow, your team click, your clients smile—that's the reward. That's the game. Enjoy the ride.

And give yourself some damn credit, too. You're the one stepping up. You're the one leaning into the hard shit instead of hiding from it. You're the one sweating it out, leading with honesty, owning the tough truths, being transparent when it would be easier to fake it. That's not easy. That's leadership.

Don't rob yourself of that acknowledgment. You're not just talking about culture; you're building it. You're not just "managing." You're leading, championing your team, your clients, your hospital, and every single pet that walks through your doors. That's real. That's rare. And leaders like you? You don't just change hospitals. You change industries. You change lives. You change the fucking world.

Leaders like you straight-up move me. You don't even realize the weight of what you're doing every single day. You're not just running appointments or keeping a hospital afloat—you're giving people like me, people who love their pets like family, a shot at more moments. More walks. More cuddles. More time.

And that matters. It matters more than you probably let yourself believe when you're exhausted, when you feel unseen. The work you do matters. You matter.

Thank you. Thank you for staying in the fight when it would be easier to give up. Thank you for showing up for people who are terrified about their pets. Thank you for carrying the emotional weight of an industry that doesn't always give you the credit you deserve.

Because for passionate, emotionally-invested pet owners—like me—you're not just "the vet" or "the hospital." You're the people we trust with our Buddy. And that's everything. You give us peace when we're scared, hope when we're unsure, and joy when our pets get one more healthy day.

You change lives every damn day. Never forget that.

Summary

Momentum isn't given. It's built, brick by brick, and it starts the second you decide to lead.

To be blunt: everything we've talked about—culture, fairness, trust, team retention—means jack if you don't execute. Ideas don't change hospitals. Action does. And that's what this six-step process is about: giving you a system to actually build momentum and keep it alive.

This isn't fluff. It's not some "feel good" exercise you do once and forget. It's heavy lifting. It's closing your hospital for a day, rolling up your sleeves with your team, and saying, "We're building the future together." It's assigning ownership. It's tracking results. It's celebrating wins. And then it's raising the bar again and again.

When you commit to this, you're not just running a workshop. You're creating a culture addicted to progress. You're building a team that feels like owners, not just employees. You're creating a place where clients walk in and feel the difference immediately. That's momentum. That's the Veterinary Trust Flywheel in action.

And don't forget: this isn't about being perfect. It's about being real, vulnerable, transparent, and relentless. Your team doesn't need a flawless boss. They need a leader who shows up, owns mistakes, and keeps pushing forward. That's what earns respect. That's what earns trust.

So here's your challenge: commit. Don't dabble. Don't wait for the "perfect time." There isn't one. The perfect time is now. Because the longer you wait, the longer your hospital stays stuck in neutral. And the second you commit, you've already separated yourself from 90% of leaders in this industry.

You've got the playbook. You've got the process. Now it's on you. Build the workshop. Lead the room. Share the wins. Keep the wheel spinning.

Because when you do? Your team will stick. Your clients will trust. Pets will thrive. And your hospital will become the one everyone else in town is chasing.

Suggested Readings

American Animal Hospital Association. *Culture Transformation Toolkit for Veterinary Practices.* AAHA, 2022, www.aaha.org

American Veterinary Medical Association. *Economic State of the Veterinary Profession Report*. AVMA, 2023, www.avma.org

Deming, W. Edwards. *Out of the Crisis*. MIT Press, 2000.

Gallup. *State of the Global Workplace Report*. Gallup, 2023, www.gallup.com

Harvard Business Review. "What Gets Measured Gets Managed." *Harvard Business Review*, Nov. 2019, hbr.org

Kouzes, James M., and Barry Z. Posner. *The Leadership Challenge*. 6th ed., Wiley, 2017.

Locke, Edwin A., and Gary P. Latham. *A Theory of Goal Setting and Task Performance*. Prentice Hall, 1990.

McKinsey & Company. "Organizational Health and Performance: Why Execution Wins." McKinsey, 2022, www.mckinsey.com

Net Promoter Network. *Using NPS for Continuous Improvement*. Satmetrix Systems, 2023, www.netpromotersystem.com

Sinek, Simon. *Start with Why: How Great Leaders Inspire Everyone to Take Action*. Portfolio, 2009.

Society for Human Resource Management. *Employee Engagement and Organizational Culture*. SHRM, 2022, www.shrm.org

Wageman, Ruth, et al. *Senior Leadership Teams: What It Takes to Make Them Great*. Harvard Business School Press, 2008.

Chapter 16
What Pet-owner Clients Want

Here's the truth, and you may have heard this before: people may forget what you did, but they'll always remember how you made them feel. In any industry, client experience is elevated when your customers FEEL that the team attending to them is on their side, has their back, and has a vested interest in helping them to achieve their objectives and get their needs met. So when we think about client or customer experience, and what that actually means, we're talking about how we make our clients or customers feel when interacting with us. Products, price, brand, layout—sure, those things matter to the experience too. But right now, we're talking *feelings*.

Every client wants to feel appreciated, valued, and like more than a number. That's the baseline.

Raise the bar a bit and you add joy, delight, convenience. Michelin service. Disney delight. Airline convenience (we can dream). Those help.

Some industries, though, a select few, are called to deliver more. More than the basics of making clients feel appreciated. More than just delivering smiles, joy, delight, and convenience. Organizations in those industries have a higher calling to establish safety and trust. And without a doubt, the veterinary industry falls into that category (as does human healthcare, by the way).

This is a higher, more difficult calling. It requires more maturity, more empathy, better communication .... And a deeper understanding of what pet owner clients really want. But for your team, it can also carry deeper rewards, deeper fulfillment, a deeper sense of meaning when delivered well.

Meeting this higher bar means that while we can incorporate tactics that deliver convenience, delight, or joy, those things alone are insufficient in meeting our pet-owner clients' innermost needs. While it certainly doesn't hurt to make the check-in or checkout process convenient, or to offer convenient appointment times or convenient parking or an easy online appointment booking experience, for example, these "convenience factors" alone are insufficient. And there are certainly opportunities to create joy and unexpected delight in veterinary care—sending clients a funny picture of their pet wearing a cute surgery cap after a successful surgery, for example, is a great way to deliver unexpected joy to a client. A spirited greeting of a new client bringing their new puppy in for their first visit, thereby bringing a smile to the client's face and pet's face, is always a good idea. But we're called to more—we're not in the business of simply making people smile. Veterinary care is serious business with clear goals: prolonging healthy pet lives, guarding the human-animal bond, guiding peaceful goodbyes. And for that to work, we have to be in the business of building trust with our clients.

As we'll talked about in detail, when we nail the client experience— when we deliver interactions that build and maintain trust— something powerful happens: clients actually follow our advice. And assuming that advice is solid medical guidance (and it damn well better be), that trust translates directly into better outcomes for pets. At the end of the day, that's why most of us are in this field in the first place. We care. We want healthier pets, grateful clients, and teams that feel proud of the impact they make.

So what does "trust" actually mean in veterinary medicine? How does a pet owner define it? What does it *look like* when a client actually feels like they can trust us?

It's tempting to reach for the clichés. "Do the right thing." "Tell the truth." "Treat people how you want to be treated." None of that is wrong, but it's surface-level. In the real world, platitudes won't cut it. We have to go deeper.

Because here's what I've learned: in the eyes of clients, trust is incredibly specific. Most can't articulate it perfectly. They're not walking into your lobby thinking, "Here are the five psychological conditions I need met in order to trust this hospital." But when you've interacted with thousands of pet owners, led dozens of focus groups, and combed through hundreds of thousands of surveys, reviews, and testimonials like I have, the patterns smack you in the face. Trust comes into focus. You start to see exactly what pet owners are looking for.

And that's what we're about to unpack. I'm going to boil down what clients need to feel in order to trust you and your team. Not theories. Not fluff. Actual, observable client needs—grounded in research, feedback, and lived experience.

So: what do clients need to feel to trust you? Let's break it down.

Feeling 1: Valued/Appreciated

We need to stop thinking of a veterinary *hospital* as simply a medical office and start thinking of veterinary *care* as a service industry. Medicine is the core, but the delivery—the *experience*—is what makes clients feel valued. As an industry, we need to start realizing that every single visit is judged not only on medical outcomes, but on how our clients felt along the way.

Clients want medical expertise, but they also want reassurance. They want to know their concerns matter. That their pets matter. That *they* matter. Meeting those emotional needs builds appreciation—and appreciation builds trust.

Client appreciation sits on two pillars: service and hospitality.

- Service is the system: check-in that runs smoothly, processes that minimize stress, a waiting area that feels cared for. Service says, "We've got our act together."
- Hospitality is the human side: genuine listening, kindness, empathy. The receptionist who notices nerves and offers comfort. The tech who remembers a kid's soccer game. The doctor who sits eye-to-eye with the client instead of towering over them. Hospitality says, "I see you."

Danny Meyer nailed it, in his book *Setting the Table*: "Service is a monologue. Hospitality is a dialogue." Service sets the stage. Hospitality creates the connection.

Clients rarely separate service and hospitality in their minds. Instead, they experience them together. When service is carefully crafted *and* hospitality is warm and genuine, clients walk away feeling not just that their pet received great care, but that *they themselves were cared for too.*

Here's where I often see hospitals stumble: they assume that delivering a differentiated service experience requires brainstorming big, flashy, creative ideas. That can feel overwhelming, so they default to business as usual.

But in reality, great service doesn't mean flashy gimmicks. It's in the small touches: the friction points that can be smoothed out, the moments where clients might feel uncertain or overlooked, the tiny touches that make them think, "Wow, they really thought about me."

Later in this book, I'll share tactical strategies that you and your team can use to design a top-notch service experience. But, I will share a quick example now to put this in context: consider follow-up calls. A hospital might establish a service standard that *every client receives a call the day after their visit*. That's great service: consistent, reliable, and designed to show that the hospital is still thinking about the client once they've left.

But hospitality transforms that routine call into something memorable. I once met a CSR named Sam who found a way to make every follow-up call personal. She never limited the conversation to, "How is your pet doing?" She also asked about the client:

"Becky, I know yesterday was stressful for you, too. How are you holding up today? Did you think of any questions last night that you didn't get a chance to ask yesterday that maybe I can answer for you now?"

Then Sam even went further, sometimes checking back several weeks later just to see how things were going. That wasn't scripted. That was just genuine care. And clients never forgot it.

This is the perfect marriage of service and hospitality. The standard creates consistency. The human connection creates loyalty.

As a hospital leader, your job is to design for both. You create service standards—for example, "Every client gets a follow-up call the next day." That ensures reliability. But then you must also invest in training your team in the principles of hospitality—active listening, empathy, and emotional intelligence—and in giving them enough leash to deliver a genuine experience their own way. But I digress, we'll get into the "How" later.

When clients experience both an organized, thoughtful service structure *and* genuine hospitality in every interaction, they feel valued. And when clients feel valued, trust deepens, loyalty grows, and your hospital becomes not just the place where their pet receives care, but the place they want to return to again and again.

Feeling 2: Known

Veterinary clients—especially returning clients—want to feel that you and your team know them and their pet. This is pivotal toward ensuring that your clients feel like more than just a number.

Feeling "known" isn't just about facial recognition. Sure, remembering a client's face or their pet's name helps. But trust goes deeper. It's about recalling details, past conversations, medical history, and showing that you actually prepared for their visit. And this standard would apply even if the team or doctor who saw a client and pet during their previous visit isn't the same team working today. Even team members seeing a client and their pet for the first time can review previous visit notes and deliver a personal greeting: "Oh, this must be Buddy! I've heard all about him and how cute he is from Dr. Melissa, who saw you last visit. And you must be Susan— so nice to meet you! How's Buddy doing on that new medication we prescribed?"

So what if the team—like perhaps the CSR and Technician—who saw Susan the pet owner and her dog Buddy during their first appointment isn't the same team that's working for today's visit? How can these team members who have never laid eyes on Susan or Buddy give the impression that they "know" them? Simple, by showing that the team, holistically, knows and understands Buddy's medical history, reason for visit, and other important details. Again, it's not just facial recognition: if the team working today didn't see the client when she came in three months ago, that visual recognition wouldn't have been established and of course shouldn't be faked.

And let's be clear: this can't be faked. You can't wing it with vague comments and hope it lands. You actually have to *know* the client and the pet. That means documenting details—both medical and personal—and reviewing them before the client's next visit.

The easiest way to feel genuine is to *be* genuine. Don't think of this as optics. Think of it as actually giving a damn. Taking notes. Preparing. Remembering. Delivering that moment of recognition that says, "We see you. We know you. You're not just a number here."

Feeling 3: Competently Supported

Here's the nonnegotiable: clients need to feel competently supported. That's obvious at the doctor level, but it has to show across the *whole team*.

Clients pick up on alignment (or the lack of it) across the team instantly. If the CSR, the tech, and the doctor all ask "What brings you in today?" (like I experienced at Linda's hospital in the previous example) confidence plummets. It screams disorganization. The second they sense the team isn't on the same page, the questions start flooding in: "If they can't even communicate basic info, are they missing something critical about my pet's care?" "I told the tech Buddy's allergic to that medication … but is the tech I told even the one doing the procedure? Did that get passed to the doctor? What if it didn't? Is Buddy at risk?"

That spiral—that pit in your stomach—is exactly what a lack of trust feels like.

The real test of whether a client feels competently supported doesn't happen during routine check-ups. It happens in the scariest moments—like when their dog needs emergency surgery.

Imagine Sarah jogging into your hospital with Max, her eight-year-old Golden Retriever, in her arms. Max collapsed at home, and she rushed him in immediately. The doctor says he needs surgery—*now*. There's no time to think. No time to shop around. Sarah has no choice but to hand Max over.

Now she's in the lobby. Waiting. For hours.

If her past visits to your hospital felt sloppy, the spiral kicks in:
"What if they missed something?"
"Did they even look at Max's records before anesthesia?"
"What if today's doctor doesn't know what the last one documented?"
"What if nobody asked me the right questions?"

That's what a lack of trust looks like. Anxiety multiplied by uncertainty. And that moment—when Max is out of sight and Sarah is left alone with her thoughts—is the *ultimate trust test*.

But now flip the script. Same Sarah. Same Max. Same emergency.

This time, the history is different. Every wellness visit before today was tight. The team remembered details. The doctor always reviewed Max's chart before walking in. The techs always communicated clearly. Sarah never had to repeat herself. The vibe was: *these people are aligned, they're competent, they care.*

So now, in the lobby, Sarah is still scared and worried about Max, but she can reassure herself:
"They've always had their act together."
"They took notes when I explained Max's allergy."
"They listen. They're on the same page. They know Max."
"I trust them."

That's a completely different emotional experience. Same situation. Same stakes. But the foundation of competence built in everyday visits becomes the safety net when things get life-or-death.

That's where trust gets tested the hardest—when the pet is out of sight, and the owner can't see what's happening, has no choice but to rely on you, and is left alone with their thoughts. Either those thoughts are calming, or they're panic-inducing. So your daily habits as a team—how well you communicate, how prepared you are, how much you *show* competence—either build that trust bank for when it matters most, or they don't.

Clients deserve that peace of mind. They deserve to feel like the team knows what they're doing, has communicated well, and is rallying together around their pet. That's not a "nice-to-have." That's a client right.

Feeling 4: Partnership—Heard and Included

Clients also need to feel like *partners*—a member of their pet's involved care team.

If the hospital comes across as rushed, disinterested, or purely revenue-driven, the client feels like they're fighting for their pet *against* the team. That's the opposite of partnership. Or in contrast, if the client feels like the hospital team IS competent and vested in the pet's care, but is seemingly making medical decisions without involving the client in the discussion or decision process, thereby not making the client feel heard, the partnership is sabotaged. In both scenarios, the client's need to feel partnered with, heard and included is absent.

If clients don't feel heard or included in discussions regarding their pet's care, trust breaks down.

Partnership requires three things: communication, listening, and transparency. Clients need clear explanations of treatment options, risks, and costs. They need space to ask questions without feeling rushed. And they need to feel empathy: that the team understands and cares about their perspective.

When partnership is present, clients feel like it's "us and them together" fighting for the pet's best outcome. That's trust. And it doesn't matter whether the pet is getting a cancer treatment or a routine rabies vaccine—the opportunity to make the client feel heard and included is always there.

Feeling 5: Affirmed

Finally, clients often need to feel affirmed.

Pets today are family. Owners see themselves as pet parents. That means they feel intense responsibility—and often, guilt or anxiety—when something's wrong. Younger owners especially adopt pets as their "test kids" or sources of connection. When their pet struggles, they often feel like *they* failed.

That's why affirmation matters. A simple, genuine comment like, "You did the right thing bringing Buddy in today" or "Buddy's lucky to have you" lifts a huge weight off a worried client's shoulders. It validates their efforts. It relieves guilt. It builds confidence.

But here's the catch: affirmation can't be scripted. You can't train your team to say, "Every client should hear their pet is lucky to have them." That's empty. Clients can smell the fake.

The right way: stay engaged. Read the client's stress level. Offer affirmation where it fits naturally. Adjust based on the situation. Done right, it feels like thoughtful reassurance—not a box to check.

When affirmation is delivered authentically, clients feel seen, appreciated, and proud. Often, it surprises them because they weren't expecting it. That surprise makes it land even harder. It shows the team took an extra beat to make the client feel good. And that's one of the simplest, most powerful ways to build trust.

So while the goal of client experience in veterinary medicine is not always to deliver unexpected delight, throwing some unexpected affirmation the client's way might just do so, and build trust too.

The Big Picture: Desired Feelings for Pet Owners

At the core, veterinary medicine is more than diagnosing and treating. It's a service industry. Clients aren't just judging outcomes. They're judging how they felt along the way.

Let's be real: clients today expect way more than just competent medicine. That's the baseline. That's table stakes. What they *really* want—and what builds actual trust—is to feel safe, valued, appreciated, known, supported, heard, and affirmed. Those aren't extras. They're not "nice-to-haves." They're emotional needs. And unless you meet those needs, trust doesn't grow. And without trust? Even the best medical advice in the world gets ignored. With trust? Clients follow your guidance, they stay loyal, and they become advocates for your hospital. That's the game.

And this is where too many in vet med miss the point: veterinary care isn't just medicine. It's a service industry. Period. Just like hospitality, retail, or dining. Clients are judging you at every single touchpoint. Was it easy? Did they listen to me? Did they remember me? Did they even care? But here's the kicker: the stakes are *way* higher here than in retail or restaurants. We're not selling jeans or tacos. Clients are handing us their family members, their pets. And that changes everything.

That's why the blend of service *and* hospitality matters so much. Service is the structure—it's how the experience is designed, the reliability of the process, the systems you put in place so things run smoothly. Hospitality is the human part: the spontaneous, genuine connection that makes people feel something. You need both. One without the other falls flat. Together, they send one clear message: "We take pride in what we do, and we care deeply about you and your pet."

And let's be clear: trust isn't built in just the big, dramatic moments in the exam room or on the operating table. It's built in the everyday stuff. It's the way the front desk greets someone. It's the thoughtful follow-up call the next day. It's remembering a pet's history or asking about a detail from a previous visit. It's in the little affirmations when an anxious pet owner needs reassurance. It's those small, human touches that pile up over time and make people *believe in you.*

When we finally own this truth—when we stop pretending vet med is just about clinical skills and accept that service excellence is baked into the profession—we unlock the real magic. That's when client experiences become unforgettable. And here's the most important part: better experiences lead directly to better outcomes. Clients who trust you follow through. They come back. They take your advice. Their pets live longer, healthier lives.

That's the power and the responsibility of working in both medicine *and* service. That's the truth of what clients actually want from us. And the hospitals who figure this out? They're the ones who crush it and win.

You want repeat business? Make your clients feel like they've got equity in your hospital. Not financial equity—emotional equity. When they leave telling their friends, 'This is *my* vet,' what they're really saying is, 'They made me feel important. They made me feel like I belong.' That's how you build loyalty at scale.

Summary

Clients don't stay loyal because of what you did for their pet. They stay loyal because of how you made them feel while doing it.

Clients aren't begging for gimmicks. They're not counting how many times you say their name or tallying up how many treats you hand out. What they actually want is much deeper: to feel valued, known, competently supported, included, and affirmed. That's the list. That's the game.

Veterinary medicine is not just about clinical expertise. That's table stakes. Clients are judging you on how you made them feel while delivering that expertise. Did you listen? Did you remember them? Did you make them feel safe? Did you give them confidence that you and your team actually give a damn? Because if the answer to any of these is no, trust dies. And once trust dies, even the best medicine in the world won't land.

But here's the flip side: when you nail this—when service and hospitality work in harmony—trust doesn't just grow, it compounds. Clients follow your advice. Pets get better outcomes. Loyalty deepens. Word of mouth explodes. Suddenly, you're not just the vet. You're *their* vet, part of their family's story.

That's the real opportunity here. To stop playing at the surface level and start owning the fact that vet med is both medicine and service. When you deliver both with authenticity, you don't just win reviews. You win trust. And trust is the currency that drives everything else.

Suggested Readings

Agency for Healthcare Research and Quality. *Patient Experience and Patient-centered Care*. U.S. Department of Health and Human Services, 2022, www.ahrq.gov

American Animal Hospital Association. *The Path to High-quality, High-value Veterinary Care*. AAHA Press, 2021, www.aaha.org

American Veterinary Medical Association. *Pet Ownership and Demographics Sourcebook*. AVMA, 2023, www.avma.org

Berry, Leonard L., and Kent D. Seltman. *Discovering the Soul of Service: The Nine Drivers of Sustainable Business Success*. Free Press, 2008.

Gallup. *Customer Experience and Emotional Engagement*. Gallup, 2022, www.gallup.com

Groth, Markus, and Angelo Ang. "The Relevance of Service Encounters in Trust Formation." *Journal of Service Research*, vol. 21, no. 3, 2018, pp. 317–331.

Haidt, Jonathan. *The Righteous Mind: Why Good People Are Divided by Politics and Religion*. Vintage, 2013.

Meyer, Danny. *Setting the Table: The Transforming Power of Hospitality in Business*. HarperBusiness, 2006.

Morgan, Robert M., and Shelby D. Hunt. "The Commitment-trust Theory of Relationship Marketing." *Journal of Marketing*, vol. 58, no. 3, 1994, pp. 20–38.

Parasuraman, A., Valarie A. Zeithaml, and Leonard L. Berry. "SERVQUAL: A Multiple-Item Scale for Measuring Consumer Perceptions of Service Quality." *Journal of Retailing*, vol. 64, no. 1, 1988, pp. 12–40.

PwC. *Experience Is Everything: Here's How to Get It Right*. PwC Global Customer Experience Survey, 2023, www.pwc.com

Serpell, James A. *In the Company of Animals: A Study of Human–Animal Relationships*. 2nd ed., Cambridge UP, 2017.

Part 4

Tactics to Improve Client Experiences and Trust

The United Airlines Wake-up Call: A Lesson in CX Failure, Culture Collapse, and Recovery

Before that infamous 2017 nightmare—the one where a paying passenger got dragged off an overbooked flight at O'Hare, the internet set United on fire, and United Airlines became a global symbol of "what not to do" in customer experience—United already had a customer experience problem.

The warning signs were blinking red. People didn't love flying with them. You know that feeling when a brand is technically "fine," but nobody chooses it on purpose? That was United.

In the early–mid 2010s, United already had a reputation problem. Not a catastrophic one yet—just a chronically underperforming, emotionally disconnected one. The numbers told the story clearly, and long before the world was watching.

- In 2014, one benchmarker placed United's Net Promoter Score (NPS) at around 10 (a solid score in most industries is above 70), one of the lowest among major carriers.
- A recent study has suggested that airlines as a category were leaving up to $1.4 billion per year in revenue on the table by failing to improve CX—and United was sitting on the wrong side of that math.

Passenger sentiment and industry commentary consistently painted the same picture: United wasn't a "hell no," but they definitely weren't a "hell yes." They were the airline you took because the timing worked, the price was okay, or you just didn't care enough to switch. This is the most dangerous kind of brand problem: not hatred—apathy. People were flying United not because they *loved* it, but because they *settled* for it.

United's operational performance didn't save them either. They ran a tight financial machine, sure, but loyalty, trust, and emotional connection lagged. This is exactly where many service businesses get blindsided: the P&L still looks fine ... right up until the culture explodes.

And United's culture was next.

United's first attempt at "fixing CX" was a Script, not a soul. They didn't start with culture. They didn't start with empowerment. They didn't start with purpose. They started with a checklist:

"Smile more."
"Say thank you."
"This is how you should 'smize'—smile with your eyes."
"Use these preapproved phrases with passengers."

Employees were even instructed to "smize"—that is, smile with their eyes (whatever that means).

It was corporate CX theater—customer experience as a performance, not a belief system. United trained its frontline workers like they were performing on Broadway instead of welcoming human beings. They were told what to *say*, not what to *mean*. They were trained to act polite, not empowered to *be* helpful.

But you can't script your way into being a loved brand. People can *feel* when the service is robotic. When the team doesn't know the "why," the customer always feels the "whatever." Passengers could smell it. Because United never gave their frontline people a deeper *why*—no lived mission, no real empowerment, no clear picture of how they actually wanted customers to *feel*—the service landed cold, stiff, and robotic. The people on the plane weren't treated like hosts; they were treated like compliance officers. And when you treat your team like compliance officers, that's exactly the energy your customers feel.

United was setting itself up for a catastrophic cultural failure; and on April 9, 2017, everything fell apart.

United Express Flight 3411 was overbooked. United needed four seats for airline employees. Nobody volunteered. They moved to involuntary removal. One of the passengers selected was Dr. David Dao, a 69-year-old physician. He refused to give up his seat, and security was called. The world watched him get dragged down the aisle, bleeding, screaming, filmed from every angle. And overnight, United transformed from a middling airline with a "meh" reputation to a global symbol of dehumanizing corporate culture.

The public response? Nuclear.

A poll of nearly 2,000 people showed:

- 79% of respondents said they would choose another airline over United in the same situation.

- 44% said they'd avoid United even if it meant paying $66 more and arriving three hours later.

Read that again. People were willing to pay more money and waste more time just to avoid the *feeling* of being treated the way they saw passengers treated on that video. That's what a culture problem looks like when it hits the open market. That's not a price objection— that's a trust objection.

Once the dust settled, United didn't just apologize. They started actually fixing the root problem: their culture, their systems, their training, and their purpose. They finally understood that scripts are useless without trust. United began investing:

- In frontline empowerment
- In technology that actually worked
- In communication systems during disruptions
- In operational reliability
- In training that taught employees *why* the work matters
- In expectations for how the airline wanted customers to feel— not just what they wanted employees to say

And you could see it in the numbers that actually track trust: United's NPS climbed from ~10 in 2014 to ~50 after several years of culture and CX improvements. In a 2024 investor update, United's leadership reported that their internal NPS had risen 24 points since Q3 2019 and was up 5 points versus the previous year—driven by investments in tech, frontline training, and operational resilience.

Think about what that means:

- They didn't just say, "Our people are smiling more."
- They said, "We rewired operations, technology, and training, and the *customer's voice* is telling us we're getting better."

By 2025, loyalty revenue was exploding. From public earnings reports: premium cabin revenue increased 6%. Basic economy revenue increased 4%, and loyalty (MileagePlus, credit card spend, repeat flyers) increased 9% year-over-year.

Today, you'll see language from United about "brand-loyal customers," "diverse revenue streams," and "unlocking the full potential" of their network—code for: we finally understand that experience and loyalty are the real product, not just the metal tube you sit in.

This is the part most leaders miss: CX improvements don't just make people happier. They make people return, spend more, and choose you even when you're not the cheapest option.

Trust is the real product in any service business—including veterinary hospitals. United's story is a giant neon sign for every veterinary hospital owner, manager, and leader, and you don't have to wait for your Dr. Dao moment to realize your culture is cracked. Learn from United's example:

1. **You cannot script your way into loyalty:** If you hand your client care team a sheet of "nice phrases to say," you're already losing. People don't want scripts. They want sincerity. CX is not just about being nice—it's about being trustworthy.

2. **Systems failures are always rooted in culture failure:** United's frontline didn't drag a passenger because they were bad people. They did it because the system taught them compliance mattered more than humanity.

3. **Trust drives revenue**: Just like airlines, veterinary hospitals make their real money not from one visit ... but from decades of loyalty, referrals, and relationship equity. When you build a culture where your team is empowered, aligned, and emotionally safe, your clients feel it—and they return, refer, and comply.

Here's the bottom line: United's story isn't a story about an airline. It's a story about what happens when a service organization ignores culture until it sets itself on fire.

United started with low trust and weak loyalty. They tried to fix it with scripts. They suffered a catastrophic culture failure. Then they rebuilt from the inside out—and the data proves it worked.

Veterinary hospitals face the same choice every day: teach your team to "smile more" ... or build a culture where the smile is real. One is a checklist. The other is a competitive advantage.

Where We're Headed Next

I'm giving you this case study now *on purpose*, because we're about to enter the part of the book everyone wants to skip to—the juicy tactics. The scripts. The step-by-step moves that make clients say, "Damn, that hospital gets it."

But I want to remind you again: none of the tactics matter if you haven't done the culture work first. You can't duct-tape "wow moments" onto a burned-out team. You can't sprinkle charm on top of resentment and call it client experience. You can't shove a script into someone's hand and expect magic.

Jumping straight to tactics NEVER works. Not in airlines. Not in tech. And definitely not in veterinary medicine.

In the chapters ahead, I'm going to lay out the exact tools and techniques I've seen explode client trust—the stuff that makes teams look polished, confident, and deeply human. Some of them will sound almost stupidly simple. You might even think, "Really? That's it?"

Exactly. That *is* it.

Because when you've actually led—when you've built fairness into the foundation, when you've invested in culture and psychological safety, when you've aligned your hospital on mission, vision, and values, when you've committed to servant leadership—the simple stuff becomes powerful. It becomes easy. It becomes *second nature*.

Without that, the tactics are empty. With it, the tactics land wildly well with your clients.

Suggested Readings

CustomerGauge. "Airline Customer Experience Net Promoter Scores." *CustomerGauge*, CustomerGauge Ltd, 2023.

CX Dive. "United Is Focused on Winning Brand-loyal Customers." *Customer Experience Dive*, Industry Dive, 2024.

Deloitte. *Airline Customer Experience: Reimagining Loyalty and Growth*. Deloitte Insights, Deloitte Development LLC, 2017.

Nasdaq. "United Airlines Holdings, Inc. (UAL) Financial Performance & Revenue Trends." *Nasdaq Market Data*, Nasdaq, Inc., www.nasdaq.com. Accessed 7 Dec. 2025.

United Airlines Holdings, Inc. *United Airlines Investor Update and Earnings Report*. United Investor Relations, 2024–2025, www.united.com/en/us/investor-relations

Victor, Daniel. "United Airlines Passenger Is Dragged from His Seat, Stirring Outrage." *The New York Times*, 10 Apr. 2017, www.nytimes.com/2017/04/10/business/united-airlines-passenger-dragged.html

Chapter 17
Setting Expectations Before Arrival

In Veterinary Medicine, Surprises Are the Enemy of Trust

Too many animal hospitals unintentionally sabotage trust before the client even steps foot in the building.

Not because the medicine is bad.
Not because the team is rude.
Not because the prices are unfair.
But because the client walks into the visit with 17 unanswered questions and 10 unspoken fears.

Veterinary care is one giant emotional unknown for most people. And the human brain hates unknowns.

Unknowns make people anxious. Anxiety makes people defensive. Defensiveness makes people assume the worst. And assuming the worst makes them interpret neutral moments as negative ones.

A 15-minute wait becomes "They don't value my time." A blood-work recommendation becomes "They're upselling me." A quiet doctor becomes "They don't care."

This is what I call Expectation Whiplash—when the client's internal expectations collide with reality and the impact fractures trust.

Here's the truth every elite hospital understands: You don't start managing client experience in the exam room. You start managing it before they walk in.

That's the heart of the *No-surprise Visit*.

This isn't hospitality fluff.
This is medicine.
This is psychology.
This is trust.

A No-surprise Visit can serve as the Flywheel's ignition point.

Part I: Why Clients Fear Surprises

There are three kinds of surprises in veterinary care:

1. **Medical Surprises**

   "We actually need X-rays."
   "We found something concerning."
   "The treatment plan will be different than expected."

2. **Financial Surprises**

   "It's going to be more expensive than I thought."
   "This procedure is out of my budget."
   "We'll need to revisit the estimate."

3. **Emotional Surprises**

   "We need to take your pet to the back."
   "There's going to be a wait."
   "That behavior is a red flag."
   "This may get serious."

Clients fear all three. But it's the emotional surprises that desta-bilize them most.

Because when people—especially anxious pet owners—lack context, their brain runs worst-case scenarios:

"He's not coming back."
"They're charging me for unnecessary stuff."
"They don't like my pet."
"They're hiding something."
"I'm failing my animal."
"Something terrible is about to happen."

It's not rational. But it's human.

The job of a high-trust hospital is not to remove the unknowns. It's to guide clients through them with clarity, empathy, and predictability. Predictability *is* psychological safety.

Part II: The No-surprise Visit Blueprint

Here is the exact operational structure that elite hospitals use to eliminate surprises and create emotionally smooth visits.

Step 1: The Pre-visit Message (Phone, Text, or Email)

The goal here is to lower anxiety, increase readiness, and prime trust. The pre-visit message should include:

- What will happen
- Who they will meet
- What they should bring
- How long the visit will take (give a range)
- Potential diagnostics (normalizing them early)
- A cost range (not exact—just a bracket)
- Anything emotionally helpful

Here's an example script you can mirror:

"Hi Sarah! We're excited to see Luna tomorrow at 3 p.m. Here's what to expect:

- You'll meet Maria (CSR) and Hannah (vet tech).
- The doctor will perform a full nose-to-tail exam.
- They may recommend bloodwork or imaging depending on what they find—we'll explain everything before moving forward.
- Most visits take 30–45 minutes.
- Please bring any medications or past records.
- If you have any concerns or emotional stress around today's visit, just let us know so we can support you.

We've got you."

This message isn't just information; it's reassurance disguised as information.

Step 2: The Warm Welcome + Expectations in the First 60 Seconds

Clients form an emotional impression within the first minute. And most animal hospitals just encourage their CSRs at the front desk to "try to flash a smile at the client as they walk in." That's not enough. A strong greeting includes:

A strong greeting includes:

- Warm eye contact
- Use of pet's name
- Confirmation of visit reason
- Setting the agenda
- Giving a time expectation

Here's another example script:

"Welcome in, Sarah! We're so happy Luna is here today. Just a heads-up, Dr. Patel will join you in the exam room in about 10 minutes. If anything changes, I'll keep you updated."

That last sentence—"I'll keep you updated"—is like oxygen to anxious clients.

Step 3: The "Road Map of Today" Speech (Tech or CSR)

Every hospital needs a 30-second script that outlines the visit.

For example, "Here's the plan for today:

1. I'll start by asking a few questions to understand what's going on.
2. Then Dr. Patel will do a full exam.
3. If she sees anything concerning, she'll talk through recommendations step-by-step.
4. You'll have full control over what we do next. Nothing happens without your okay.
5. And I'll let you know exactly what things cost before you decide."

You can feel the anxiety melting.

Step 4: The "Prep Clients for the Back Room" Moment

The "back" is where trust goes to die ... if the client doesn't understand what's happening.

Narration fixes this.

Script Example: "We'll take Luna to our treatment area for X-rays. It usually takes 8–10 minutes. If it takes longer, I'll pop in for an update. You're welcome to wait in the exam room or lobby, whatever feels best."

Notice the clarity: What. Where. Why. How long. What the client can choose.

This level of transparency prevents 90% of panic-based frustrations.

Step 5: The "Before You Leave" Summary

The last 60 seconds determine what the client remembers. The visit should end with:

- A recap of findings
- Clear next steps
- How the client will receive results
- When to return
- Exactly who to contact for questions
- A moment of gratitude

For example, "Today we identified early kidney changes. Thanks for trusting us with labs—we'll call you with results within 24 hours. If anything worries you tonight, just text or call us. And we'll see you in three months for the recheck. You're doing an amazing job with Luna. We're grateful for you."

Clients walk out feeling in control, not confused.

Part III: Why No-surprise Visits Boost Revenue (Without Trying)

Data shows that when clients know what to expect, they:

- Approve more diagnostics
- Ask better questions
- Believe your intentions
- Complain less and leave fewer negative reviews
- Rebook more consistently
- Trust estimates
- Feel more confident in your expertise
- Refer more friends
- Show up on time
- Follow treatment plans

And here's the big one: Expectation-setting increases compliance by 20–40% in most hospitals.

That's revenue.
That's outcomes.
That's loyalty.
That's Flywheel acceleration.

Part IV: Case Study—The Hospital That Eliminated Surprises and Transformed Their CX

Let's call the hospital **Riverbend Veterinary Center**.

They had all the classic problems:

- Long waits
- Clients upset about cost
- A tense front desk
- Doctors feeling attacked
- Reviews referencing "miscommunication"
- High team turnover

They implemented a No-surprise Visit protocol for 60 days. Then, here's what changed:

- On-time arrivals improved 28%.
- Upset-client escalations dropped from 20/week to 4/week.
- Bloodwork compliance rose 35%.
- Recheck appointments jumped dramatically.
- Doctors reported "less emotional fatigue" from defensive clients.
- Team morale improved because clients were calmer and kinder.
- Revenue increased—but with no price changes.
- Their Google rating increased from 4.0 to 4.6.
- The hospital became known locally as "the gentle place."
- Client trust skyrocketed.

The secret? Predictability. Clarity. Narration. No surprises.

Psychological safety for clients starts with predictability. Psychological safety for the team gets easier when clients aren't in fight-or-flight.

This is how culture meets CX meets medicine meets business.

Summary

The Five Laws of a No-surprise Visit:

1. Start the visit before the visit.
2. Narrate the flow of the day.
3. Normalize diagnostics early.
4. Communicate time expectations constantly.
5. End with clarity and connection.

The Result: A calmer client. A more confident team. Higher compliance. Better medical outcomes. Stronger loyalty. More revenue. And a flywheel that spins with ease instead of friction.

Suggested Readings

Agency for Healthcare Research and Quality (AHRQ). *Improving Patient Safety Through Communication and Teamwork*. U.S. Department of Health and Human Services, 2022, www.ahrq.gov

American Animal Hospital Association (AAHA). *Communication Skills in Veterinary Practice*. AAHA Press, 2023, www.aaha.org

Berger, Charles R., and Richard J. Calabrese. "Some Explorations in Initial Interaction and Beyond: Toward a Developmental Theory of Interpersonal Communication." *Human Communication Research*, vol. 1, no. 2, 1975, pp. 99–112.

Bitner, Mary Jo, Amy L. Ostrom, and Felicia N. Morgan. "Service Blueprinting: A Practical Technique for Service Innovation." *California Management Review*, vol. 50, no. 3, 2008, pp. 66–94.

CustomerGauge. "How Customer Expectations Impact Net Promoter Score." *CustomerGauge*, CustomerGauge Ltd., 2024, www.customergauge.com. Accessed 7 Dec. 2025.

DiMatteo, M. Robin. "Evidence That Patient Adherence Is Associated with Provider Communication Skills and Relationship Quality." *Medical Care*, vol. 42, no. 3, 2004, pp. 297–306.

Kahneman, Daniel. *Thinking, Fast and Slow.* Farrar, Straus and Giroux, 2011.

Levinson, Wendy, et al. "Physician–patient Communication: The Relationship with Malpractice Claims among Primary Care Physicians and Surgeons." *JAMA*, vol. 277, no. 7, 1997, pp. 553–559.

Maister, David H. "The Psychology of Waiting Lines." *Harvard Business School Working Paper*, Harvard Business School, 1985.

Montague, Enid, and Paul J. Asan. "Trust in Technology-mediated Collaborative Health Encounters." *Human Factors*, vol. 54, no. 5, 2012, pp. 829–844.

Chapter 18

Doctor Communication That Builds Unshakable Trust

Veterinarians massively underestimate their role in client experience. Too many vets hide behind the medicine. They think, "If I'm great at diagnosing, if I do the right treatment plan, if I help the pet, then I've done my job." Wrong. That's table stakes. That's the minimum requirement for even being in the game.

Let's face facts: medicine matters ... a lot. If you're not doing all you can to practice best-quality medicine, just leave the industry. But medicine doesn't build trust by itself. The *moment-to-moment* interactions matter a hell of a lot: the way you look a worried pet parent in the eye and explain things in plain language, the way you pause to acknowledge their fear, the way you treat them like a partner instead of a problem. That's where trust is won ... or lost.

As I've covered many times in this book (but STILL think it's worth repeating), trust is EVERYTHING in veterinary medicine. Clients are not just buying medicine, they're buying belief. They're buying into the fact that YOU, the doctor, care about them and their pet as much as they do. They don't have your degree. They don't understand the labs, the imaging, the jargon. They're scared, they're vulnerable, and they're making decisions about hundreds, sometimes thousands of dollars of care in real time. If you don't earn their trust, they're likely to decline the very plan that could save their pet.

So here's the punchline: your job isn't just chief medical officer. You are the chief trust builder.

The hospital manager can coach CX, the CSRs can be warm and welcoming, the techs can bring empathy; but at the end of the day, the client primarily looks to YOU, the veterinarian, as the ultimate source of credibility and care. If you don't step into that responsibility, the whole system collapses.

This isn't optional. It's not "nice to have." It's your responsibility as a leader, as a healer, as the voice the client looks to in their scariest, most emotional moments. You are literally holding their family member's life in your hands. So don't just deliver medicine. Deliver trust.

Because when you do? The client says yes. They follow through. They come back. They tell their friends. They become lifelong advocates for you and your hospital. And when you don't? They walk, they second-guess, they distrust. It doesn't matter how great the medicine is if it never gets accepted.

So stop underestimating yourself. Stop thinking CX is someone else's job. It's YOU. Own it. Embody it. Be the chief trust builder your clients need.

So let's talk about how you, as a veterinarian, can win that game— whether it's a nail trim, a vaccine, or a life-or-death ICU stay.

Clients aren't complicated. Strip away the jargon, and clients want to *feel confident their pet is in good hands, that you actually care about them and their pet, to understand what's happening, to be included in decisions around their pet's health, and to feel supported throughout and after their visit to your hospital.*

That's it. Hit these notes, and you're building loyalty and trust.

What Clients Are Telling Us About Doctor Communication

I've spent hours—I mean, literally hundreds of hours—reviewing pet-owner reviews of animal hospitals in search of themes, understanding client needs and opportunities to better serve them, and best practices to earn client trust and heighten the quality of their experience. Here are five findings that I thought were particularly interesting to me over the past few years of analysis:

1. Clients who can recall their Doctor's name after their visit rate their review much higher than those who can't. Whether it's a review on Yelp or Google, or a response to an online survey, the same pattern emerges: when clients use the name of the veterinarian (e.g., Dr. Smith) in their review rather than generically saying "the Doctor," their ratings go up—like, way up.

2. Satisfied clients will very often mention that the Doctor "took the time." I mean, it was literally eyebrow-raising to me to see how often I saw that exact "took the time" phrase. It was an interesting learning for me that clients actually understand that hospital teams—particularly doctors—keep a busy schedule. Many of them have sadly learned from experience that hospital teams are often rushed, under pressure, and balancing a lot at once. If their visit feels rushed, that can make a client feel like a number: obviously not a great formula for building trust. So they're pleasantly surprised when the doctor takes that extra beat of time to make sure the client's questions are answered, checks to see if anything else is on their mind about their pet, etc. In practice, the truth is that, usually, a doctor "taking the time" requires very little additional TIME at all, but that

EXACT phrase "took the time" literally appears word-for-word in thousands of positive pet owner reviews every year in veterinary medicine.

3. Clients don't care much about how doctors greet THEM upon entering the exam room, but they REALLY care about how the doctor greets and handles their pet. A doctor who walks into the exam room, crouches down on the floor to give Buddy a gentle head scratch, and asks, "How are we feeling today, Buddy? I heard we haven't been eating much lately?" has taken a huge step toward earning trust with the client—because that doctor is showing the care they have for the pet. Often, highly satisfied clients will discuss this pivotal little moment as the one that means the most to them in their hospital experience. Clients also perceive "value" with perceived attention given to their pet, by the way. At the end of the visit, a client is far more likely to feel gypped or frustrated by price if they felt the doctor didn't give them or their pet the time of day.

4. And speaking of price, the biggest driver of whether a client complains about price is whether or not they perceive the doctor to be transparent and whether or not the doctor invited the client into the conversation about the pet's care. More often than not in reviews or surveys, complaints about price are accompanied by mention of feeling "surprised" by the price or feeling omitted from that conversation. In other words, clients rarely complain about price alone: they complain that the doctor didn't warn them about the estimated price ahead of time and/or obtain their buy-in to proceed with treatment with an agreed-upon price (even if that price is a price range).

5. Clients don't appreciate the doctor making them feel dumb. You might be surprised to learn how often this happens for pet owners, and it happens one of two ways. Either (1) the doctor talks DOWN to the client or (2) the doctor doesn't simplify medical jargon, essentially speaking in verbiage that goes over the client's head. In either scenario, the client feels disrespected or robbed from a productive conversation about their pet's treatment. That's a sure-fire way to burn client trust.

Strategies for Elevating Your Client Interactions

So let's unpack these a bit. What do these mean for doctors, in practice?

1. **Take pride in how you enter the exam room, and how you introduce yourself.**

   As mentioned above, your entrance into the exam is one of the most pivotal points in any client's experience in the hospital. Take extra care to greet the pet with love and care. Express concern about what the pet is in for, if there's a concern ("I've heard you've been scratching yourself a lot, Buddy!") or show delight and excitement to meet a new pet who's in for a wellness visit (or a new puppy or kitten visit). The key here is to show the client how much of a "dog person" or "cat person" you are—how much you love and care about pets. You might assume that's an obvious, foregone conclusion (you've committed your life to treating animals, after all) but not necessarily. Greeting the pet with warmth and a gentle touch, and talking directly to the pet the way any pet owner would, builds immediate rapport.

   In my experience training doctors, when they hear that "when a client remembers the doctor's name, they rate the visit better" they assume that that means they should work extra hard to repeat their name over and over again to make sure the client remembers their name. Nope—that's not the strategy. While I certainly encourage you to introduce yourself by name, and perhaps remind a client of your name if they come in for a second visit, clients will actually remember your name WILLINGLY and PURPOSELY if they have a great experience with you (in other words, if you earned their trust). Why? To make sure they get to see you again. Clients will literally say to themselves, "Okay, I have to remember Doctor Smith's name so that I can request them when I make Buddy's next appointment." I've seen many clients actually ask the receptionist on their way out the door, "Hey, remind me again the name of the doctor we saw today? I want to continue seeing her, she was amazing." That's the magic. Deliver such a solid experience that clients WANT to remember your name for the purpose of seeing you again. Then, try not to blush when you see your name in their next Google review.

2. **Don't make clients feel dumb**.

I described earlier in this book about how many pet owners are at least a little insecure and sensitive to feeling judged by the doctor or hospital team. They love their pets so much and take so much pride in their pet's health that they'll immediately feel guilty and responsible if their pet has a health problem. They may feel embarrassed about mistakes they made, "obvious" things they forgot to do, etc. Your job as a doctor is to provide comfort, reassurance, and affirmation—not pile onto insecurities. And talking down to clients, or confusing them by using detailed medical jargon, is a sure-fire way to heighten client embarrassment, make clients feel like they can't ask questions, and break trust when clients are at their most vulnerable.

Looking to crush clients' spirits and make them feel dumber than a dog chasing parked cars? Here are some guaranteed phrases you can say to make your clients feel like shit:

- *"It's really simple…"*
  Clients may feel like, "If it's so simple, why don't I understand it?" Instant insecurity.
- "Don't worry about that, I'll take care of it."
  This shuts the client out of the decision-making process, leaving them powerless and without a voice.
- "That's not really accurate. What you read online isn't correct."
  This makes the client feel dismissed, even though they were trying to be informed.
- "We already explained this earlier."
  This suggests the client wasn't smart enough to get it the first time.

- "This is standard, everyone does it."
  This implies they should just accept your recommendation without asking questions. It's a great way to make the client feel pressured while erasing their individuality, dismissing their concerns, and completely removing them from the conversation about their pet's care.
- "You wouldn't understand the details."
  The ultimate shutdown. It alienates the client immediately. For efficiency, it's often just quicker to just call them an idiot.

In contrast, if your goal is to elevate clients rather than making them feel dumb, here are some better alternatives:

1. Replace "It's really simple" with "Let me break this down step by step, so it's clear."
2. Replace "Don't worry about that" with "Here's how I'd recommend handling it, and here's what it means for you and for Buddy."
3. Replace "That's not accurate" with "I see why that article said that. Here's how it applies to your pet's situation and here's what I would add."

You get the gist. Invite clients into a collaborative, two-way discussion about their pet's health. Don't ostracize and judge. Acknowledge their feelings.

3. **Invite clients into conversation about treatment plan options. Discuss alternatives, medical implications, and financial impacts**.

When it comes time to discuss treatment options, and ultimately presenting a treatment plan, it's absolutely crucial to keep the client feeling informed, valued, and included.

What are some best practices to do this? Here are a few great practices that you should consider making habits:

- Ask open-ended questions. In other words: Ask, don't assume. Asking, "How has Buddy been acting at home?" opens doors.

While yes or no questions have their place, open-ended questions invite conversation and build more rapport.

- Embrace "The River to Stream" approach. Start with broad questions, then narrow down. In other words: listen first, then zero in. Approaching interactions this way helps clients feel included, as the two of you work together as a team to uncover what Buddy might be experiencing. The idea behind the name: Start wider, like a river, and then hone in more narrowly—the stream.

- Practice "Signposting" and "Serve and See." As you're describing the steps involved in Buddy's care, lay out the roadmap: "Here's what we'll do next." This helps clients feel anchored, not lost. Then "Serve and See" is all about breaking information down into small pieces: serve up some information, and then see if it lands. After each bit of information is delivered, check in: "Does that make sense?"

- Balance confidence with openness. Clients need to see that you believe in your plan *and* that you're honest about what's uncertain. Confidence builds safety, openness builds authenticity.

- Make it personal. No one wants cookie-cutter care. Use names. Notice details. Show them you see *their* pet, not just another chart.

- Explain so people actually get it. Drop the medical jargon. Break things down into plain, everyday language. If a 13-year-old could understand you, you're on the right track.

- Summarize choices and next steps. Don't just throw options at the wall. Lay them out clearly, talk through pros and cons, and make the path forward obvious.

- Work with clients, don't talk at them. Invite them into the decision-making. Treat them like partners. People support what they help build.

These aren't tricks. They're tools to make the client feel included and to ensure that the information is landing clearly.

When you strip it down, the veterinarians who consistently earn client trust all practice the same habits. Call them skills, call them mindsets, call them best practices, call them whatever. They're the moves that transform a medical interaction into a *human* one:

Routine Visits: The Everyday Trust Builders

I discussed earlier how the true test of client trust is when the client is left with their thoughts when their pet is undergoing an intense procedure or being treated in a high-stakes, emergency situation. There, I shared this really important secret: That the routine visits are where you *bank* trust. I like to call them "trust deposits." When you crush the basics, you create a reservoir of goodwill that pays off during the big, scary moments. Here are some great ways to do that:

- Smile when you walk in. Your energy sets the tone.
- Sit at eye level. Standing over clients screams hierarchy; sitting signals partnership.
- Review notes from prior hospital visits. Then, during the visit, recall details and ask questions—both about the pet and the client: "Now I remember Buddy was here a couple of months ago because he was scratching a lot. How's he doing with that?" And "Kim, I remember you telling me last time that you were getting ready to head to Italy. I have to ask: how was it? Is it as beautiful there as everyone says it is?"
- Narrate the physical exam. Don't be a silent robot. "Her heart sounds great, lungs are clear. I love hearing that."
- Celebrate the good. Point out "the healthy," not just "the problem." "His teeth look great. Whatever you're doing at home is working!"
- Express gratitude. "Thanks for trusting us with Buddy's care. We love seeing him" goes a long way.

- Acknowledge potential frustrations. "Hey I know our wait was a little longer today. I'm so sorry it took us a little while to get you seen today. Here's what happened ..." This makes clients feel seen, and reassures them that they're a priority (see Chapter 13 for more details.)
- Reassure, to release client guilt or anxiety. This might sound like, "Lots of pets develop this at Buddy's age. You caught it early, which is great."
- Affirm the client (this goes directly back to one of the feelings clients crave): "You did the right thing in bringing Buddy in today" or "Buddy is so lucky to have you. You're taking such great care of him."
- Summarize next steps clearly, by ending with a concise recap. "So today we updated vaccines, and we'll recheck that skin in two weeks." This signals you're organized and dependable.

Do this consistently, and clients will never see you as transactional. They'll see you as *their* vet.

Critical Care Visits: The Stress Test

When the stakes are high, your communication either builds unshakable trust, or it breaks everything.

Here's how servant-minded vets show up when emotions are raw:

- Slow it down. You may be in crisis mode, but the client is in *panic mode*. Match their pace with clarity, not chaos.
- Acknowledge emotions. "I know this is overwhelming. I'm here with you." Don't gloss over feelings.
- Give structured choices. "Here are the three options. Here's what each means for Bella. Here's what I recommend." That clarity is oxygen when they're drowning in fear.
- Be present at the hard moments (especially with euthanasia). Sit. Hold silence. Let your humanity show. That's servant leadership.

Team Communication = Client Confidence

Clients watch how you talk to your team. If you bark orders, roll your eyes, or contradict your tech, you're burning trust in real time. On the flip side, when you model respect, collaboration, and clarity with your staff, clients feel it. It's contagious.

Best Practices Beyond the Exam Room

- Follow up. A quick call the next day is a trust multiplier.
- Set communication goals. Don't wing it—practice like it's a clinical skill.
- Seek feedback. Ask your team, "How did I come across?" Self-awareness is a weapon.
- Keep learning. Communication isn't a one-and-done skill. It's a craft.

Quick-hit Guide for Every Vet

- Walk in with warmth.
- Use the pet's and client's names.
- Explain simply, check understanding.
- Summarize options and guide, don't dictate.
- Partner, don't preach.
- Respect your team in front of clients.
- Follow up like you mean it.

I want to close this chapter, and really drive my points home, with a few quick (and real-life) case studies.

Story 1: The Nail Trim That Wasn't About Nails

Max was just a little dachshund, but to his owner, Emily, he was family. A rescue with a rough past, Max hated the vet. The second he saw the lobby, he'd start trembling, tail tucked, eyes darting like he was searching for an escape route. And Emily—already nervous herself—would tense up right alongside him. Most visits turned into a wrestling match.

On this particular Tuesday, it was "just a nail trim." But here's the thing: nothing is *just* a nail trim to the client. Every interaction is a test of whether you care. The veterinarian walked into the room, but instead of diving straight in, she sat on the floor. She let Max come to her. She spoke softly, called him by name, and asked Emily, "Does he usually get this anxious at home? What works for him when he's scared?"

That five-minute pause changed everything. Max crept forward, sniffed, and slowly relaxed. The vet clipped one nail, then another, narrating gently the whole time. By the end, Max wasn't shaking. Emily wasn't fighting back tears.

When they left, Emily said, "That's the first time I haven't felt guilty bringing him here." Do you understand how massive that is? That wasn't a nail trim: it was a trust deposit. Emily didn't just see a vet who cut nails. She saw someone who cared about her dog's soul.

Next time Max needs vaccines—or heaven forbid, surgery—Emily won't shop around for the cheapest option. She won't hesitate. She already knows: *this is our vet.*

Story 2: The Middle-of-the-night Phone Call

It was 2:07 a.m. when the doors slammed open. A family rushed in, cradling their golden retriever, Daisy. She was gasping, sides heaving, eyes wide. Their teenage daughter was sobbing, her dad's hands were shaking, and mom was whispering "please, please" like a prayer.

The veterinarian on call could have gone straight into clinical mode—oxygen mask, IV line, diagnostics. But he stopped for two seconds, looked that family in the eye, and said: *"I know this is terrifying. I promise I'm going to explain everything we do. You won't be left in the dark."*

That mattered more than any machine in the room.

He talked them through every step: "We're putting her on oxygen now so she can breathe easier. Next, we'll take X-rays to see if her lungs are clear. I'll come back in five minutes to update you." He didn't sugarcoat the seriousness, but he didn't dump jargon either. He kept them in the loop, minute by minute, because in moments like that, silence feels like abandonment.

By sunrise, Daisy was stable. Exhausted but alive. And when the family went home to shower and cry it out, their phone rang that afternoon. It was the vet, calling just to check: "How's Daisy doing? How are you holding up?"

That phone call meant more than the medicine. Think about it: the family had already paid, already left, the "job" was technically done. But that one call told them, "We still care. She still matters. You still matter."

Years later, that family still tells the story. They don't start with the diagnosis. They start with: "That doctor called us the next day. He cared about us as much as our dog."

Story 3: The Hardest Goodbye

The room was quiet except for the muffled sobs of Mr. and Mrs. Carter. Their shepherd mix, Rosie, was 15 years old. Her hips had finally given out, and her once-bright eyes were clouded with pain. They had put off this day as long as they could, clinging to every extra sunrise with her. But now, sitting in the exam room, they knew it was time.

This is the moment where communication either heals or destroys. And the veterinarian knew it. She didn't barge in with forms and needles. She sat down, eye level with the Carters, and started with the simplest, most human words: "I'm so sorry you're facing this. Rosie has been so lucky to have you."

Then she walked them gently through what would happen, step by step, using calm, plain language. No jargon. No rush. "First, she'll get a small injection that makes her very sleepy. She won't feel scared. She'll just feel like she's drifting off. When you're ready, I'll give the final injection. She won't feel pain. She'll just ... fall asleep in your arms."

She paused. "You can hold her the whole time. Take as much time as you need. This room is yours."

Rosie's head rested in Mrs. Carter's lap as the sedation set in. Mr. Carter whispered stories from when she was a puppy: how she used to steal socks, how she'd run circles in the yard until she collapsed. The vet didn't interrupt. She sat quietly, a hand on Rosie's side, creating space for memory, for grief, for love.

When it was over, the Carters stayed in the room for almost an hour. The vet didn't push. She didn't hover. She simply said, "When you're ready to say goodbye, we'll take care of everything."

Two weeks later, the Carters received a handwritten card in the mail. The vet had written: "Rosie touched all of us here. Thank you for letting us be part of her life. She was special, and she will be missed."

The Carters tell people that their vet gave them the gift of a "beautiful goodbye." Not because of the medicine, but because of the compassion, the clarity, the willingness to sit in the grief with them.

That's trust at its deepest level. That's servant leadership in action.

Conclusion: Your Responsibility Is Bigger than Medicine

Here's the truth nobody tells you in vet school: communication isn't a soft skill. It's the hardest damn skill you'll ever have to master. It's harder than surgery. Harder than pharmacology. Harder than memorizing every obscure parasite under the microscope. Why? Because people don't judge you by what's in your head. They judge you by how you make them *feel*.

Think about Emily and Max. That dachshund didn't just need a nail trim—he needed a safe place, and his owner needed to see a vet who cared enough to slow down. That moment wasn't about nails. It was about trust.

Think about Daisy's family in the middle of the night, holding onto hope by a thread. They didn't remember the dosage of oxygen or the model of X-ray machine. They remembered the doctor who looked them in the eye and said, "I know this is scary. I'm here with you." That was the medicine that mattered most.

And think about the Carters with Rosie, facing the hardest goodbye. What stayed with them wasn't the injection protocol. It was the vet who sat in silence, cried with them, and mailed a handwritten card two weeks later. That's what turned an unbearable moment into a beautiful memory.

These aren't outliers. These are the everyday moments you get to step into. This is the job. This is the privilege.

You get a rare opportunity—one of the rarest in all of healthcare—to build trust in moments people will remember for the rest of their lives. And make no mistake: they *will* remember. They'll remember if you brushed them off, if you hid behind jargon, if you treated them like just another Tuesday appointment. And they'll damn sure remember if you sat with them in their fear, made space for their emotions, and showed them you gave a shit.

This is the responsibility. This is the game. And here's the kicker: medicine alone won't win it. You can be the most brilliant diagnostician in the world, but if clients don't trust you, none of it matters. They'll leave. They'll find someone else who earns their trust, even if that vet isn't as sharp as you are.

So own it. Build trust in the easy moments: when it's "just" a nail trim, "just" a vaccine, "just" a check-up, because those reps compound. They stack like deposits in a bank account. Then, when the hardest moments come: the midnight emergencies, the euthanasia decisions, you'll have the capital to guide them through it.

You are not just a provider of medicine. You are a builder of trust. And if you take that responsibility seriously, you won't just keep clients—you'll create raving fans, loyal families, and a legacy that outlasts any single appointment.

Summary

If you can't build trust with your words, your medicine will never matter—because clients won't follow what they don't believe.

Medicine matters, but it's table stakes. If you can't diagnose well and deliver sound treatment, you shouldn't be in the game. But medicine alone doesn't build loyalty. Trust does.

And trust is won or lost in the micro-moments: the way you greet the pet before the client, the pause you take to check if they actually understood you, the space you create for them to ask questions without feeling dumb. These little choices are the difference between "just another doctor" and "our doctor for life."

Clients don't walk out remembering the dosage you prescribed. They remember how you made them feel when their world was spinning. Did you sit down at eye level? Did you explain things like a partner instead of preaching like a professor? Did you acknowledge their guilt and fear, or pile onto it with jargon and dismissiveness?

The data backs it up:

- Clients rave when doctors "take the time."
- Trust skyrockets when doctors invite clients into the treatment conversation.
- Price complaints tank when clients feel informed, not blindsided.
- And the single most powerful move you can make? Show real care for the pet in front of the client.

This is the hardest skill in vet med. Harder than surgery. Harder than pharmacology. Because people don't judge you by what's in your head. They judge you by how you make them feel.

Here's the bottom line: you are not just the Chief Medical Officer. **You are the Chief Trust Builder**. And if you own that role—if you consistently make "trust deposits" in the easy visits—then when the critical, gut-wrenching moments arrive, your clients will lean on you instead of second-guessing you.

That's how you move from transactional care to transformational impact. That's how you turn clients into lifelong advocates. That's how you create legacy.

So stop hiding behind the medicine. Step into the role. Deliver trust. Every damn day.

Suggested Readings

Agency for Healthcare Research and Quality. *Improving Patient–Provider Communication for Better Outcomes.* U.S. Department of Health and Human Services, 2022, www.ahrq.gov

Back, Anthony L., et al. "Approaching Difficult Communication Tasks in Oncology." *CA: A Cancer Journal for Clinicians*, vol. 55, no. 3, 2005, pp. 164–177.

CustomerGauge. "Why Trust and Time Drive Higher Net Promoter Scores." *CustomerGauge*, 2024, www.customergauge.com

DiMatteo, M. Robin. "The Role of Effective Communication in Improving Patient Adherence to Medical Recommendations." *Medical Care*, vol. 42, no. 3, 2004, pp. 297–306.

Epstein, Ronald M., and Richard L. Street. *Patient-Centered Communication in Cancer Care.* National Cancer Institute, NIH Publication No. 07-6225, 2007.

Kashiwagi, David T., et al. "The Impact of Sitting vs Standing on Patient Perception of Provider Presence and Satisfaction." *Patient Experience Journal*, vol. 5, no. 1, 2018, pp. 105–110.

Levinson, Wendy, et al. "Physician–patient Communication: The Relationship with Malpractice Claims among Primary Care Physicians and Surgeons." *JAMA*, vol. 277, no. 7, 1997, pp. 553–559.

National Institutes of Health. *Clear Communication: An NIH Health Literacy Initiative.* NIH, 2023, www.nih.gov. Accessed 7 Dec. 2025.

Street, Richard L., Jr., et al. "How Does Communication Heal? Pathways Linking Clinician–Patient Communication to Health Outcomes." *Patient Education and Counseling*, vol. 74, no. 3, 2009, pp. 295–301.

Chapter 19
Speak Human, Not Medical

Here, I want to talk about the communication decoding system that makes clients actually understand you.

Veterinary medicine is fluent in a language almost no client speaks:
"Bilateral otitis externa."
"Increase to BID dosing."
"Grade II/VI systolic murmur."
"Stomatitis."
"Dermatophytosis."
"Reactivity vs. aggression."
"Diagnostic differentials."

It's clean. It's accurate. And it often confuses the hell out of clients.

Confusion lowers trust.
Confusion lowers compliance.
Confusion makes clients Google your advice to double-check it.

Speaking "medical" might make the doctor feel competent, but speaking *human* makes the client feel confident.

This chapter delivers a full communication decoding system:

- The *Translation Rule*: no phrase leaves your mouth without a human translation.
- The *"Because" Bridge*: medical fact → human relevance ("We recommend bloodwork because it tells us what your pet can't.")
- The *15-Second Rule*: every explanation should pass the "Could a tired parent at 6 p.m. understand this?" test.
- The *Visual Metaphor Method*: kidneys = filters, cortisone = dimmer switch, diabetes = thermostat.
- The *Check-for-understanding Script*: "How does that explanation land? Want a simpler version?"

Your language shouldn't prove your intelligence. It should prove your partnership.

Clients don't remember Latin terms. They remember how you made the problem feel solvable.

Intro: You're Not Dumbing It Down. You're Making It Land

Veterinary professionals speak two languages:

1. Medical language: precise. Technical. Efficient. Perfect for records. Perfect for clinicians.
2. Human language: emotional. Relatable. Visual. Perfect for clients. Perfect for trust.

Many hospital teams confuse the two: they talk to clients using the language they use in SOAP notes. Then they wonder why clients hesitate, panic, reject recommendations, or spiral into Google at 2 a.m.

Here's the truth every elite communicator knows: clients don't judge you for simplifying your language. They trust you for it. Because the goal of communication in veterinary medicine isn't to sound smart. It's to make the client feel informed, included, and empowered.

You're not performing a monologue. You're guiding a human through uncertainty.

This chapter is a deep masterclass on how to translate medical expertise into human clarity, without losing authority, accuracy, or confidence.

When you speak human, trust skyrockets. When trust skyrockets, compliance becomes easy. When compliance becomes easy, outcomes improve. And when outcomes improve, everything - from client loyalty to team morale to hospital financials—begins to flywheel upward.

Communication, in other words, is medicine.

Why Medical Language Breaks Trust (Even If the Medicine Is Perfect)

Clients process visits emotionally first, intellectually second. When you speak in medical jargon, the client experiences:

1. Confusion: "What does this mean?"
2. Shame: "Am I supposed to know this?"
3. Fear: "Is it serious?"
4. Distrust: "Why can't they just tell me what's wrong?"

And here's the kicker: confused clients rarely ask clarifying questions. They just sit quietly and feel stupid. Then they leave the hospital and tell someone, "I don't really know what happened."

Or worse: "They're not telling me something."

In veterinary medicine, confusion is not neutral—it's dangerous.

Confusion kills compliance.
Confusion kills trust.
Confusion kills revenue.
Confusion kills outcomes.

The 15-second Clarity Rule

A client should be able to understand any explanation within 15 seconds, even if:

- They're stressed.
- They're emotional.

- They're exhausted.
- They're overwhelmed.
- They're not medically knowledgeable.

If you can't explain something in 15 seconds, it's not because the concept is too complex. It's because you're explaining it wrong.

Human clarity is a skill.

The Translation Rule

Here's the core principle: no medical phrase leaves your mouth without a human translation immediately after.

Here are a few examples:

Medical:	"Bilateral otitis externa."
Human:	"Both ears are inflamed and painful, like a really bad swimmer's ear."
Medical:	"Diabetes reduces insulin production."
Human:	"His body isn't processing sugar correctly, like a thermostat stuck on the wrong setting."
Medical:	"We need abdominal imaging."
Human:	"We're taking a picture of what's going on inside so we're not guessing."
Medical:	"A dental prophylaxis is recommended."
Human:	"He needs a deep-clean under anesthesia—like when humans get the tartar removed below the gumline."

You're not simplifying the medicine. You're simplifying the emotion, because translation makes clients feel safe.

The "Because" Bridge

This one strategy will change your entire exam room experience, because clients trust recommendations they understand. And they approve recommendations they feel emotionally connected to.

Your explanation must always start with **why**, not just **what**.

Wrong: "We recommend bloodwork."

Right: "We recommend bloodwork *because* it tells us what your pet can't say—how their organs are functioning on the inside."

Wrong: "We should get X-rays."

Right: "We should get X-rays *because* they show us whether this is a minor issue or something more serious. It helps us avoid guessing."

Wrong: "We want to do a recheck."

Right: "We want to do a recheck *because* catching things early is the best way to avoid emergencies and keep them comfortable."

The "because" bridge transforms compliance. It shifts the client from "Do I need that?" to "Of course that makes sense."

The Visual Metaphor Method

The human brain understands stories and images, not medical terminology. In other words: if they can picture it, they can understand it.

Here are some examples of metaphors that land instantly:

Kidneys = Coffee Filters: "When the filters get clogged, toxins build up."

Liver = Water Treatment Plant: "It processes everything that goes into the body."

Diabetes = Broken Thermostat: "The sugar levels can't regulate themselves."

Antibiotics = Firefighters: "They put out the infection flames but don't rebuild the house."

Steroids = Dimmer Switch: "They turn down inflammation, like lowering a bright light."

Arthritis = Rusty Hinges: "Things get stiff and painful when they move."

Dental disease = Rotting floorboards: "Things look okay on top, but underneath there's damage you can't see."

When you use metaphor, clients stop feeling overwhelmed and start feeling informed.

The Teach-back Checkpoint

This might be the most underused tool in vet med. After a medical explanation, ask:

"How does that explanation land? Want me to go simpler, or go more detailed?"

OR

"Can I check, what's your understanding so far of what's going on?"

If the client can't repeat it back simply, you haven't communicated effectively.

Case Study: The Doctor Who Changed One Sentence and Changed an Entire Hospital

Dr. Kelsey was clinically brilliant, but her clients often left confused.

Her compliance was low. Her callback complaints were high. She saw "difficult clients" everywhere. So her manager asked to sit in on a visit.

Within five minutes, the issue was obvious: she spoke perfect veterinary medicine, but zero human language.

So they implemented one small rule: every medical explanation must have a human metaphor.

Within 30 days:

- Her client complaints dropped by 80%.
- Her diagnostic compliance increased.
- Her appointments ran smoother.
- Clients specifically said, "Dr. Kelsey explains things so well."
- Her confidence skyrocketed.

Nothing changed medically. Everything changed emotionally. Because she finally spoke the language her clients lived in.

Summary

The Communication Decoding System

1. Translate every medical term.
2. Use metaphors clients can see.
3. Always start with "why."
4. Keep explanations under 15 seconds.
5. Check for understanding.
6. Ask, "How does that land?"
7. Validate emotions before explaining facts.

Why It Works

- Clients feel respected
- Clients feel smart
- Clients feel safe
- Clients trust more
- Clients comply more
- Pets get better care
- Teams get fewer escalations
- Hospitals grow loyalty + revenue

Speaking human is not a soft skill. It's a clinical skill. It's the bridge between your brilliance and their belief.

Suggested Readings

Agency for Healthcare Research and Quality. *The Teach-Back Method: A Tool for Improving Patient Understanding.* U.S. Department of Health and Human Services, 2023, www.ahrq.gov. Accessed 8 Dec. 2025.

American Animal Hospital Association (AAHA). *Client Communication Guidelines for Veterinary Practices.* AAHA Press, 2023, www.aaha.org. Accessed 8 Dec. 2025.

American Medical Association. *Health Literacy and Patient Safety: Help Patients Understand.* AMA Foundation, 2022, www.ama-assn.org. Accessed 8 Dec. 2025.

DiMatteo, M. Robin. "The Role of Effective Communication in Improving Patient Adherence to Medical Recommendations." *Medical Care*, vol. 42, no. 3, 2004, pp. 297–306.

Epstein, Ronald M., and Richard L. Street. "The Values and Value of Patient-centered Care." *Annals of Family Medicine*, vol. 9, no. 2, 2011, pp. 100–103.

Houts, Peter S., et al. "The Role of Pictures in Improving Health Communication: A Review of Research on Attention, Comprehension, Recall, and Adherence." *Patient Education and Counseling*, vol. 61, no. 2, 2006, pp. 173–190.

National Academy of Medicine. *Health Literacy: Improving Health, Health Systems, and Health Policy Around the World.* National Academies Press, 2013.

National Institutes of Health. *Clear & Simple: Developing Effective Print Materials for Low-Literacy Audiences.* NIH, 2021, www.nih.gov. Accessed 8 Dec. 2025.

Paasche-Orlow, Michael K., and Donald A. Wolf. "The Causal Pathways Linking Health Literacy to Health Outcomes." *American Journal of Health Behavior*, vol. 31, suppl. 1, 2007, pp. S19–S26.

Street, Richard L., Jr., et al. "How Does Communication Heal? Pathways Linking Clinician–Patient Communication to Health Outcomes." *Patient Education and Counseling*, vol. 74, no. 3, 2009, pp. 295–301.

Chapter 20
The "Narrate Everything" Method

Introduction: Silence Is Where Fear Lives

If you've spent five minutes in veterinary medicine, you know this truth: a quiet room is rarely a calm room.

Silence makes clients wonder.
Silence makes clients assume.
Silence makes clients catastrophize.
Silence makes clients misinterpret neutral moments as negative ones.
Silence makes clients feel forgotten.
Silence makes clients lose trust.

And yet, hospitals are full of silence. We've all seen it: the tech leaves to run a test. The doctor steps out for X-rays. The client waits alone in the exam room. The pet is taken "to the back." A 10-minute delay feels like 40. A shift in tone feels like bad news. A pause before speaking feels like danger.

In human psychology, the brain hates a void. So when clients don't know what's happening, their brain fills in the blanks with fear.

NEO—Narrate → Empathize → Offer—is the antidote.

This simple method transforms the emotional tone of your entire hospital.

NEO eliminates ambiguity, reduces conflict, builds compliance, creates calm, and prevents escalation. NEO is one of the highest-ROI CX tools in all of veterinary medicine.

This chapter will give you the scripts, frameworks, examples, case studies, and team exercises to make NEO instinctive across your entire hospital.

Why Narration Works (The Neuroscience)

Clients walk into the hospital with elevated cortisol and decreased cognitive processing, because:

- They're worried about their pet.
- They're scared about cost.
- They're unsure what you'll recommend.
- They don't understand the medical terms.
- They don't know what will happen next.

This creates what neuroscientists call "prediction error": when your brain doesn't know what's about to happen, it shifts into vigilance mode.

Vigilance = fear.
Fear = reactivity.
Reactivity = conflict.

Narration fixes the prediction error.

Narration tells the brain: "You are safe. You know what's happening. Nothing bad is happening without your awareness." Just by narrating what you're doing, you change the client's emotional state.

This is not a "customer service trick." This, literally, is brain science.

The NEO Framework

1. **Narrate**: Tell them what's happening, what you're doing, and what to expect next.
2. **Empathize**: Validate their emotional experience, out loud.
3. **Offer:** Give them clarity, options, or a next step.

Simple. Fast. Repeatable. Powerful.

How NEO Works in Real Moments

Let's break down how NEO transforms the most common anxiety-triggering moments in a hospital.

Scenario 1: Taking the Pet to the Back

This is the biggest trust-loss moment in veterinary medicine.

Without NEO

"We're taking her to the back for X-rays." (No timeline. No reassurance.)

Clients think:

- "What's happening back there?"
- "Why can't I be with them?"
- "Are they doing something I didn't approve?"
- "Does something bad usually happen in the back?"

With NEO

Narrate: "We'll take Bailey to our treatment area for X-rays. It usually takes about 8–10 minutes."

Empathize: "I know it can feel stressful when they go out of sight, so we'll keep everything gentle and slow."

Offer: "If it takes longer than 10 minutes, I'll come update you. You're welcome to wait here or step out—whatever feels best."

The difference is profound.

Scenario 2: Diagnostics or Treatment Delays

Without NEO

Silence. Client spirals.

With NEO

Narrate: "Bloodwork is running now—it typically takes 20 minutes."
Empathize: "I know waiting is the hardest part."
Offer: "I'll check in halfway through so you're never wondering."

This is the emotional oxygen clients crave.

Scenario 3: Giving Bad News

Without NEO

Medical terms. Flat effect. Clinical distance. Client feels blindsided or alone.

With NEO

Narrate: "I want to walk you step-by-step through what we found."
Empathize: "I know this is hard to hear. You're not alone in this."
Offer: "Here are our next options, and we'll go at your pace."

Scenario 4: Presenting an Estimate

Without NEO

"This is the estimate."

Client experiences sticker shock and silence.

With NEO

Narrate: "I'm going to walk you through the plan line by line."
Empathize: "I know costs can feel overwhelming."
Offer: "We'll talk about what's essential for today and what can wait."

Watch compliance jump.

The Micro-narration Script Library

Here are short, powerful narration phrases that can be used anywhere:

Narration Phrases

- "Here's what happens next ..."
- "Let me walk you through the plan ..."
- "Before we move forward, here's what to expect ..."
- "I want to keep you in the loop ..."
- "I don't want you wondering, so ..."
- "I know this part can feel stressful."
- "You're doing great."
- "A lot of people feel nervous during this step."
- "We're right here with you."

Offer Phrases

- "Would you like the simple version or more detail?"
- "We can slow down—no rush."
- "Here are your options ..."
- "What questions can I answer for you?"

Teach the team these and your hospital becomes emotionally elite.

Case Study: The Hospital That Eliminated 80% of Escalations with NEO

A hospital in the Pacific Northwest was drowning in client escalations:

- Long waits
- Angry clients
- Doorway confrontations
- Negative reviews referencing "communication issues"

The leadership team implemented a simple rule: **Narrate Every Transition. Every Time**.

Within 45 days:

- Angry-client escalations dropped by 80%
- Compliance improved significantly
- Front desk stress fell
- Doctors said visits felt "calmer and easier"
- Google reviews shifted from three to four stars to four to five stars
- The medical team felt "more in sync"
- Clients mentioned "clarity," "communication," and "updates" constantly

Nothing else changed. Not staffing. Not pricing. Not scheduling. Just narration. That's the power of emotional predictability.

Summary

The NEO Formula is rooted in three deceptively simple but profoundly powerful behaviors: Narrate, Empathize, and Offer. To Narrate is to tell clients exactly what's happening and what will happen next—eliminating the mystery that fuels anxiety. To Empathize is to acknowledge and validate their emotional experience out loud, signaling that you see them, not just the medical problem. And to

Offer is to provide clear next steps, choices, or reassurance so the client never feels directionless or powerless.

NEO works because it reaches the core of client psychology. It reduces uncertainty, which is the engine behind fear and defensiveness. It calms anxious clients by giving their brains something predictable to hold onto. It prevents escalation by addressing confusion *before* it becomes frustration. It builds trust because clients feel guided rather than abandoned. It increases compliance because people say "yes" when they feel understood and safe. It also makes teams feel more in control, because narration creates emotional structure in moments that otherwise feel chaotic. Ultimately, NEO improves outcomes and strengthens long-term loyalty by turning scary moments into collaborative ones.

This approach matters most during transitions—the moments where silence or ambiguity sneaks in and rattles clients. NEO should be used every time the emotional terrain shifts: when entering or exiting the room, when taking a pet to the back, when bringing them back, when waiting for diagnostics, when reviewing results, when presenting estimates, and when closing out the visit. These are the fault lines where clients either lose trust or deepen it.

And above all, remember this truth: clients don't fear diagnosis—clients fear silence. Your job is not just to deliver medical care, but to protect them from the emotional freefall that happens when they don't know what's happening. You eliminate fear by filling the silence with clarity and compassion.

Suggested Readings

Agency for Healthcare Research and Quality. *The Role of Communication in Patient Safety*. U.S. Department of Health and Human Services, 2023, www.ahrq.gov

American Academy of Pediatrics. *Family-centered Care and Communication in Clinical Practice*. AAP Press, 2021.

American Animal Hospital Association. *Client Communication Guidelines for the Veterinary Practice*. AAHA Press, 2023, www.aaha.org

Balint, Michael. *The Doctor, His Patient, and the Illness*. International Universities Press, 2000.

Coan, James A., Hillary S. Schaefer, and Richard J. Davidson. "Lending a Hand: Social Regulation of the Neural Response to Threat." *Psychological Science*, vol. 17, no. 12, 2006, pp. 1032–1039.

Harvard Medical School. *Understanding the Stress Response*. Harvard Health Publishing, 2022, www.health.harvard.edu.Kahneman, Daniel. *Thinking, Fast and Slow*. Farrar, Straus and Giroux, 2011.

Levine, Peter A. *In an Unspoken Voice: How the Body Releases Trauma and Restores Goodness*. North Atlantic Books, 2010.

National Institutes of Health. *Stress and the Brain: How Uncertainty Triggers the Fear Response*. NIH, 2022, www.nih.gov

Patient Safety Network (PSNet). *Communication Breakdowns and Patient Harm*. Agency for Healthcare Research and Quality, 2023, psnet.ahrq.gov

Rosenberger, Kendra J., et al. "Patient Uncertainty and Emotional Distress During Diagnostic Waiting Periods." *Journal of Behavioral Medicine*, vol. 41, no. 5, 2018, pp. 564–72.

Street, Richard L., Jr., et al. "How Does Communication Heal? Pathways Linking Clinician–Patient Communication to Health Outcomes." *Patient Education and Counseling*, vol. 74, no. 3, 2009, pp. 295–301.

Chapter 21
The Anti-whiplash Rule

One message. One standard. One team. How consistency becomes the ultimate trust multiplier in veterinary medicine.

Introduction

Let's start with the truth nobody in veterinary medicine wants to say out loud:

Clients can handle bad news.
Clients can handle long waits.

What they cannot handle is inconsistency.

The fastest way to destroy trust in a hospital is not cost, or policies, or even mistakes ... it's **whiplash**.

Whiplash is what clients feel when:

- One doctor says one thing, another says something totally different.
- One tech says, "We always do bloodwork," another says, "You don't really need that."

291

- One CSR says rechecks are important, another doesn't mention them at all.
- One staff member uses shame-based messaging around preventatives, another is gentle.
- One doctor spends 20 minutes explaining a diagnosis, the other one—on the next visit—bolts out of the room.
- One team member says, "We can do that today," and the next says "We don't offer that."

Whiplash is emotional turbulence. Turbulence erodes trust. And trust erosion is the death of compliance, loyalty, and long-term revenue.

This chapter is about eliminating that turbulence. It's about building a hospital where clients know exactly what standard of care they'll get: every time, from every person, on every visit.

One message. One standard. One team.

What Client Whiplash Looks Like (And Why It's So Damaging)

When a client gets mixed messages, they don't think: "Wow, there seems to be slight variability in internal medical protocols."

They think:

"Someone is wrong."
"Someone is hiding something."
"Someone is upselling me."
"Someone is guessing."
"These people aren't aligned."
"This feels like a red flag."

Whiplash triggers three dangerous emotions:

1. Confusion—"If the hospital doesn't agree with itself, how am I supposed to decide?"

2. Distrust—"If they can't align on something this basic, how do I trust them with serious things?"
3. Anxiety—"What else are they inconsistent about that I can't see?"

Confusion → distrust.
Distrust → resistance.
Resistance → noncompliance.
Noncompliance → poor outcomes.
Poor outcomes → emotional blame.
Emotional blame → negative reviews, leaving the hospital, or both.

It's a domino effect. And it starts with the small stuff.

The Anti-whiplash Rule Explained

The Anti-whiplash Rule is simple:

If one person on the team says it, everyone says it.
If one person believes it, everyone believes it.
If one person recommends it, everyone recommends it.

Not because you're robots. Not because you're removing individuality. But because clients need consistency to feel safe.

Consistency = competence.
Competence = trust.
Trust = compliance.
Compliance = outcomes.
Outcomes = loyalty.
Loyalty = financial health.
Financial health = reinvestment.

This is the Trust Flywheel at full speed.

The Three Types of Whiplash You Must Eliminate

To build a truly high-trust hospital, there are three categories of inconsistency you must remove from your culture. Each one creates a different type of client confusion, a different form of emotional friction, and a different kind of trust erosion. Even if the medicine is excellent, whiplash makes your hospital feel unpredictable; and unpredictability is the opposite of psychological safety.

Below is a deeper look at each type of whiplash, why it happens, how clients interpret it, and why eliminating it is one of the most powerful CX upgrades a hospital can make.

Medical Whiplash: Different Providers, Different Recommendations

Medical whiplash is the #1 trust destroyer in veterinary medicine. It happens when the hospital feels like five different hospitals depending on who's working that day.

Examples:

One doctor says, *"We recommend annual bloodwork."*
The next says, *"He's young, you don't really need it."*

One doctor says, *"Dental care is essential."*
Another says nothing.

One tech says, *"All dogs should be on year-round preventatives."*
Another says, *"It's optional."*

Why whiplash happens: Because medicine is personal. Doctors practice differently. Techs explain things differently. CSRs emphasize different points based on their comfort level. Nobody is wrong individually, but collectively the hospital sounds disorganized.

How clients interpret it: Not like clinicians. Not like scientists. Not like people who understand nuance. They interpret it like humans under emotional stress:

- "Someone's wrong."
- "Someone's hiding something."
- "They're guessing."
- "These people are not aligned."
- "If they can't agree on this, how do I trust anything else?"

Medical whiplash instantly creates doubt—about competence, about integrity, about motives. Doubt kills compliance. And when compliance dies, outcomes suffer.

Medical Whiplash is deadly because it attacks the very thing clients are hiring you for: your expertise.

Financial Whiplash: Inconsistent Explanations of Cost

Financial whiplash happens when the hospital sends mixed signals about pricing, estimates, or the necessity of recommended care.

Examples:

One CSR says, "This will be around $450."
Another says, "No idea—it depends on what the doctor finds."

One doctor says, "This is essential."
Another says, "You should think about it."

Why whiplash happens: Because money conversations are uncomfortable. Some team members overshoot, some undershoot, some avoid specifics completely. Without standardized language around cost, every conversation becomes inconsistent and emotionally risky.

How clients interpret it: Clients don't think, "Ah, yes, each staff member simply has a slightly different communication comfort zone." They think,

"They're hiding the real price."
"I'm being upsold."
"They're making it up as they go."
"I can't trust this estimate."

Financial whiplash triggers defensiveness because ambiguity around money feels like danger. Even when the actual prices are fair, the lack of clarity feels threatening.

This is why clients sometimes say, "It's too expensive" when what they really mean is,
"I'm confused, and I don't feel safe."

Financial clarity isn't about affordability. It's about trust.

Emotional Whiplash: Inconsistent Tone, Empathy, and Communication

Emotional whiplash happens when the experience shifts unpredictably from warm → cold, patient → rushed, clear → silent.

This form of whiplash is deeply destabilizing because clients are already vulnerable, already emotional, already in protective mode.

Examples:

One team member is warm and gentle. The next is blunt and clinical.

One tech narrates beautifully. The next disappears with the pet for 20 minutes without a word.

One CSR is calm and patient. Another is visibly stressed and short.

Why whiplash happens: Because people have different personalities, different stress loads, different communication habits—especially during busy days. Without a unified emotional standard, clients ride a rollercoaster of tone and energy.

How clients interpret it: Clients don't think, "The tech must be overwhelmed today; totally understandable."

They think:

"Am I annoying them?"
"Am I being judged?"
"Is something wrong with my pet?"
"Why is everyone acting differently?"
"Do they even care?"

Emotional whiplash creates uncertainty, and uncertainty is poison for anxious people.

This form of inconsistency makes the hospital feel unsafe—not medically, but emotionally. And again, when clients don't feel emotionally safe, trust collapses.

How to Build a One Message, One Standard, One Team Culture

This isn't about scripts. This is about identity. Elite hospitals do these four things:

They Build a Culture that Celebrates Clear Standards

We talked about the importance of culture, and of having a clear direction for your hospital in the form of mission, vision and values. This is foundation upon which standards are built and upheld.

High-trust hospitals don't get lucky. They get aligned. They build a culture where clarity isn't optional, it's celebrated. Instead of letting each individual operate from their own comfort zone, preferences, or personal philosophy, they create shared standards that everyone is proud to uphold. These standards aren't rules; they're your identity. They are the collective promise you make to every client and every pet that walks through your doors.

In a hospital with true cultural alignment, every team member knows exactly what "good medicine" looks like here. They understand *why* certain recommendations are made. They use language that supports clients rather than confuses them. They know what the hospital stands for and what it will never compromise on. They know how to communicate in a way that protects psychological safety. They know how to explain care in human terms. They know how to uphold the emotional experience with as much intention as the medical one.

These aren't scripts. These aren't rigid mandates. These are *shared beliefs* about how your team shows up for clients and for each other. This is the difference between a hospital that "lets people do their own thing" and a hospital where everyone is rowing in the same direction with the same emotional and medical clarity.

When a team is aligned around clear standards, the hospital becomes predictable in the best possible way. Not boring—trusted.

Not robotic—consistent. Not restrictive—empowered. Clear standards don't limit individuality; they give it direction. They ensure that every client, no matter who they interact with, receives the same level of care, compassion, communication, and confidence.

This isn't rigidity. This is integrity in action.

They Train Cross-role Consistency

In elite hospitals, consistency isn't an accident; it's a discipline. Every role in the building, from CSR to assistant to tech to doctor, becomes part of *one unified voice* speaking on behalf of the hospital. Not because they're parroting lines, but because they understand the *why* behind the messaging and carry it forward with confidence.

A high-trust hospital doesn't allow each role to operate like a separate department with its own vocabulary, tone, beliefs, or emotional approach. They cross-train like a championship team. CSRs learn how doctors explain common diagnoses. Doctors learn how CSRs set expectations at the front desk. Techs learn the metaphors doctors use. Assistants learn the emotional anchors CSRs rely on during tough moments. Everyone learns how everyone else communicates—so they can reinforce it, not contradict it.

This type of alignment makes the hospital feel coherent, predictable, and deeply safe.

What cross-role consistency actually looks like:

Same metaphors. If the doctor uses the "coffee filter" metaphor for kidneys, the tech uses the same one. The CSR uses it on follow-up calls. The assistant uses it during care instructions. Clients hear one story, not ten versions.

Same medical rationale. If the hospital believes annual bloodwork protects pets by catching early disease, *everyone* explains it that way—not "some doctors do it" or "it depends who you get."

Same emotional anchors. Whether it's validating fear, reducing shame, or narrating transitions, every team member knows how to ground a client emotionally in the same consistent, calming way.

Same tone. Warm. Clear. Compassionate. Confident. Not one person gentle and the next abrupt. Not one narrator and the next silent. Tone becomes a standard, not a personality quirk.

Same sequence of explanations. Everyone follows the same flow:

1. Why it matters
2. What you're recommending
3. What the options are
4. What comes next

When everyone follows the same structure, clients stop feeling like the hospital is improvising.

Clients talk to multiple people during a visit. If each person delivers a different message, tone, metaphor, or level of confidence, the client starts connecting dots that aren't there. They lose clarity. They lose trust. They lose the sense that the hospital knows what it's doing.

But when everyone sounds aligned—even with different personalities—the message becomes unshakably stable. It becomes the hospital's truth, not just one person's opinion.

To give you an example: When a client asks a tech, *"Do I really need the recheck?,"* the answer carries enormous weight.

If the doctor says, "This recheck helps us make sure we're controlling inflammation early," but the tech says, "Some people skip it; it's up to you," the client experiences whiplash. Trust fractures. Compliance tanks. And the doctor's credibility evaporates.

But if the tech instead says, "Yes, because it helps us confirm the treatment is working and catch anything early," the hospital suddenly feels aligned, competent, and trustworthy.

Cross-role consistency turns the entire team into a unified front of clarity, confidence, and compassion—exactly what anxious clients need. This is not about everyone memorizing the same script. It's about everyone communicating the same mission. That's when consistency becomes a culture, not a task.

They Create "Unity Scripts" (Not Robotic Scripts)

High-performing hospitals don't rely on improvisation when it comes to client communication. They don't leave messaging up to chance, personality, or whoever happens to be working that day. Instead, they create Unity Scripts: not memorized lines, not canned dialogue, but *shared frameworks* that ensure every team member hits the same emotional and informational beats, in the same order, with the same clarity.

Unity Scripts are about structure, not sameness. They aren't meant to strip away personality—they're meant to build consistency. They give every team member the confidence to communicate in a way that feels natural, but still aligns with the hospital's values and standards.

In other words: everyone sings their own melody, but follows the same sheet music.

Clients don't need identical wording from every staff member. But they absolutely need identical clarity.

Without Unity Scripts, communication varies wildly:

- One person starts with price.
- One starts with options.
- One starts with the diagnosis.
- One forgets to emphasize urgency.
- One makes it sound optional.
- One uses jargon.
- One uses metaphors.

- One rushes.
- One over-explains.

This inconsistency doesn't feel like "different communication styles" to clients; it feels like different standards of care. And that's terrifying.

Unity Scripts eliminate mixed messages by ensuring the *flow* stays the same, even when the delivery changes. They give clients the sense that the hospital knows exactly what it's doing, and that everyone is on the same page.

That psychological stability is priceless.

So what do Unity Scripts actually look like? Unity Scripts are frameworks with specific anchors that must always appear in the conversation, no matter who's speaking. Below are examples with expanded rationale:

Example: Bloodwork Unity Script Framework

1. *Why bloodwork matters*—The hospital must start in the same place: with meaning, not medicine. For example, "Bloodwork lets us see what your pet can't tell us—how their organs are functioning on the inside" or
2. *What it tells us*—For example, "It helps us catch problems early, before they become painful or expensive."
3. *What might change depending on results*—Example: "We usually have results within 24 hours. If anything looks off, we'll adjust medication or treatment."
4. *Next steps*—Example: "We usually have results within 24 hours. Then, after we review the results, we'll reach out with a personalized plan."

This is the skeleton. Each team member gives it flesh with their own personality, but the bones stay the same.

Estimate Presentation Unity Script

Money conversations only feel safe when the messaging is unified. Here are some phrases that I very commonly recommend that hospitals put to good use:

1. *"Let's walk this together."* Signals partnership—not pressure.
2. *"Here's what's essential today."* Creates clarity and prioritization.
3. *"Here's what we can plan for later."* Shows flexibility and respect for financial reality.
4. *"You're in control."* Restores agency, lowers fear, strengthens trust.

Every team member—from CSR to tech to doctor—uses this same emotional sequence so clients never feel blindsided or cornered.

The Magic Behind Unity Scripts: Structure + Personality

Unity Scripts do NOT turn your team into robots. They do the opposite. They give your team permission to relax, to be themselves, to speak with authenticity—because the *framework* carries the weight of consistency. The script holds the structure; the person provides the heart.

One team member can deliver the script with warm humor. Another with calm reassurance. Another with confident efficiency.

Different personalities. Same experience. Same clarity. Same hospital identity. That's the magic.

The Result: Predictability, Safety, Trust

Unity Scripts eliminate the most dangerous sentence a client can think: *"I don't know what to expect from this place."*

When the messaging feels unified:

- Clients relax.
- Compliance rises.
- Upset interactions drop.

- Your values become visible.
- Your team becomes aligned.
- Your hospital's brand becomes stronger.

Unity Scripts are not about communication. They're about trust engineering.

Because a hospital that speaks with one voice becomes a hospital clients believe in, even when the news is hard, the cost is high, or the stakes are emotional.

This is clarity. This is culture.

They Practice "Unified Debriefing"

Elite hospitals don't assume their messaging stays aligned. They actively *maintain* alignment. They understand that communication naturally drifts over time. People pick up habits. New hires bring old scripts from previous hospitals. Doctors develop their own phrasing. Techs simplify in ways that accidentally strip meaning. CSRs try to help but end up improvising. What starts aligned slowly becomes fragmented unless the team intentionally realigns.

That's where Unified Debriefing enters the culture.

Unified Debriefing is not a meeting. It's not a training. It's a muscle, one that must be exercised regularly to stay strong. It's the practice of gathering as a team regularly, to make sure the hospital still speaks with a single, confident, consistent voice.

How Unified Debriefing Actually Works

The team picks one common clinical scenario, something that happens constantly and affects every role. For example:

- A dog limping suddenly
- A senior cat losing weight
- A dental disease conversation
- A vomiting puppy

- A chronic condition recheck
- A heart murmur newly detected
- A preventative-care explanation

Once the scenario is chosen, each role takes a turn presenting how they would explain the situation to a client. No notes. No scripts. Just their honest, real-world communication.

The doctor explains it how they'd explain it.
Then the tech explains it their way.
Then the CSR explains it their way.
Then assistants or other team members share how they'd support that same client.

And here's where the magic happens: As each person shares, the team suddenly sees the gaps—the subtle inconsistencies that cause client whiplash:

- The tech gives more detail than the doctor.
- The CSR sounds unsure.
- The doctor uses jargon the others aren't repeating.
- The assistant explains something essential the doctor forgot.
- Someone unintentionally makes a recommendation sound optional.
- Someone explains cost differently.
- Someone uses a metaphor nobody else uses.
- Someone leaves out the emotional empathy piece.

These inconsistencies are invisible in the day-to-day chaos, but they show up the moment people speak their messaging aloud. In other words, Unified Debriefing forces the invisible to become visible.

Once all roles have shared, the team works as a unit to refine, unify, and tighten the messaging.

- Which explanation was clearest?
- Which metaphor landed the best?
- Which emotional anchor made the client feel seen?
- Which phrasing captured the hospital's values most effectively?

- Which order of explanation felt natural and calming?
- Which gaps could confuse a client?
- Which parts need to become nonnegotiable?

Together, the team creates one unified communication flow—the hospital's shared "North Star" for that scenario.

This is where alignment is born. The goal is not to bulldoze individuality. The goal is to protect clarity.

Everyone leaves with the same foundation, the same framework, the same emotional architecture, while still using their own voice.

This practice really matters. Why? Hospitals without this ritual drift. Slowly. Quietly. Unintentionally.

One doctor starts soft-pedaling dentals.
A new tech starts overselling diagnostics.
A CSR starts saying "I'm not sure" when asked about cost.
Assistants start skipping narration.
Doctors start using totally different phrases for the same condition.
People fill in communication gaps with their best guesses.

And suddenly, the hospital feels unpredictable, even though nobody meant for that to happen.

Unified Debriefing prevents that drift.

It keeps the culture sharp.
It keeps the messaging aligned.
It keeps the emotional experience consistent.
It keeps the hospital feeling safe—for clients *and* for the team.

It's a tune-up for the hospital's communication engine.

And yes, it strengthens culture, psychological safety, and operational excellence in one move. When hospitals practice Unified Debriefing:

- Messaging becomes tighter.
- Recommendations sound unified.

- Clients hear the same story from every role.
- The hospital feels predictable and trustworthy.
- Team members understand each other's roles better.
- New hires get onboarded into alignment immediately.
- Senior staff stay accountable to clarity.
- Complicated cases are explained more consistently.
- Upset-client interactions drop dramatically.

This is how you build a hospital that sounds like one team, not 20 individuals.

This is communication excellence.
This is culture in motion.

What Unified Messaging Feels Like to a Client

When a hospital follows the Anti-whiplash Rule, clients experience:

- Calm instead of confusion
- Predictability instead of anxiety
- Confidence instead of hesitation
- Trust instead of doubt
- Consistency instead of contradiction
- Safety instead of stress

They stop questioning your recommendations.
They stop shopping around for other hospitals.
They stop spiraling emotionally.
They stop writing harsh reviews.

They feel held. They feel guided. They feel understood. And when clients feel understood, the entire hospital thrives.

Case Study: The Hospital That Eliminated Whiplash and Exploded Compliance

Let's call them Maple Hill Veterinary Center: a solid hospital with good doctors, caring techs, and a loyal client base. But behind the scenes, they were dealing with the same invisible friction that slows down so many well-intentioned practices. Each doctor practiced in their own style, using different language, different metaphors, and even different standards for when to recommend diagnostics or follow-ups. Techs explained things however they had learned at previous jobs or from whomever had trained them first. CSRs gave vague pre-visit instructions because they weren't sure what each doctor preferred.

Clients felt the inconsistency immediately. They asked questions like, *"Why didn't the last doctor mention this?"* or *"Is this new?"* or *"Do I really need this if no one else brought it up?"* Compliance swung wildly from one provider to the next, with no predictable pattern. Doctors complained about having "noncompliant clients," not realizing that mixed messaging was driving fear and hesitation. Techs felt stuck in the middle, trying to translate different medical philosophies on the fly without stepping on anyone's toes. The team worked hard—no one could deny that—but it felt like everyone was paddling in different directions.

Then Maple Hill implemented the Anti-whiplash system: One Message, One Standard, One Team. And the transformation was dramatic.

Within just 90 days, diagnostic compliance increased by 22%—not because clients suddenly had more money, but because they finally heard one clear, unified message across the entire staff. Recheck adherence rose, preventative sales climbed, and upset-client interactions dropped significantly. Doctors began trusting each other more because they could count on consistent communication backing their recommendations instead of unintentionally undermining them. Techs, for the first time, reported feeling confident explaining *anything* because they knew their messaging matched the doctor's. CSRs felt empowered instead of unsure—they finally had clarity about what to say, how to set expectations, and how to guide the flow of the visit.

Clients noticed, too. The hospital felt calmer. Smoother. More predictable. Leadership described the entire operation as "easier to run"—not because the medicine changed, not because workloads decreased, not because staffing improved, but because communication finally worked in harmony instead of chaos.

Nothing else changed.
Not pricing.
Not staffing.
Not scheduling.

Just messaging.

That's the power of a unified hospital: One Message, One Standard, One Team.

Summary

The Anti-whiplash Rule is simple but transformative: One Message. One Standard. One Team. It's the backbone of a hospital that clients trust, teams feel proud of, and leaders can actually breathe inside. When every member of the team speaks with the same clarity, the same rationale, and the same emotional stability, the hospital becomes predictable—not in a boring way, but in a *safe* way. Predictability is the foundation of psychological safety, and psychological safety is the soil where trust grows.

Consistency is not a "nice to have." It's the force multiplier that separates elite hospitals from chaotic ones. When your messaging is aligned, you build trust because clients feel like everyone is rowing in the same direction. You reduce confusion because no one contradicts the person before them. You increase compliance because clients feel confident, not conflicted. You improve outcomes because care plans are clearer and follow-through becomes easier. You decrease escalations because mixed messages are the #1 spark of frustration and panic. You strengthen team morale because people stop feeling like they're constantly cleaning up someone else's communication mess. And yes, you boost the hospital's financial health because clarity is the gateway to loyalty, repeat business, and smooth operational flow. In short: consistency accelerates the entire Veterinary Trust Flywheel.

But consistency doesn't happen by accident. It must exist across every touchpoint where trust is built or broken: medical recommendations, diagnostic explanations, preventative-care conversations, estimate presentations, emotional tone, visit narration, warmth during hard moments, and the follow-up communication that closes the loop. Every one of these moments is either reinforcing the hospital's identity or fracturing it.

The ultimate goal is a hospital where it doesn't matter who you talk to—the receptionist, the tech, the assistant, the doctor—you get the same clarity, the same compassion, and the same standard of care. Clients don't feel like they're entering a lottery every visit, hoping they get "the good doctor" or "the helpful tech." Instead, they experience a unified team delivering a unified message with a unified heart. When your hospital operates like that, trust becomes automatic, loyalty becomes inevitable, and your culture becomes unstoppable.

Suggested Readings

Agency for Healthcare Research and Quality. *TeamSTEPPS® 2.0: Strategies and Tools to Enhance Performance and Patient Safety.* U.S. Department of Health and Human Services, 2023, www.ahrq.gov. Accessed 9 Dec. 2025.

American Animal Hospital Association. *Client Communication Guidelines for the Veterinary Practice.* AAHA Press, 2023, www.aaha.org. Accessed 9 Dec. 2025.

American Medical Association. *Improving Communication for Better Patient Outcomes.* AMA Press, 2022, www.ama-assn.org. Accessed 9 Dec. 2025.

Bodenheimer, Thomas, and Christine Sinsky. "From Triple to Quadruple Aim: Care of the Patient Requires Care of the Provider." *Annals of Family Medicine*, vol. 12, no. 6, 2014, pp. 573–576.

Edmondson, Amy C. *The Fearless Organization: Creating Psychological Safety in the Workplace for Learning, Innovation, and Growth.* Wiley, 2018.

Gittell, Jody Hoffer. *High Performance Healthcare: Using the Power of Relationships to Achieve Quality, Efficiency and Resilience.* McGraw-Hill, 2009.

Institute of Medicine. *To Err Is Human: Building a Safer Health System.* National Academies Press, 2000.

Joint Commission. *Advancing Effective Communication, Cultural Competence, and Patient- and Family-centered Care.* Joint Commission Resources, 2022.

Kahneman, Daniel. *Thinking, Fast and Slow.* Farrar, Straus and Giroux, 2011.

Makoul, Gregory, and Traci H. Curry. "The Value of Assessing and Addressing Communication Skill Deficits in Medical Practice." *Journal of the American Medical Association*, vol. 298, no. 9, 2007, pp. 1057–1059.

Patient Safety Network (PSNet). *Communication Failure and Patient Harm.* Agency for Healthcare Research and Quality, 2023, psnet.ahrq.gov. Accessed 9 Dec. 2025.

Street, Richard L., Jr., et al. "How Does Communication Heal? Pathways Linking Clinician–Patient Communication to Health Outcomes." *Patient Education and Counseling*, vol. 74, no. 3, 2009, pp. 295–301.

Wolever, Ruth Q., et al. "Effective and Efficient Communication Across Healthcare Teams: A Mixed-Methods Study." *Journal of Healthcare Management*, vol. 63, no. 4, 2018, pp. 249–263.

Chapter 22
How to Handle Mistakes and Near Misses

Intro: The Moment Every Hospital Fears, and Why It Doesn't Have to Ruin You

In veterinary medicine, mistakes and near misses aren't hypothetical. They're reality.

Samples get mislabeled.
A treatment gets delayed.
A note gets missed.
A client hears one thing while the doctor meant another.
A pet reacts unpredictably.
A voicemail goes unreturned.
A critical lab value slips through the cracks.

Every team has "Oh shit" moments.

But here's the truth the best hospitals understand: **mistakes themselves rarely destroy trust. Avoidance, defensiveness, and silence do.**

Clients don't expect perfection.
They expect ownership.
They expect honesty.
They expect accountability.
They expect partnership.

When a hospital recovers from a mistake with transparency and grace, something profound happens: **the client trusts you more than before the mistake**.

Because now they've seen your character. Your integrity. Your humanity. Your commitment to doing right when it's hardest.

The difference between a one-star reviewer and a lifelong advocate is not whether something went wrong. It's what you do in the *five minutes after* something goes wrong.

This chapter is your blueprint.

PART I: The Psychology of a Client During a Medical Mistake

When something goes wrong—or even feels like it might have—clients move instantly into one of three emotional states:

1. Fear: "Is my pet in danger?"
2. Shame: "Did I do something wrong?" "Are they judging me?"
3. Betrayal: "I trusted them. Are they hiding something?"

Fear, shame, and betrayal are explosive emotions. But transparency disarms all three.

When you say, "We caught something, and here's what we're doing," the client's brain moves from:

Danger to safety
Uncertainty to direction
Abandonment to partnership

That shift is the heart of psychological safety—both for the client and the team.

PART II: The Five-minute Medical Recovery Framework (FMMR)

This is the exact, step-by-step framework elite hospitals use.

Step 1: State the Reality Clearly (No Euphemisms)

Clients do NOT want soft language. Soft language feels like hiding.

Use:

"I want to be fully transparent with you."

Avoid:

"There was a little mix-up ..."
"We had a small issue ..."
"It's not a big deal but ..."

Step 2: Own What Happened (Without Blame or Deflection)

Clients want to know ONE thing above all: "Does someone here take responsibility?"

Use:

"This is on us."
"This was our error."
"I want to walk you through exactly what happened."

Avoid:

"The system glitched."
"We've been really busy."
"Someone must have ..."
"Your paperwork didn't include ..."

Blame erodes trust faster than the mistake itself.

Step 3: Empathize with the Emotional Impact

Not the medical impact, the *emotional* impact.

Most hospitals skip this step. And most hospitals struggle with client relationships.

Use:

"I can imagine how stressful this feels."
"Your trust really matters to us."
"I know this must have been upsetting to hear."

This resets the emotional temperature. It tells the client, "We see you, not just the issue."

Step 4: Outline the Correction Plan (With Absolute Clarity)

Clients calm down when they understand what you're doing, why you're doing it, and how quickly it starts.

For example, "Here's what we're doing right now:

1. We're rerunning the bloodwork at no charge.
2. Dr. Nguyen will call you personally with the results today.
3. We've flagged your file so this doesn't happen again."

This is the moment trust rebuilds.

Step 5: Offer Fair Resolution (Even If Small)

Not "compensation." Resolution.

Resolution says: "We value this relationship enough to invest in it."

Examples:

- Waive a fee
- Provide complimentary recheck
- Provide a complimentary follow-up test

- Give a discount on future visit
- Add a grief resource or educational resource
- Add priority scheduling
- Cover a medication refill

Small gestures build enormous loyalty.

PART III: The Script Library (Your Team's Verbal Armor)

Here are ready-to-use scripts for the most common scenarios in an animal hospital.

Scenario 1: A Lab Sample Was Lost

"Sarah, I want to be completely transparent with you. We made an error and your sample wasn't processed correctly. This is on us. I'm so sorry for the stress this creates.

And here's what we're doing right now: we'll redo the sample today at no cost, and Dr. Patel will call you as soon as the results are in. Your trust in us matters a lot, and we're committed to keeping you informed every step."

Scenario 2: A Client Receives Conflicting Information

"Thank you for bringing this to our attention. You're right. What you heard yesterday and what was said today don't align. That's on us, and I'm sorry for the confusion it caused.

Here's what's true: [Unified answer].

And here's what we're doing to make sure this doesn't happen again: our team is regrouping to make sure we're aligned before communicating next steps. We appreciate your patience, and your trust."

Scenario 3: A Pet Had a Tough Experience or Injury at the Hospital

"Before anything else, I want you to know your pet's safety is our top priority. Something happened today that you deserve to know about. During the procedure, Luna became stressed and bumped her nose on the kennel. She is stable and comfortable now, but I want to be fully transparent.

Here's what we're doing: we cleaned the area, started monitoring, and she's doing well. We'll keep a close eye on her and update you frequently.

I know hearing this feels scary. Thank you for letting us share openly and honestly."

Again, clients do not abandon hospitals for moments like these. They abandon hospitals that hide moments like these.

PART IV: The Internal Side: How Teams Should Handle Mistakes Without Shame

Mistakes don't only destabilize clients—they destabilize teams. Shame, fear, gossip, and defensive culture follow hospitals that treat mistakes as moral failures.

High-performing hospitals treat mistakes the way aviation does: as data. Not judgment.

These hospitals:

- Debrief quickly
- Separate emotion from process
- Look for system gaps
- Identify training needs
- Praise early reporting
- Celebrate catches
- Do NOT punish honesty

The team needs to feel psychologically safe to speak up. And clients need to feel psychologically safe to forgive.

When teams debrief without shame, they become tighter, smarter, and calmer. Clients feel that energy. This is how the Trust Flywheel accelerates internally and externally.

PART V: Case Study—The Hospital That Turned Mistakes into Loyalty

Let's call the hospital Lakeside Animal Health. Before implementing this framework, they had:

- Defensive doctors
- Techs terrified to admit errors
- Clients frequently escalating online
- A 3.9-star Google rating
- Low staff morale
- Confusion around who speaks to clients after a mistake

After implementing the Transparency + Grace Blueprint for 90 days:

- Mistake reporting increased
- Actual mistakes decreased
- Client escalations dropped by 70%
- Doctors said they felt "relief" because they didn't have to hide anything
- Team trust went up
- Google ratings started to climb steadily
- Twice as many five-star reviews mentioned "honest" or "transparent"
- Fewer clients left the hospital
- Rechecks and diagnostics improved

And the biggest win? Team members began to say, "We trust each other more now."

The recovery process didn't just improve CX. It improved culture.

PART VI: Workshop Exercise—"The Five-minute Recovery Drill"

Get everyone into small cross-role teams of three to four. Give each team a scenario:

- Lost sample
- Missed note
- Miscommunication
- Back-room injury
- Angry client call
- Dosage near miss

They must write:

1. The exact words they'd say to the client
2. The internal debrief steps
3. The resolution they would offer

Then teams present to each other and vote on:

- Most empathetic
- Most transparent
- Most psychologically safe
- Most clear and concise

Summary

The Transparency + Grace Blueprint

1. State reality clearly.
2. Own what happened.
3. Validate the client's emotion.
4. Outline next steps.
5. Offer resolution.
6. Debrief internally without shame.

Why It Works

- Transparency builds trust.
- Trust builds compliance.
- Compliance builds outcomes.
- Outcomes build loyalty.
- Loyalty fuels revenue.
- Revenue allows reinvestment.
- Reinvestment strengthens team experience.
- Strong team experience reduces errors.

The Trust Flywheel spins because mistakes become opportunities—not fractures.

Suggested Readings

Agency for Healthcare Research and Quality. *Communication and Optimal Resolution (CANDOR) Toolkit.* U.S. Department of Health and Human Services, 2023, www.ahrq.gov. Accessed 10 Dec. 2025.

American Animal Hospital Association. *Client Communication Guidelines for the Veterinary Practice.* AAHA Press, 2023, www.aaha.org. Accessed 10 Dec. 2025.

American Medical Association. *Disclosing Medical Errors to Patients: Ethical and Practical Issues.* AMA Journal of Ethics, 2021, journalofethics.ama-assn.org. Accessed 10 Dec. 2025.

Dekker, Sidney. *Just Culture: Restoring Trust and Accountability in Your Organization.* 3rd ed., CRC Press, 2016.

Edmondson, Amy C. *The Fearless Organization: Creating Psychological Safety in the Workplace for Learning, Innovation, and Growth.* Wiley, 2018.

Gallagher, Thomas H., et al. "Patients' and Physicians' Attitudes Regarding the Disclosure of Medical Errors." *Journal of the American Medical Association*, vol. 289, no. 8, 2003, pp. 1001–1007.

Institute of Medicine. *To Err Is Human: Building a Safer Health System.* National Academies Press, 2000.

Joint Commission. *Sentinel Event Data Summary 2023.* Joint Commission Resources, 2024, www.jointcommission.org. Accessed 10 Dec. 2025.

Leape, Lucian L. "Errors in Medicine." *Clinical Chemistry*, vol. 43, no. 5, 1997, pp. 691–696.

Mazzucco, Wendy, et al. "Disclosure of Adverse Events and Patient Safety: A Systematic Review." *International Journal of Quality in Health Care*, vol. 29, no. 1, 2017, pp. 8–17.

Reason, James. *Human Error*. Cambridge University Press, 1990.

Sutcliffe, Kathleen M., and Karl E. Weick. *Managing the Unexpected: Resilient Performance in an Age of Uncertainty*. 2nd ed., Wiley, 2015.

Vincent, Charles. *Patient Safety*. 2nd ed., Wiley-Blackwell, 2010.

Wachter, Robert M. *Understanding Patient Safety*. 3rd ed., McGraw-Hill Education, 2017.

Chapter 23

Use the "Page Method" to Stop Client Frustration in Its Tracks

I want to talk about what I think is my BEST strategy for preventing complaints from pet owners. And what I'm not going to say is, "Well, just don't screw up and clients won't complain." Life doesn't work that way. Shit goes wrong. Tech breaks. Emergencies throw the schedule off. A truck blocks your parking lot. You can't control it all.

When clients get upset, like any of us, psychologically it's usually because they have an unmet emotional need—they feel like nobody cares about them, or their pet, or their problem. We've all been there, of course. But there's a simple technique I've learned that, in my experience at least, usually prevents clients from boiling over and truly becoming frustrated to the point where they complain. And often, it creates trust and gratitude from the client at the same time. I call it Proactive Gratitude. And once you get the hang of it, it's a total game-changer.

The key to the Proactive Gratitude strategy—as the name suggests—is to be *proactive* rather than *reactive* to client complaints. In other words, get ahead of a complaint early, even before the client has the chance to verbalize it.

Aight. Story time—I'll tell you how I first became aware of this strategy.

A few years ago, I moved from my place in Westwood, Los Angeles, to Venice Beach. For several reasons I needed a change of scenery in my life, but this was genuinely an exciting move for me; I'd be living steps from the sand, which was really attractive given my not-so-secret obsession with beach volleyball. I was stoked about the move, but not so stoked about ... uh ... moving. Most of us have had to move from one home to another in the past, and like many people, I'd had my share of horrible moving experiences. (When I moved from Boston to California back in 2018, for example, ONE of my plates survived the move. One. Out of about 30.)

My move to Venice Beach wasn't really that painful, though, until ... It was time to call the cable company. The company I had in Westwood didn't serve my new neighborhood in Venice Beach so I had to call and cancel my internet service. You know where this is going ...

I'm not here to bash any particular company, so I'll keep the company's name generic. I'm nice like that. But I called my internet provider to cancel my internet plan, and immediately hit a phone tree where "change your current service" was option number 8, which took so long to get to that it might as well have been option number 800. I was immediately put on hold. Thirty-seven minutes of elevator music—the same awful, three-minute song on repeat. I listened to that song so many damn times that I literally heard it in my sleep that night. But finally, the company rep picked up my call and asked who she had "the pleasure of speaking with." I told her my name and that I was calling to cancel my internet plan, to which she said that she had to transfer me to cancellations. "Well, wait" I said.

"I thought I selected "change my current service"—am I in the wrong place?" "Yeah," she said, "Canceling your plan would have been option number 9—*cancel service*. You pressed option 8—which is to *change service*." Back on hold, same friggin' song, for another 26 minutes.

Of course, at this point I've lost my patience. Then the next agent answers the phone and opens with a sales pitch: to bundle my home, internet, and cable services and take advantage of some blah blah blah promotion they were running.

"No, thank you. I've been on the phone waiting for over an hour now. I really just need to cancel my service."

"Oh, well sorry to hear that, sir. Luckily, you called at a great time. We have some great bundle deals going on right now, and ..."

"Please stop!" I shouted over her. I got heated and sarcastic: "And by the way, who needs phone service anymore? It's not 1972!" Clearly, at this point, I'd lost it. I felt a little guilty about raising my voice to the innocent phone operator, but ... only a little. Long story short, I was eventually able to finally cancel my internet package.

I left the call feeling so, just ... mad. Defeated, even. I literally grunted as I hung up the phone and had to go for a walk around my neighborhood just to relieve some stress.

Now more relaxed, I geared up for my next call, to the NEW cable company where I'd be getting my new internet plan. Commence the torture, right?

Well actually this call went much, much better. For a lot of reasons: I wasn't transferred from one agent to the other. The woman answering the phone, Page, was friendly, not pushy. I still had to navigate a phone tree and sit on hold for about 20 minutes or so, and yet I left the call feeling relaxed and almost thankful to give this new company my money. Odd! So I reflected back to try to figure out why I left call number two with Page feeling so satisfied, after call number one had left me frustrated and needing to blow off steam.

I have an answer, I think. It wasn't just that call number two had fewer transfers, or that the hold music was slightly less annoying. It was how Page ADDRESSED my long wait. She asked my name, then said, "Hello, Ryan. My name is Page. Now before we get started, I just want to say thank you so much for your patience. I know there was a bit of a wait there. One of our systems unexpectedly broke down this morning, and we've just been swamped with calls from people looking for tech support. We just weren't staffed enough to take so many calls at once, so I really appreciate you bearing with us today. I know that must have been frustrating."

This was so much better than call number one, where I told the Agent about my long wait and was given an empty, kind of disingenuous, "Well okay, sorry." Page didn't need me to *tell* her I'd had a long wait; she made herself aware of it, and acknowledged it right off the bat before I even had the chance to complain. And she didn't apologize for it; instead she THANKED ME for my patience and my understanding, and then explained WHY it happened. Even though the experience wasn't a perfect one, this left me feeling ... Great. Respected. Considered. Valued. I actually felt like Page cared. She wasn't defensive and didn't come off as making excuses. Instead, she basically insinuated that I had done something kind in waiting for her, and she thanked me for being patient. It was *so disarming*, and kind of made me think, "Wow, Page seems to think pretty highly of me. I don't want to disappoint her by lashing out!" And, I didn't. She had completely disarmed me and calmed me down. All of a sudden, my long wait no longer seemed like that big of a deal.

Unexpectedly, when visiting an animal hospital I was advising a few weeks later, I saw a similar approach being taken by one of the CSRs, Kate. I'd sometimes pop into the hospital to talk to pet owner clients, see how things are going with the team, maybe try some new ideas. While sitting in the waiting room, I saw this older woman who had brought her cat in, and who was clearly getting agitated by her wait. You could just see it on her face and in her demeanor. Now, I'd had clients complain to me about wait times in the past, as we all have, and my usual response when I received a complaint about the wait was to say something like: "Oh, I'm so sorry. Let me take a look for you and see how much longer it's going to be. Thank you for letting me know." That approach always felt good enough; and it was certainly well intentioned. But my response—"Oh sorry, let me look"—never seemed to actually help that much. It usually just got a response like, "Okay" or "huff ... alright, thanks."

But the CSR, Kate, used a different approach, which seemed a lot like how Page engaged me on my service call. Kate went into the computer to see how long this woman had been waiting—25 minutes—and also checked her name: Nancy, and her cat's name, Butters. She took the initiative to walk right up to Nancy, crouched down to her eye level, and said, "Hi, Nancy. I'm Kate. I know you've been waiting for over 25 minutes now and how frustrating that is. Thank you so, so much for your patience. We had an unexpected emergency case come in the door, which threw our team behind schedule. But we'll be right with you and Butters. It should only be a few more minutes, and I really appreciate you bearing with us today. Can I get you a glass of water while you wait?"

Nancy's face lit up, from a sunken frustration to a gentle, understanding smile. Her face showed her genuine concern for the emergency case Kate mentioned, and she warmed right up to Kate. She gently grabbed and squeezed Kate's hand with both of hers, which Kate later told me hurt a little bit because Nancy was wearing a LOT of rings, and said, "Oh my gosh. Of course! I understand! That's just fine. Thank you so much for coming by to see us. I hope everything is okay with the emergency." Talk about effective. Nancy was disarmed, felt informed and valued, and even grateful—despite her frustrating wait time.

The team got her and Butters into an exam room about 5 minutes later. But here's what's cool: On her way out of the hospital a little while later, Kate and Nancy bumped into each other again. Nancy extended her arm to give Kate a quick one-armed hug and a warm, genuine thank you.

Intrigued, I went to work experimenting with this strategy myself and used it anytime I was able to identify a potential emerging concern for a pet owner client—a long hold time on the phone, a longer the ideal wait in the lobby, an overcrowded lobby or overcrowded parking lot, when we run out of something, when the checkout process takes longer than it should, times like that. I found that this simple little approach works wonders in preventing frustration for clients suffering an inconvenience, who might have soon complained if they continued to feel inconvenienced.

I've since studied this "Unexpected gratitude" technique in more detail. It's so effective because it acknowledges the person's frustration before they have a chance to boil over. Being proactive *feels* to them that you notice them, you care about them, and you value their time. It also shows them genuine appreciation when they're not expecting it.

Proactive gratitude disarms people. It shows you *see* them before they have to demand to be seen. It gives them dignity. And it frames them as patient and kind, which makes them want to live up to that. Nobody wants to blow up at the person who just thanked them for their grace.

I've used it outside hospitals too. Last year while leaving a Luke Combs concert, stuck in a nightmare parking lot exit, I tried it on a couple ready to yell at me for merging into their lane in front of them. I rolled down my window and said, *"I know you've been waiting forever, and this sucks. We're not trying to cut—just stuck in the wrong lane. I'm so sorry to ask, but we'd really appreciate it if you let us in."* They smiled and laughed, said they'd been prepared to flip me off, and waved me in. During our wait, we engaged in deeper conversation and go to know each other. Two weeks later, we had dinner together. True story.

PAGE's Proactive Gratitude Strategy—Summarized

Here's how to practice Proactive Gratitude to stop a client from getting upset when they're inconvenienced. It's four simple steps:

Step 1: Proactively identify potential client frustration BEFORE the client has a chance to bring it up or complain. This is key. If you wait for the client to complain, you've lost your golden opportunity. You've gotta get to them before they get to you by staying aware of your surroundings and staying on the lookout for clients that may have a growing reason to be upset.

Step 2: Approach and address the client by name, and acknowledge their inconvenience. And if you can include the pet's name in your dialogue, even better. It shows that you know them and their pet, and (as we discussed in Chapter 3) pet owners LOVE that.

Step 3: Express genuine gratitude and appreciation for their patience and understanding.

Step 4: Explain WHY the mistake/inconvenience happened. And be honest.

I tried to come up with an easy way to remember this strategy. Here's what I came up with: Just remember Page—PAGE—from the cable company:

P—PROACTIVE. Keep tabs on potential client frustration points, and get ahead of the complaint before it happens.

A—ACKNOWLEDGE the inconvenience and (second "A"), ADDRESS the client and pet by name

G—GRATITUDE. Thank and affirm the client for being so understanding, patient, etc., and then

E—EXPLAIN WHY.

There's also an optional Step 5 that I think is a nice "extra touch." Offer the client a small gift—water or treats, a free coffee from the coffee shop next door, maybe a complimentary nail trim, something like that. A small gesture of goodwill shows that extra ounce of appreciation.

To summarize this again, by revisiting our example: "Hi, Nancy. I'm Kate. I know you've been waiting for over 25 minutes now and how frustrating that is. Thank you so, so much for your patience. We had an unexpected emergency case come in the door, which threw our team behind schedule. But we'll be right with you and Butters. It should only be a few more minutes, and I really appreciate you bearing with us today. Can I get you a glass of water while you wait?"

Apologies can be fine when you actually screw up. But when life throws an unavoidable curveball—emergencies, systems down, long waits—apologizing just makes it sound like you're guilty. Proactive gratitude reframes the whole experience. It tells the client: *You matter. We see you. We appreciate you.*

Do this consistently, and you'll not only head off complaints. You'll earn trust and maybe even the occasional hug or dinner invite.

Summary

Every hospital has screwups. The winners aren't the ones who avoid them; they're the ones who know how to flip those moments into trust.

Look, shit's gonna go wrong in your hospital. Period. You can't control every emergency, every delay, every broken piece of tech. But you *can* control how you show up when it happens. And that's where the PAGE Method comes in.

Most clients don't lose their cool because of the wait or the bill. They lose it because they feel invisible. They feel like nobody gives a damn. PAGE flips that. You jump in *before* they blow up. You call them by name. You acknowledge the inconvenience. You thank them for their patience. And you explain what's going on. Boom. Frustration defused. Trust built.

Here's the truth: apologies often feel weak. Gratitude feels strong. One says, "We screwed up." The other says, "You matter, and we appreciate you." That's a whole different vibe.

The PAGE Method isn't some corporate playbook. It's human. It's raw. It's how you take a moment that could tank your relationship with a client and turn it into one that earns you respect, loyalty, and maybe even a little hug in the lobby.

So don't wait for complaints to hit you in the face. Get ahead of them. The hospital that consistently shows clients they're seen, valued, and appreciated? That's the hospital people rave about. That's the hospital clients trust.

Suggested Readings

American Animal Hospital Association. *Client Communication Guidelines for the Veterinary Practice*. AAHA Press, 2023, www.aaha.org

Baker, Matthew A., and Michael D. Magnini. "The Effects of Proactive Versus Reactive Service Recovery." *Journal of Services Marketing*, vol. 30, no. 5, 2016, pp. 528–539.

Bies, Robert J. "Interactional Justice: Communication Criteria of Fairness." *Research on Negotiation in Organizations*, vol. 1, 1987, pp. 43–55.

Davidow, Moshe. "The Bottom Line Impact of Organizational Responses to Customer Complaints." *Journal of Hospitality & Tourism Research*, vol. 27, no. 4, 2003, pp. 473–514.

Edmondson, Amy C. *The Fearless Organization: Creating Psychological Safety in the Workplace for Learning, Innovation, and Growth*. Wiley, 2018.

Frederickson, Barbara L. *Positivity: Top-Notch Research Reveals the 3 to 1 Ratio That Will Change Your Life*. Crown, 2009.

Gallup. *State of the American Consumer: Emotional Engagement Predicts Loyalty*. Gallup Press, 2014.

Heskett, James L., et al. *The Service Profit Chain*. Free Press, 1997.

Maister, David H. *The Psychology of Waiting Lines*. David Maister Associates, 2005.

McCullough, Michael E., et al. "Gratitude as a Moral Affect." *Psychological Bulletin*, vol. 127, no. 2, 2001, pp. 249–266.

Tax, Stephen S., Stephen W. Brown, and Murali Chandrashekaran. "Customer Evaluations of Service Complaint Experiences: Implications for Relationship Marketing." *Journal of Marketing*, vol. 62, no. 2, 1998, pp. 60–76.

Tucker, Amy L., and Amy C. Edmondson. "Why Hospitals Don't Learn from Failures: Organizational and Psychological Dynamics That Inhibit System Change." *California Management Review*, vol. 45, no. 2, 2003, pp. 55–72.

Zeithaml, Valarie A., Ananthanarayanan Parasuraman, and Leonard L. Berry. *Delivering Quality Service: Balancing Customer Perceptions and Expectations.* Free Press, 1990.

Chapter 24

Client De-escalation Strategies and the "ALARM" Method

Let's get one thing straight: if you work in veterinary medicine, you are going to deal with upset clients. It's not an "if," it's a "when." This is part of the job. People walk into your hospital carrying fear, anxiety, and love and concern for their pets that is so deep that it can feel like life or death. Add in money, time pressure, and a sense of helplessness, and boom: you've got a recipe for blowups. Some of those blowups are small just a client venting. Some escalate into complaints that need addressing. And sometimes, clients go nuclear. Yelling. Swearing. Verbal abuse. It's ugly, and it's not right, but it's reality.

Here's another reality: In those moments when a client is upset, you don't get to control their behavior. You only get to control your own. How you show up matters more than anything else. Do you pour gas on the fire by getting defensive, folding your arms, and rolling your eyes? Or do you de-escalate, take the oxygen out of the flames, and protect the hospital, your team, and yourself?

The number one rule in any interaction with an upset client is this: stay calm and actually listen. I don't care how ridiculous the complaint sounds, or how unfair the client is being—you've got to hold steady. That means making eye contact, keeping your posture open, and not hiding behind a desk or a screen. It means shutting your mouth long enough to hear them out. It means listening for the *why*. Because trust me, it's rarely about the $22 nail trim charge or the fact they had to wait fifteen minutes. It's about fear: Fear that their pet is suffering, fear that they aren't being heard or valued, fear that they're losing control. If you can see past the yelling to the fear underneath, you've got the leverage to handle it.

Now, not all client frustration is created equal. I like to think of it in three levels.

Level 1: Dropping Hints of Frustration

They're pointing something out or dropping hints that they're potentially getting agitated. At Level 1, the client is still reachable and reasonable. They haven't blown up, and often they don't want to. But if their cues are ignored, they can slip into Level 2 (Angry) fast. This is the moment to lean in with curiosity and empathy.

How can you tell if a client is in Level 1? It's not always obvious, and it's easy to miss clues. It could sound like a subtle sigh, eye rolls, or quick glances at their watch or the clock. You might hear simple statements like "That's not what I was expecting" or "I thought you said this would only take a minute." Or questions like "Why is this taking so long?," "Is the Doctor running behind again?" or "Are you sure that's right, on the bill?" It might even show up in a passive-aggressive tone: "Well I guess I'll just wait here ... again" or "That's fine, whatever." Level 1 clients, in other words, haven't come out to bluntly express frustration, but they're dropping hints.

The easiest fire to put out is the one that hasn't spread. At Level 1, pay attention to body language: the crossed arms, the silence when they'd normally ask a question, and the confused look. This is your chance to lean in with curiosity:

- "Tell me how you're feeling about this."
- "Do we have an error on the invoice?"
- "Is something wrong? I can't quite tell what you're thinking."

That kind of gentle probing shows you care and can stop frustration from snowballing into rage.

Level 2: Complaining

Here, the client is undoubtedly angry or upset, but they are still manageable. So there's still a chance to turn things around.

So how do you handle upset clients? You've got options.

- Remind them you're here to help and want the same things they do. "I want the same thing you do—to help Buddy feel better." This is atop the list for a reason. By far, I've found this to be the most effective way to calm down an upset client in veterinary care—reminding them that you're on the same team.
- Shift the stage. Pull them out of the lobby and into a private space. Nobody calms down when they feel like they're on stage.
- Use nonverbal calm. Sit, turn your body at a 45-degree angle, keep your palms open, and slow your tone and blinking. You're broadcasting safety.
- Be curious. Let them vent. Do not interrupt.
- Paraphrase and mirror back. "What I'm hearing is ..." Even if you don't agree, validate the feeling.
- Ask if there's more. "Is there anything else that didn't feel right?"
- Share your side—only if they invite it. "I'd like to explain my perspective. Is that okay?"
- Offer options. Don't trap yourself in one solution. Present a few paths forward.
- Close with thanks. "I appreciate you sharing this. Even when it's hard to hear, your input matters."

Even if you don't agree with their reasoning, validate what they're feeling. Keep your body language neutral. No crossed arms. No sighs. No sarcasm. Your energy sets the tone.

Done right, this approach doesn't just solve the problem. It prevents things from escalating further. But perhaps most importantly, it builds trust in the middle of chaos.

Level 3: Verbal Assault

Here, the client has gone off the rails. Yelling, swearing, maybe threatening. Reason goes out the window. They're not looking for a solution in that moment—they're looking to unload. At this point, you're not solving the problem; you're just trying to defuse the bomb.

Level 3 is where most people screw it up: they argue back. They defend themselves. They explain policy. And all of that is useless. Once someone is screaming, the goal is no longer to solve the problem. The goal is to de-escalate. Period.

Because let's be real: when someone crosses into verbal assault, those tools won't cut it. That's when you need to flip to a different playbook: the ALARM method. When someone crosses into verbal assault, you flip the switch (or maybe I'll be cheeky and say *raise the ALARM*):

- **A—Area Change.** If the client is open to it and if you feel SAFE doing so, take the conversation off the lobby floor. Invite him or her into an open exam room for a private conversation so that they're not making a scene and stressing out other clients. (If this client is not open to this option, or if you fear for your safety by being alone with the client, skip this step.)
- **L—Listen.** Shut up and stop talking. Don't try to reason with a screaming person. Hear what they have to say.

- **A—Acknowledge.** Give cues that you're listen: "Uh huh." "Okay." Nod along. Make it clear to you're hearing them (but still without interrupting or chiming in).
- **R—Reset & Remind.** You're okay. Reset yourself. Remind yourself that the client isn't made at you; they're mad at the situation and usually acting emotionally, out of fear. Take a breath, and then:
- **M—Move on.** Calmly say:

"I hear you. I so badly want to help you and your pet, but I cannot do that while you're yelling at me because all I can focus on is you yelling at me. So this isn't productive for either of us right now. I want to help you, and I need some time to process what you've shared and figure out the best path forward. I'm going to respectfully ask you to leave for now, and I promise we'll get back to you later today."

That's it. That's the move. That's your closer. No more explaining. Just done. You're not trying to win. You're not trying to change their mind. You're not trying to solve the problem, at least not yet. You're trying to safely end the chaos so you can live to fight another day—to move on and close the interaction before things get worse. Sometimes, the best you can do is not end on a good note, but simply end. Calmly, respectfully, firmly. Then, you have time to work with your team to figure out the best path forward. And of course, you won't be able to make every client happy every time. Sometimes you'll be calling the client back to tell them you've already done all you can, or that the decision your team made won't be changing. But better to deliver that once they've had to process and calm down, and in a setting where they're not making a scene in front of other clients.

And if they keep yelling? You repeat yourself. Calmly. If it still doesn't stop? You escalate to a manager. If it gets threatening? You remove yourself and you call the police. Nobody—not a doctor, not a CSR, not a tech—deserves to be belittled or abused. Ever.

General Phrases to Avoid and Lean On to Encourage Client Calm

Now let's talk language, because words matter. There are phrases that pour water on the fire, and phrases that pour gasoline. Gasoline phrases to avoid sound like:

- *"Don't take it personally."*
- *"Calm down."*
- *"Don't be mad"* or *"Don't get angry"* (telling people how to feel)
- *"Stop being emotional"* or *"You're getting emotional."*
- *"This isn't my fault."*
- *"No offense, but ..."*
- Use of always or never *"You always do this ..."* or *"You never do this ..."*
- Bringing up the past: *"Last week you ..."* or *"Last visit you ..."*
- *"That's ridiculous."*
- *"I don't care"* or *"You don't care"*
- Blaming "corporate" or the computer. That's weak, excuse-making. And clients smell it from a mile away.
- In general, using the word "you": *"You did this,"* *"Here you go again,"* *"You are exaggerating,"* *"Here you go again,"* *"You calm down"*

Instead, use water phrases:

- *"I'm glad you told me."*
- *"I'm sorry you've had such a frustrating experience."*
- *"This isn't acceptable to us either."*
- *"Here's what I can do for you."*

These phrases don't mean you're rolling over; they mean you're in control. You're owning the interaction, you're showing empathy, and you're moving things forward.

Whenever possible, pull the client off the stage. The waiting room lobby is the worst place to hash things out. Take them into an exam room if you can. Listen intently. Mirror back: "You're upset because ..."

Summary

De-escalation isn't about keeping the peace. It's about proving you're the kind of leader who can take the punch, keep your composure, and still protect the trust that feeds your hospital.

Upset clients are inevitable in veterinary medicine, but chaos doesn't have to be. The way you show up in those heated moments determines whether you protect trust or destroy it.

- Level 1 frustration is your easiest win: catch the subtle cues early, lean in with curiosity, and stop problems before they escalate.
- Level 2 complaints demand calm leadership: validate emotions, remind clients you share the same goals, and offer paths forward. Done right, you not only resolve the issue, you deepen trust.
- Level 3 verbal assaults require strength, not defensiveness. That's when the ALARM Method is your playbook: change the area if safe, listen fully, acknowledge, reset yourself, and move on. You're not trying to "win" the fight or solve the problem (yet). You're protecting yourself, your team, and the other clients who are watching.

The bottom line: de-escalation isn't weakness, it's power. It's the art of diffusing tension, protecting your culture, and keeping the hospital safe for everyone—pets, clients, and staff. When you master these skills, you don't just avoid blowups; you build credibility as a leader who can stay calm under fire. And that credibility translates into the one thing you need most: trust.

Suggested Readings

American Animal Hospital Association. *De-escalation and Client Conflict Management in Veterinary Practices*. AAHA Press, 2023, www.aaha.org

American Veterinary Medical Association. *Workplace Safety and Client Aggression in Veterinary Medicine*. AVMA, 2022, www.avma.org

Bies, Robert J., and Joseph S. Moag. "Interactional Justice: Communication Criteria of Fairness." *Research on Negotiation in Organizations*, vol. 1, 1987, pp. 43–55.

Edmondson, Amy C. *The Fearless Organization: Creating Psychological Safety in the Workplace for Learning, Innovation, and Growth.* Wiley, 2018.

Goleman, Daniel. *Emotional Intelligence: Why It Can Matter More Than IQ.* Bantam, 2006.

Korn, Joseph H., and Jeffery W. Bremer. "Anger, Aggression, and Control: When Clients Become Verbally Abusive." *Professional Psychology: Research and Practice*, vol. 25, no. 1, 1994, pp. 64–72.

Maister, David H. *The Psychology of Waiting Lines.* David Maister Associates, 2005.

Occupational Safety and Health Administration. *Guidelines for Preventing Workplace Violence for Healthcare and Social Service Workers.* U.S. Department of Labor, 2016, www.osha.gov

Rogers, Carl R. *On Becoming a Person: A Therapist's View of Psychotherapy.* Houghton Mifflin, 1995.

Tax, Stephen S., Stephen W. Brown, and Murali Chandrashekaran. "Customer Evaluations of Service Complaint Experiences: Implications for Relationship Marketing." *Journal of Marketing*, vol. 62, no. 2, 1998, pp. 60–76.

Tucker, Amy L., and Amy C. Edmondson. "Why Hospitals Don't Learn from Failures: Organizational and Psychological Dynamics That Inhibit System Change." *California Management Review*, vol. 45, no. 2, 2003, pp. 55–72.

Zeithaml, Valarie A., Ananthanarayanan Parasuraman, and Leonard L. Berry. *Delivering Quality Service: Balancing Customer Perceptions and Expectations.* Free Press, 1990.

Chapter 25
Navigating Difficult Pricing Discussions

Let's not sugarcoat it—talking about price in veterinary medicine sucks. It's messy, it's emotional, and sometimes it's heartbreaking. But if you're in this field, it's part of the gig. Clients will complain about prices. Not "maybe." Not "someday." It's inevitable. And how you handle those conversations will either further build trust or nuke it.

Here's the thing: everything is expensive right now. Groceries, gas, housing—you name it. Inflation has been hammering people for years. So when pet owners walk through your doors, they're already primed with financial anxiety before you even say "Hello." Add in the fact that their pet is sick—their family member is hurting—and you've got the perfect storm for a meltdown.

I'll give you an example that crushed me. I was advising a specialty hospital who had taken in a 13-year-old Labradoodle, Caesar. The poor guy had an intestinal blockage from a rawhide, and emergency surgery was the only shot. The doctor, a friend of mine and one of the most compassionate people I know, did what every doctor has to do: she explained the urgency and the cost. The client flipped.

She screamed that the doctor was greedy, soulless, and even evil. Later, she wrote a brutal online review saying our hospital "profits from sick pets" and that "unless you're rich, don't bother."

When my doctor friend saw that review, she called me in tears. And you know what? She wasn't crying because someone insulted her. She was crying because she *wanted* to save Caesar's life and hated being painted as someone who didn't care. That's the paradox of veterinary medicine. You love animals so much that you've made it your life's work, but to keep the lights on, you *have* to charge for care.

So let's cut to the chase: you can't stop all price complaints. Sometimes, they're inevitable. But you can learn to navigate them without losing your sanity, your confidence, or your compassion.

I want to start by showcasing some "truths" I've learned about price increases, and then get specific for you—how to handle difficult conversations about pricing when clients push back on a treatment plan estimate or bill.

Five Truths About Client Price Increases and Strategies That Work

Truth #1: Price Complaints Are Rarely About Price

In a study I ran several years ago, specifically looking at why people complain about prices, here's what I found: less than 2% of clients who report having a great experience complain about cost. And the vast majority of survey responses and online reviews that include a complaint about price (e.g., "too expensive," "costs too much," "price gouging," etc.) also shared that something else had gone wrong during their hospital visit. That means most "it's too expensive" conversations are actually about something else: a long wait time, a cold interaction, a breakdown in communication. Price becomes the scapegoat.

The truth is, as we've increased prices across the veterinary industry, expectations from clients have risen as well. They expect superior care, as well as great experiences and service. We've discussed how clients want to feel during their hospital visit, and as we raise prices, clients increasingly EXPECT to have their wants and needs realized.

To be honest, I don't think that's unfair. Whenever I'm a customer of any company—especially a service industry—my expectations are high if they're charging what I perceive to be a high price. Whether I'm taking my car to be serviced, dining at a 5-star restaurant, or paying for a premium seat on an airplane, if I'm paying high prices, I'm expecting high-quality service that warrants that price. And if something goes wrong—if I feel undervalued, overlooked, and unconsidered as a customer—my mind immediately goes to asking, "What the hell am I paying for, here?"

Now, you might be thinking, "Well, Ryan, the fact that veterinary care has become so expensive nowadays is not my fault or the fault of my team. Why should we be responsible for having to raise our game and improve our service to warrant higher prices that we never wanted to charge in the first place?" My answer: because there's no alternative. Price increases in our industry, frankly, are what they are. You can't control inflation, higher vendor costs, increases to rent and taxes, etc.—I get that. But either you challenge your team to up their standards to warrant the higher prices that are beyond all of our controls, or you'll lose to the hospital up the street who does. But this is also a mute point: if you truly understand the Veterinary Trust Flywheel, you won't need to motivate your team to better serve clients "because client expectations have increased as prices have increased." They'll be motivated to better serve clients and earn client trust because they understand the value of doing so: a healthier culture, better service to clients in their moment of need, better pet outcomes, and a healthier future for the hospital. If you follow this principle and up your client experience game, you'll be delighted by how many fewer price complaints you get—because again, they're often accompanied by shitty client experiences.

So fix the experience. Deliver warmth, eye contact, empathy, and gratitude. Make people feel heard. If they leave thinking, "Yeah, that bill stung, but damn, they treated me and my pet like gold," then you've done your job.

Truth #2: No Surprises. Ever

The fastest way to piss off a client? Hand them a bill that's way higher than they expected. That's betrayal 101.

Always—always—share a treatment plan with the client before you touch their pet. Lay out the options, walk through the costs, and let them decide what works for their budget and their values. Clients don't need cheap; they need choice. They need to feel like *they* are in control of the decisions around their pet's care. This goes directly back to the client's need for partnership—to be heard and included.

Truth #3: Kill Anger with Kindness, Not Business Details

When someone's yelling about price, your instinct might be to defend yourself with logic: "Well, inflation ..." or "Well, our rent went up ..." or "Well, meds cost more now." Stop. Clients don't care about your overhead. They don't want a TED Talk on CPI trends. That's just noise to them. They'll see it as an excuse.

What they want is to feel like you still care about their pet more than you care about the invoice. So stay calm. Listen. Thank them for their honesty. Acknowledge their stress. Kindness disarms faster than facts. Don't fight fire with fire; fight fire with water. We'll talk more about HOW to do that later in this chapter.

Truth #4: Never Apologize for Your Prices

This is the one that gets most teams tripped up. You want to be empathetic, so you say, "Sorry it's so expensive." Don't. That one little word—*sorry*—undermines everything. It implies guilt, like you're charging unfairly.

Instead, stand tall in your value. "Thank you for trusting us with Buddy's care. Our priority is to deliver the highest standard of medical care so that Buddy receives the best care possible. Our fees reflect the training, equipment, and expertise it takes to deliver that."

And here's the kicker: it's not spin or bullshit. It's actually true. Every fair dollar that comes into your hospital fuels more staff, better tools, higher wages, and ultimately more lives saved. Charging fairly isn't greedy. It's the only way to keep delivering the care you love.

Truth #5: Some People Just Complain. Let Them

While most price complaints come from dissatisfaction about something else—a poor experience or surprise on the bill—you can do everything right and still get slammed sometimes. That's life. Don't let it get to you. One angry review doesn't cancel out the hundreds of quiet clients who are deeply grateful but never say a word. Anchor yourself in the reality that your work matters, your care is priceless, and your hospital deserves to thrive.

Here's the raw truth: there are clients who will complain no matter what you do. You could comp the bill, carry their dog to the car, hand them a Starbucks gift card, and they'd still find something to torch you for in a review. Some clients have reasonable concerns and are providing feedback that we ought to listen to in pursuit of improvement—that's great, and that's fair. But here, I'm talking about those few clients who will complain no matter what you do, who are offering nothing constructive or actionable and just want to complain for the sake of complaining.

How do you handle those clients? Well, if you have a client who's really violently complaining and objecting to price, start by following the advice I give in Chapter X about managing conflict. There, I talk about the importance of staying calm, listening, and diffusing the situation.

But I also want to add this, here: this past summer I read Mel Robbins' "The Let Them Theory." I highly recommend it, and some of the advice in her book is directly applicable here. Mel's advice? When people do what they do—gossip, nitpick, criticize, complain—your job isn't to fix them. Your job is to let them. Let them complain. Let them stew. Let them be who they are. Because the second you try to change their behavior, you hand them the keys to your own energy.

In her words, "Let them" is freedom. It's not surrender; it's strategy. You can't control what people say or do, but you can control what you give your attention to and whether or not you allow other people's actions to ruin your mood or your day.

So when Mrs. Jones is red-faced, calling you greedy for charging money to save her dog's life, take a breath and just remember: let her. Let her vent. Do what you can to diffuse the situation, then redirect your energy where it actually matters: to the hundreds of other clients who deeply appreciate your care. Don't let unreasonable, ungrateful people ruin your day.

In other words, stop playing defense against the 5% of clients who complain no matter what. Play offense with the 95% who love you. Mel's "let them" isn't weakness—it's a power move. It's how you protect your mindset so you can keep showing up for the clients and pets who actually deserve your energy.

The Bottom Line

Price conversations aren't about money. They're about trust. If clients trust you, the price becomes tolerable—even if it hurts. If they don't trust you, even a fair price will feel like a rip-off.

So stop apologizing, stop over-explaining, and start leading with transparency and unapologetic confidence in your worth. Your hospital isn't just selling "services." You're selling peace of mind. You're giving families more time with the creatures they love most. And be assured—that's worth every damn penny.

Your Irate-price Conversation Playbook

Let's be real: nothing knots your stomach faster than the moment a client looks at your treatment plan and says, "Are you kidding me? That's outrageous." You can feel the air shift, you can see their face tighten, and suddenly it's not just about a number on paper—it's about whether they trust you at all. That's where people crack. But this is also where leaders separate themselves from the pack. Handling these moments isn't about being slick or manipulative. It's about holding your ground, keeping your humanity, and refusing to let someone else's anger derail your hospital's mission.

Here's how to handle it when these (unfortunately, sometimes inevitable) situations arise:

Step 1: De-escalate and Anchor to the Pet

When a client first verbalizes a concern about price, the first 30 seconds matter more than anything. Your goal is to lower the temperature without lowering your standards. That means you don't match their volume if they're getting agitated. You don't roll your eyes. You don't get defensive. You stay calm, and you bring it back to the one thing you both actually care about: the pet.

What does that sound like? Let's say a client is objecting to a treatment plan estimate, and immediately exclaims, "This is the actual cost? This is outrageous!" Your move is to respond with something simple: "Thank you for being straight with me about how you're feeling. I can hear the stress in your voice. Remember that we're on the same side—both of us want Buddy to be comfortable and safe. Give me a minute to walk you through the plan so you can decide what works best."

Boom. You validated their stress, you made it clear you're aligned, and you put a boundary on the conversation. No apology, no flinch, and no lecture. Just empathy and control.

Step 2: Set the Frame: Intention, Not Justification

Here's how some hospital teams blow it: they start explaining overhead—"our rent went up, our meds cost more, inflation blah blah blah." Guess what? Clients don't give a damn about your rent. They care about their cat bleeding on the table and how they're going to get that cat the care he needs.

So instead of justifying costs, set the frame around intention. Lay it out like this: "This plan is built to do two things: relieve Bella's pain now, and rule out the dangerous stuff early so we don't miss anything. I've got three versions of this plan—gold, silver, and essentials—so you can decide what feels right for you and Bella."

Notice what happened? You reframed the conversation around outcomes, not invoices. You handed them a choice, rather than forcing them into a corner.

Step 3: Put the Options on the Table

Never, ever hand a client a single estimate like it's a ransom note. Options are your secret weapon: "Gold covers everything today. Silver tackles pain and the top risks first. Essentials stabilize now and plans the rest later." You put them all down in writing. You walk the client through them side by side. You circle or point out the key differences. You invite them to choose.

And here's the line that closes the loop: "We'll only move forward on what you feel most comfortable with and authorize."

That one sentence kills 80% of price blow-ups because it gives clients control. The fear of being railroaded is eliminated.

Step 4: Ride Out the Eruption

Okay, let's say you do all that and the client still loses it. They call the price outrageous, accuse you of being greedy, maybe even drop the "you don't care about animals" bomb. This is the moment where your stomach flips and you want to either fight or flee. But don't.

Instead, run a quick loop: "Reflect, Align, Redirect."

- Reflect: "I hear you; It feels like a lot."
- Align: "Your priority and our priority is getting Buddy help today."
- Redirect: "So do you want the gold plan that covers everything now, or the silver plan that gets pain under control and rules out the biggest risks today?"

You see the move? You acknowledge the heat, you center on the shared goal, and then you immediately redirect back to options. You don't leave the conversation sitting in complaint mode. You keep it moving.

What about when clients really go for the gut punch? They tell you, "you're greedy," "you're price gouging" or "you're only in it for the money." That hurts—a lot. I've been there; I've had clients say this to my face, too. So I get it. It hurts because it's the opposite of who you are. You got into this field to help animals and pet owners, not to make a quick buck. But you can't show that pain on your face. Instead, answer with calm conviction.

The "Reflect, Align, Redirect" strategy works here, too:

"I get how scary this is. We're here because we care about Buddy. We charge what we do so our doctors and nurses can deliver the highest level of care with the best tools and training. That's how we keep helping families like yours tomorrow, too."

Then, redirect: "Which option feels right for you today?"

Notice: no apology, no defensiveness, no lecture. Just steady confidence in your value and a hand back to the client.

Step 5: Close the Loop with Consent

Once the client picks an option, don't just say "Great" and disappear. Close with crystal clarity: "Perfect—silver plan it is. Total today is $____. With your okay here, we'll start pain control in the next

10 minutes, then move to [next step]. If anything changes, medically, or cost-wise, we'll pause and talk before doing anything else."

That "pause-if-things-change" line is magic. It reinforces transparency and continues to build trust.

Those are my five steps, and they've proven to be the most effective steps I've seen in these unfortunate situations.

But What About When They Truly Can't Afford It?

Here's the reality check: sometimes the client flat-out cannot afford even the essentials. This sucks, but it happens. And when it does, your job is to preserve the relationship and still offer a medically-responsible path.

Say this: "Thank you for telling me. We've got two paths: essentials today to keep Max comfortable and safe, then stage the rest over time; or financing, which we can check now and, if approved, gets us started today while spreading payments out."

If neither works, you don't abandon them. You point to safety-net options in the community. It's not ideal, but it's honest.

Summary

Price conversations aren't about money. They're about trust, control, and whether clients believe you actually care. If you can stay calm, frame care around outcomes, show options, give the client a say in their pet's care, and never apologize for your worth, you have the best chance to turn even the ugliest moments into trust-building opportunities.

The client doesn't walk out saying, "That was cheap." They walk out saying, "That price stung, but damn, they took incredible care of Max." That's the win. That's how you survive the price war: by never making it a war in the first place. If your client trusts you, they'll appreciate your candor and care even if the bill stings. If they don't, even the fairest estimate will feel like robbery.

So stop playing defense. Stop apologizing for your prices. Stop hiding behind inflation charts or your rent going up. None of that matters in the moment. What matters is how you make people feel. Do they feel heard? Do they feel like they had a choice? Do they feel like you gave a damn about their pet first and the invoice second? That's the game.

Your playbook is simple:

- No surprises—ever.
- Anchor every tough convo to the pet, not the price.
- Give options, not ultimatums.
- Stay calm, kind, and confident in your worth.
- And when the outliers show up—the clients who just want to complain no matter what? Let them. Don't waste your energy trying to fix the unfixable. Pour your energy into the 95% of clients who see your heart and trust your care.

And again, for those unreasonable clients who complain for the hell of it or don't have reasonable expectations? Remember what Mel Robbins suggests: let them. Let them complain, let them rant, let them be who they are. Because the moment you try to win them over at the expense of your own energy, you lose. And if you let these people get to you and ruin your energy or your mood, you'll have a harder time remaining calm, balanced, and rational when dealing with the next client—so the next client loses too. "Let them" isn't giving up or giving in. It's freedom. It's choosing to pour your energy into the 95% of reasonable clients who are grateful and appreciate your efforts and intentions, not the 5% who will never see the good you do.

Suggested Readings

American Animal Hospital Association. *The Cost of Care: Communicating Value and Addressing Financial Barriers in Veterinary Medicine.* AAHA Press, 2022, www.aaha.org

American Veterinary Medical Association. *Economic State of the Veterinary Profession: Costs, Inflation, and Client Affordability.* AVMA, 2023, www.avma.org

Cialdini, Robert B. *Influence: The Psychology of Persuasion.* Rev. ed., Harper Business, 2021.

Edmondson, Amy C. *The Fearless Organization: Creating Psychological Safety in the Workplace for Learning, Innovation, and Growth.* Wiley, 2018.

Maister, David H. *The Psychology of Waiting Lines.* David Maister Associates, 2005.

Robbins, Mel. *The Let Them Theory.* Hay House, 2024.

Tax, Stephen S., Stephen W. Brown, and Murali Chandrashekaran. "Customer Evaluations of Service Complaint Experiences: Implications for Relationship Marketing." *Journal of Marketing*, vol. 62, no. 2, 1998, pp. 60–76.

Thaler, Richard H., and Cass R. Sunstein. *Nudge: Improving Decisions About Health, Wealth, and Happiness.* Rev. ed., Penguin, 2021.

Chapter 26
Embrace the Small Moments That Matter

People don't remember the grind of everyday details. They remember the "spikes"—the highs that made them feel special, the "lows" that crushed them, and the "moments of change" where something shifted. Chip and Dan Heath described this in their book *The Power of Moments*, a book I referenced often when advising clients on their customer experience strategies while working as a CX consultant. The Heath brothers call these moments "defining moments," and the crazy thing is, they're not accidents. You can design them.

Think about that for a second. Every single client walking into your hospital is primed for an emotional memory: their dog's first check-up, their cat's scary illness, their kid's tears in the lobby. These are moments they'll think and talk about for years. The question is: are you going to let those moments happen by chance, or are you going to create them with intention?

And here's the best part: it doesn't take balloons, champagne, or some huge budget. It's not about grand gestures. It's about the smallest details done consistently and with heart. Asking, "Anything else on your mind before we wrap up?" That's a defining moment. Making a follow-up call the next day—defining moment. Walking a client to their car—ditto.

This chapter is about those micro-moves. The tiny actions that don't cost you much time but build loyalty like nothing else. The Heath brothers would say these are your chances to create "peaks" in a client's memory. I'd say they are your opportunity to stop being forgettable and start being legendary.

Because in veterinary medicine—hell, in life—the little things aren't little. They're everything. In veterinary medicine, the big stuff often gets all the credit: the lifesaving surgeries, the complex diagnoses, and the heroic overnight shifts. And yeah, those are incredible. But the secret to winning a client's trust for life isn't typically in the big things. It's in the *tiny*, everyday touches—like Carla from Ryan Veterinary Hospital getting me to crack a smile while Buddy was undergoing lifesaving surgery after being attacked.

Here's my list of "micro-moves" strategies that take almost zero extra time, cost nothing, and yet hit your clients straight in the heart. A lot of these might look familiar to you. They're so simple, yet so many animal hospitals overlook them. Absolutely zero of them are complex or difficult, but stack them up consistently, and suddenly your hospital feels like home.

The "Anything Else?" Pause

Most doctors wrap a visit with something like, "Alright, we'll see you in six months." Boom. Done. Transaction over. But here's the kicker: nine times out of ten, the client is still sitting there with something else on their mind. They just don't want to "bother you."

That's where the magic happens. Just pause for two seconds and say: *"Anything else on your mind before we wrap up?"* or *"Any other questions for me about Buddy before we finish for today?"*

That single line stops clients from walking out the door with doubts, unasked questions, or lingering fears. It tells them: I've still got time for you. You matter.

It's tiny. It's free. And it screams care. And if the client does have additional concerns, sometimes it leads to a conversation that elevates patient care. It also has the potential to save both you and the client time later on: it eliminates the risk that the client leaves regretting that they didn't get to ask that extra question, which can often lead to them making an additional phone call to the hospital the next day to get that question answered.

The Pet AND Client Day-after Check-in

I'm a huge proponent of calling clients the day after an appointment, even if it was just a basic wellness exam.

In Chapter 4, I described a strategy I noticed a CSR named Sam adopting in her animal hospital, where she turned a usually routine call into a peak micro-moment by making the call feel more personal and genuine. As you might remember, she didn't limit the conversation to, *"How is your pet doing?"* but also asked about the client.

After checking in on the pet, Shadow, she followed up and went a little above and beyond: *"Becky, I know yesterday was stressful for you, too. How are you holding up today? Did you think of any questions last night that you didn't get a chance to ask yesterday that maybe I can answer for you now?"*

Now, the exact verbiage may obviously be more appropriate for higher-stakes visits and more serious medical concerns where the client had a reason to feel stressed (which may not be the case for a basic wellness exam). But the point still holds: take the opportunity to consider the client's feelings and needs during your follow up calls, rather than limiting the conversation to ONLY be about the pet. That's the point.

This extra step takes a few extra seconds. But to the client, you've just gone above and beyond. They'll tell their friends, their coworkers, and their neighbor at the dog park.

The Pet Name Sprinkle

Clients love hearing their pet's name. Not just once at check-in. Sprinkle it throughout the whole damn visit. "Buddy looks great." "How's Buddy's appetite been?" "Buddy was such a champ for his vaccines."

It's not about theatrics. It's about respect. Pets are family. And when you use their name, you're saying: I see your family member, not just your invoice.

The Pet Compliment

Similarly, find opportunities to compliment the pet. This is simple, but money: "Wow, Buddy's coat looks incredible—What's your secret?" Pet owners light up. This will earn you massive goodwill.

The Client Affirmation

This one will come at no surprise given the detail I've given throughout this book about how clients crave to feel affirmed by their hospital team. But it's so important that it's worth repeating, and here, I'll give some tangible examples on what client affirmations might sound like:

Affirming Their Care and Commitment:

- "You're doing such a great job with Buddy. We can tell he's loved and cared for."
- "I can see how much time and energy you put into keeping Buddy healthy."

- "Buddy's coat/weight/energy shows the effort you've been putting in. Really nice work!"

Affirming Their Decisions:

- "You did the right thing by bringing Buddy in today—catching this early makes a huge difference."
- "I know this decision wasn't easy, but you're making the best choice for Buddy."
- "It's clear you've been thinking carefully about what's best for Buddy, and that matters."

Affirming Their Love and Bond:

- "It's obvious how much you love Buddy. He's lucky to have you."
- "I can tell the bond between you and Buddy is strong. He trusts you."

Affirming Their Advocacy:

- "Thank you for speaking up for Buddy. You know him best, and your input helps us care for him better."
- "We appreciate the questions you're asking. It shows how much you want the best for Buddy."
- "You've been such a strong advocate for Buddy's health. That makes a huge difference in his care."

Affirming Their Patience and Understanding

This relates directly back to the PAGE strategy of Proactive Gratitude, too.

- "Thank you so much for your patience today—we know waiting isn't easy, and it means a lot."
- "We appreciate how understanding you've been, especially with that emergency we had."
- "Thanks for rolling with us today. You've been awesome."

The Milestones Celebrations

Why do hospitals wait until something bad happens to show emotion? Flip it. Make the good moments loud. Clients will never forget joy delivered with enthusiasm.

First puppy visit? Put it on a whiteboard in the lobby: *"Congrats to Max—first check-up today!"* Cancer-free anniversary? Hand the client a tiny "certificate of bravery" for their pet. Here are a few more examples:

- Adoption Day/Gotcha Day. First visit after a client adopts a pet? Celebrate like a birthday. Snap a photo, give a "Welcome to the Family" certificate, or post a quick shout-out (with permission).
- Weight-Loss or Health Goal Achieved. If a dog drops those extra 10 pounds, or a diabetic cat's glucose levels stabilize, make it a big deal. "Charlie crushed his weight goal—healthier and happier!"
- Graduating from Puppy/Kitten Series. Last vaccine in the series? Hand out a "Big Kid Now" bandana or snap a "Graduation" picture.
- First Senior Exam. When a pet officially enters "senior" care, mark it as a celebration of longevity, not a sad milestone. "Rocky just joined our Senior Wellness Club!"
- Celebrate Health Victories. Removed sutures? Call it a "healing graduation" or give a little "Bravery Certificate." After a dental cleaning, hand out a "Fresh Smile" photo card or sticker. Or if an at-risk pet's bloodwork comes back clean, announce it with joy: "Great news! Bella's results are clear!"
- Annual Loyalty Recognition. Some hospitals do a little "Happy Anniversary" message when a client has been with them for 1 year, 5 years, and 10 years. Low effort, huge payoff.
- Pet Birthday or Half-Birthday. If you've got the date on file, drop a quick text or email: "Happy Birthday, Luna! Thanks for letting us celebrate another year with you."

- "Cancer-Free" or Chronic-Illness Milestones. Acknowledge remission anniversaries or 1-year milestones living with a chronic illness. Clients treasure that recognition.
- Client Milestones. Sometimes it's not about the pet. Congratulate the family on life events they mention: a new baby, retirement, graduation. It shows you're listening beyond the exam room.

Like all of the tactics in this chapter, none of these cost more than a minute or two of effort, but they make a family feel like their pet just graduated Harvard.

The Gratitude at Checkout

Here's one that's criminally underused. At the desk, don't just slide a receipt across. Look the client in the eye and say: "Thanks for trusting us with Daisy today. We loved seeing her."

It's such a basic human move, but it transforms a transaction into connection.

The Photo Op and Social Shoutout

Take 10 seconds to snap a pic of the puppy with their first vaccines. Text it to the client or, with permission, tag them on your hospital's social feed.

That photo isn't just cute; it's a digital memory you created for them. They'll keep it forever, and they'll remember who gave it to them.

One of my favorite strategies is to text a client a picture of their pet when they've completed a successful surgery. You can make it fun—put a medical cap on the pet and snap a quick photo. Same idea: a simple step that brings joy (and relief) that will live forever in the client's memory.

The Human Stuff Recollection

Similar to the client milestones above, remember tidbits about your clients and their lives. When Mrs. Lopez tells you her kid has a soccer final, jot it down. Next visit, ask how it went. That little recall tells the client, "I see you as more than a credit card. I actually care about your life."

And the client thinks: "This place is different."

The Help to the Car

It's five steps. That's all. But when a client is juggling a leash, a carrier, and a bag of meds, offering to walk them to their car is five-star service. Hospitality lives in those little offers.

Summary

In vet med, the small stuff isn't small. It's the whole game.

Client trust isn't earned in the big, flashy moments. It's won in the small ones. The two-second pause where you ask, "Anything else on your mind?" The check-in call the next day that feels anything but routine. Saying the pet's name like it actually matters, because it does. Walking a client to their car when their hands are full. That's the shit people remember.

The truth? Clients expect the big stuff. Surgery, diagnostics, treatment. That's the baseline. That's table stakes. What they tell their neighbor at the dog park, what makes them write a five-star review? The micro-moves. The everyday touches that scream: *we see you, we value you, you matter to us.*

So eliminate the misconception within your team that successful client experiences require big, bold grand gestures or crazy-unique ideas that nobody has thought of before. While big, bold ideas can be great, start with the small stuff. Because in this business—and frankly, in life—the little things aren't little. They're everything. Stack these little moments day after day, client after client, and your hospital becomes legendary, because of how people feel when they walk out your door.

The little things *are* the big things. Stop chasing gimmicks. Double down on the micro-moves. That's how you turn ordinary visits into defining memories. That's how you build trust that lasts.

Suggested Readings

American Animal Hospital Association. *Clients as Partners: Strengthening the Human–animal Bond Through Communication.* AAHA Press, 2021, www.aaha.org

Fredrickson, Barbara L. "The Role of Positive Emotions in Positive Psychology." *American Psychologist*, vol. 56, no. 3, 2001, pp. 218–226.

Gallup. *The HumanSigma Framework for Emotional Engagement.* Gallup Press, 2019, www.gallup.com

Heath, Chip, and Dan Heath. *The Power of Moments: Why Certain Experiences Have Extraordinary Impact.* Simon & Schuster, 2017.

Kahneman, Daniel. "Objective Happiness." In Daniel Kahneman, Ed Diener, and Norbert Schwarz (Eds.), *Well-being: The Foundations of Hedonic Psychology* (pp. 3–25). Russell Sage Foundation, 1999.

Keller, Ed, and Jon Berry. *The Influentials: One American in Ten Tells the Other Nine How to Vote, Where to Eat, and What to Buy.* Free Press, 2003.

Maister, David H. *The Psychology of Waiting Lines.* David Maister Associates, 2005.

Pine, B. Joseph, and James H. Gilmore. *The Experience Economy.* Updated ed., Harvard Business Review Press, 2019.

Chapter 27
Take Pride in Your Hospital's Design and Feel

You want to talk about trust? Okay, let's get real: trust isn't just what you say, how you treat clients, or what your specialists do. Trust is what people *feel* when they walk through the door. That includes what they see, smell, and hear—before you even say a word. That first impression can lock in trust or shatter it.

If you're a hospital leader or owner, your hospital design is one of the best places to invest. Because you can't always change personalities or budgets overnight, but you *can* change the design of your hospital. And that change *can pay off*: in client confidence, referrals, loyalty, outcomes, and word-of-mouth. Let's dive in.

What the Research Says

Here are the facts. Multiple studies, recent architectural research, and evidence-based design in both human and veterinary settings show that the built environment has real, measurable effects on outcomes. Not just aesthetic. Actual outcomes. Reduced stress. Better compliance. More trust.

Here are the key findings:

- Evidence-based design (EBD) principles: Things like access to daylight, nature views, good lighting, acoustics, materials don't just look good. They help reduce stress for animals, reduce staff fatigue, reduce errors, improve patient rest, and improve satisfaction.
- In veterinary hospital design, species-specific needs matter. What feels safe for a cat is different from what a dog tolerates. The waiting room, the smells, the sightlines. If dogs bark right next to cats, you're creating anxiety. If possible, have separate waiting areas for dogs and cats. If that's not possible, encourage pet owners to wait comfortably in their car (weather-permitting) until you're ready to see them, then usher them directly to the exam room when it's their turn.
- Layout, workflow, and space planning mat ter. A poor layout can create bottlenecks, staff inefficiencies, elevated noise, and more stress all around—for clients and your team. Better layout supports smoother operations, faster responses, and less animal agitation. Pet owners shouldn't have sight into surgery rooms, animals under anesthesia, or anything else even remotely graphic. That's simple respect.
- Lighting, color, finishes—even flooring—matter. Natural light, softer lighting, and biophilic elements (plants, wood tones, and nature views) calm people and animals. Harsh lighting, loud colors, and clashing finishes—those send subconscious signals: "medical, cold, stressful."
- Waiting rooms and front-of-house design are super important. The moment a pet parent walks in: smells, reception desk lay-out, visibility, and waiting room comfort—these all affect how safe, trusted, and calm the client feels.
- Animal welfare informs design. For instance, noise control, sightlines that reduce fear, dedicated species-specific zones, safe transport from car to exam room, and "buffer" zones so animals don't get unnerved by each other.

- Look, this one's not from a study—it's just something I've always felt strongly about. Cut the crap off your walls and front desk. I know pharma reps and vendors love to throw posters and displays at you, but trust me: nobody wants to walk into a waiting room and be greeted by giant photos, displays, or live TV images of fleas, ticks, and parasites. It's gross. It's not welcoming or trust-building. In my opinion, if it's not something you'd proudly hang in your living room, it doesn't belong in your lobby. Your waiting room should feel calm and inviting, not like a flea circus. And for the love of God, clear off the front desk. If clients can barely make eye contact with the CSR or find a spot to sign a form because of all the tchotchkes and branded materials piled up on the front desk, you're doing it wrong. Keep it clean. Keep it human. Prioritize connection, not clutter.

Why Design Is a Trust Multiplier (Not Just a Nice-to-Have)

Here's where I get fired up: too many hospitals treat the building like wallpaper. "Yeah, we'll put nice tiles, paint it calming colors." But design is a trust multiplier. It *amplifies* everything you do well, and it *exposes* everything you don't.

If your clinical outcomes are great, but your hospital feels stressful, noisy, and confusing, that drags down everything. Clients leave uneasy. On the other hand, if your hospital feels safe, warm, and thoughtful, clients are emotionally primed to believe you, to follow your recommendations, to refer you.

In short: design isn't decoration. It's part of the promise you make. It is *nonverbal communication* saying: "We respect you. We understand your pet. We've thought about your stress. We want you to feel safe, comfortable, and considered here."

Action Plan: How Hospitals Can Use Design to Earn Trust

This is your checklist. Don't get stuck in dreaming. Make moves.

1. Walk your hospital as if you're a client. Park, walk to the door, wait, and go into the exam room. What hits you first? How's the smell, the sound, the light? Take notes.

2. Map the flow. From reception to treatment to discharge. Where are choke points? Long corridors? Noisy intersections? Where are clients exposed to animal stressors (other animals, smells, noise)?

3. Invest in lighting and natural light. If windows are possible, maximize them. If not, get LED lighting that mimics daylight. Use softer lighting in waiting rooms and exam rooms.

4. Design or reconfigure waiting rooms. Separate species if you can. Use comfortable furniture. Clean surfaces. Visual barriers if needed. Access to water, treats. Calming materials.

5. Make exam rooms both functional and comforting. Adjustable tables. Provide places to put carriers safely. Have lighting that's not harsh, surfaces that are clean and safe.

6. Create private, compassionate spaces. A room where staff can deliver bad news, talk about euthanasia, or hold after-hours grievances. Don't force such moments to happen in public view.

7. Consistent aesthetic and finish quality. If your front door looks nice but the corridors are peeling paint, and have flickering lights and worn floors, you're losing trust. Keep your finishes, materials, and surfaces looking cared for.

8. Choose materials with durability AND comfort in mind. Surfaces that clean easily but don't look harsh. Flooring safe for paws. Wall colors that feel warm, not clinical. Scent control and ventilation that neutralize odors.

9. Noise control and sensory management. Use sound-absorbing materials, create quiet zones, reduce mechanical noise, separate louder work areas from quieter ones.

10. Get feedback & iterate. Ask clients what made them anxious in your space. Survey them about lighting, waiting, and comfort. Use those insights to make small but meaningful changes.

Challenges & How to Overcome Them

Because I know what you'll say: "Ryan, this all sounds expensive," or "We've got limitations: an old building, budget constraints." Cool, but here's how you still win:

- Prioritize low-cost/high-impact fixes first. Paint, furniture, lighting, rethinking waiting room layout. These can move trust a lot.
- Phased improvements. Don't try to rebuild the whole building at once. Do sections (like, do exam rooms or do reception). Then move out in waves.
- Use temporary/mobile design hacks. Curtains, room dividers, plants, and calming panels. These can make an immediate difference while you plan bigger redevelopment.
- Engage your team. Let staff point out pain points in flow, lighting, smells. They live in the space. Their observations often uncover high-return fixes.
- Use the research to build your case. When you propose budget for design improvements, show data: stress reduction, faster healing, better client retention, and staff satisfaction. Use proven studies (EBD, etc.) so leadership sees ROI.

Summary

If you nail design, you don't just get a pretty building. You get *credibility*, *confidence*, *calm*, *trust*. Every client who walks in already has fear, worry, hope. Your design can help them lean toward hope. Design can become a key part of your brand and reputation. It can yell (silently): "You're in the right place." Your exam rooms, your corridors, your waiting room—all of that becomes part of the reputation they are trusting you with.

Suggested Readings

American Animal Hospital Association. *Veterinary Facility Design Guide*. AAHA Press, 2018, www.aaha.org

Benedetti, Francesca, et al. "Effects of Light on Health: The Role of Daylight and Artificial Lighting." *Neuroscience and Biobehavioral Reviews*, vol. 113, 2020, pp. 180–199.

Bringslimark, Tina, Terje Hartig, and Grete G. Patil. "The Psychological Benefits of Indoor Plants." *Journal of Environmental Psychology*, vol. 29, no. 4, 2009, pp. 422–433.

Hansen, Bjarke V., et al. "Influence of Acoustics on Patient Recovery and Staff Performance." *Building and Environment*, vol. 95, 2016, pp. 68–77.

Institute for Healthcare Improvement. *Evidence-based Design for Healthcare Facilities*. IHI, 2017, www.ihi.org

Kazemzadeh, Nima, et al. "Environmental Stressors and Their Effects on Companion Animals in Veterinary Clinics." *Journal of Veterinary Behavior*, vol. 45, 2021, pp. 1–8.

Pine, B. Joseph, and James H. Gilmore. *The Experience Economy*. Updated ed., Harvard Business Review Press, 2019.

Ulrich, Roger S., et al. "A Review of the Research Literature on Evidence-based Healthcare Design." *HERD: Health Environments Research & Design Journal*, vol. 1, no. 3, 2008, pp. 61–125.

Wells, Nancy M. "The Effect of School Design on Student Performance." *Journal of Environmental Psychology*, vol. 20, no. 2, 2000, pp. 173–181.

Chapter 28
Designing the End-of-life Experience with Intention

INTRO: The Final Visit Defines the Entire Relationship

There is no moment in veterinary medicine more emotionally charged, more delicate, or more defining than end-of-life care.

It's the moment that lives forever in a client's memory.
It's the moment they replay in their mind for years.
It's the moment they talk about whenever your hospital's name comes up.
It's the moment that either becomes a story of pain or a story of gratitude.

Often, it's the moment that dictates whether the client adopts another pet in the future or not.

Clients don't always remember the thousand small things you did right for their pet. But they do remember the final thing.

This chapter is about intentionally designing the end-of-life experience—not reacting to it, not improvising it, not hoping it goes smoothly, but *engineering* it with dignity, compassion, emotional clarity, and trust.

End-of-life care is not "just another appointment." It is the emotional Super Bowl of veterinary CX. This is where reputations are made. This is where the Trust Flywheel compounds like nothing else. This is where lifelong loyalty is born, often in the middle of heartbreak.

And if you design it with intention, your hospital becomes not just a medical facility, but a sanctuary.

The Six Pillars of an Intentional End-of-life Experience

These pillars are the difference between transactional and transcendent.

Pre-visit Guidance (So Clients Don't Feel Alone Before They Arrive)

Clients are terrified before EOL visits. They're asking:

"Will my pet suffer?"
"How long will it take?"
"What will it look like?"
"Can I hold them?"
"Will I regret something?"
"Will the team judge me?"

A simple pre-visit message dissolves 70% of their fear.

Here's a sample Pre-visit Message: "I'm so sorry you're facing this. We'll take gentle care of you and Milo every step of the way. Here's what to expect during the process, what to bring, and how we honor this moment with you."

This creates emotional safety before they walk in the door.

The Sacred Room Setup

The room (many hospitals call it a *comfort room*) must communicate warmth, compassion, and softness.

Here's what to include:

- Soft blankets
- Dimmed lighting
- Tissues
- Water bottles
- Privacy sign
- Soft music option
- Comfortable seating
- A symbolic object (candle, pawprint stone, or small plush)
- No medical clutter in sight
- No "clock-watching" items
- No stainless-steel coldness
- No interruptions

If possible, have a separate exit from your comfort room directly to the hospital exterior, so that your clients who just said their goodbye don't have to walk back through the lobby looking emotionally devastated.

This is not about aesthetics. This is about *permission*—permission to feel, to cry, to say goodbye without fear of being watched or rushed.

The Emotional Check-in (The First 30 Seconds)

You set the entire tone with your first words. Never open with paperwork. Never open with logistics.

Use this: "I'm so sorry you're going through this. Before we begin, how are you holding up? What support do you need from us today?"

Then be silent.
Let them cry.
Let them breathe.

This moment matters more than any medication.

The Gentle Medical Roadmap (Clarity Removes Fear)

Clients fear the unknown. The process should be explained with extreme gentleness and transparency.

Script Example: "I'm going to walk you step-by-step through what will happen so nothing feels sudden. We'll go at your pace, and you can stop me anytime."

Outline:

1. Sedation
2. Time to say goodbye
3. Final injection
4. Peaceful passing
5. Aftercare options

This reduces panic. It builds trust. It honors their emotional bravery.

The Ceremony (Yes, Ceremony—This Is a Ritual)

The best hospitals create rituals that turn grief into connection.

Ideas include:

- A soft candle with "This flame honors your love."
- A final pawprint made
- A farewell blanket
- A memory stone
- A fur clipping given in a small envelope
- A comfort basket with tissues and chocolate
- Writing the pet's name on a tile, leaf, or wall
- A "moment of silence" led by the doctor
- A "final walk" exit where team members lower their voices

These rituals don't cost much. But they mean everything.

The Follow-up (The Moment That Creates Lifelong Loyalty)

Most hospitals stop caring once the appointment ends. Elite hospitals continue caring.

Follow-Up Options:

- A handwritten sympathy card
- A phone call 24–48 hours later
- A memorial donation in the pet's name
- A digital memorial photo
- A grief-support resource list
- An email acknowledging their loss and offering support

This one gesture creates seismic emotional loyalty. Clients never forget who cared for them in their darkest hour.

The Power of a Dedicated EOL Team (The "Comfort Crew")

Some hospitals create a Comfort Crew, team members who are:

- Emotionally intelligent
- Calm under pressure
- Gifted with grief support
- Skilled at narration
- Able to hold emotional space

These team members:

- Prepare the room
- Greet the family
- Walk them through the process
- Handle aftercare
- Provide tissues
- Provide quiet presence

This reduces doctor overwhelm and elevates the entire experience.

Summary

Intentional end-of-life care rests on six core pillars that transform a heartbreaking moment into one filled with dignity, connection, and peace. It begins with pre-visit guidance, giving families clarity about what to expect before they even walk through the door—reducing fear and setting the tone for a supportive, predictable experience. Once they arrive, the environment matters deeply; compassionate room design creates a safe emotional space where grief feels held rather than exposed, replacing clinical coldness with warmth, softness, and privacy.

The experience continues with an emotional check-in, a moment where team members acknowledge the family's pain and ask what support they need. This alone can transform panic into trust. Families then need a gentle, step-by-step roadmap, ensuring nothing feels rushed, sudden, or unexplained. Every stage of the process should be narrated with care so that no one is left wondering or fearing what comes next.

Intentionality continues through ceremonial touches—small but meaningful rituals that honor the life of the pet and the love behind the decision. These moments become some of the most cherished memories for grieving families. Finally, meaningful follow-up ensures your compassion doesn't end when the appointment does. A heartfelt card, a phone call, or a memorial gesture reinforces that their loss mattered to you long after they left the hospital.

And above all, remember this: you're not just helping a pet pass—you're helping a family heal. The way you handle this moment becomes part of the emotional legacy of your hospital. Families will remember your presence, your gentleness, and your care for the rest of their lives.

Suggested Readings

American Animal Hospital Association. *End-of-Life Care Guidelines*. AAHA, 2020, www.aaha.org

Cooney, Kathleen A. *The Veterinary Guide to Pet Loss: A Comprehensive Resource for Supporting Clients and Staff*. Wiley-Blackwell, 2012.

Corr, Charles A., Clyde M. Nabe, and Donna M. Corr. *Death and Dying, Life and Living*. 7th ed., Cengage Learning, 2013.

Hafen, Brenda Q., et al. *Counseling Strategies for Loss and Grief*. 4th ed., Prentice Hall, 2007.

Hoad, Jody, et al. "Owner Experiences with Companion Animal Euthanasia." *Journal of Veterinary Behavior*, vol. 49, 2022, pp. 1–9.

Institute for Human-Animal Connection. *The Human-animal Bond and Grief Support in Veterinary Medicine*. University of Denver, 2019.

Kogan, Lori R., et al. "Grief and Bereavement Support in Veterinary Medicine." *Veterinary Clinics of North America: Small Animal Practice*, vol. 46, no. 3, 2016, pp. 541–556.

Norberg, Amy L., et al. "Pet Loss and Human Bereavement: A Qualitative Study." *Omega: Journal of Death and Dying*, vol. 80, no. 3, 2020, pp. 402–424.

Quackenbush, Judi E., and Jeff K. McCutcheon. *Pet Loss Support Hotline Training Manual*. Purdue University Press, 2000.

Relf, P. Diane. "Ritual and Healing in Grief and Loss." *Journal of Therapeutic Horticulture*, vol. 20, 2010, pp. 5–15.

Rollin, Bernard E. *An Introduction to Veterinary Medical Ethics: Theory and Cases*. 3rd ed., Wiley-Blackwell, 2011.

Shanan, Alan. "The Veterinarian's Role in End-of-Life Care." *Veterinary Clinics of North America: Small Animal Practice*, vol. 43, no. 3, 2013, pp. 515–525.

Ulrich, Roger S., et al. "The Role of the Physical Environment in the Hospital of the 21st Century." *The Center for Health Design*, 2008.

Chapter 29
Crush the Review Game

Listen, let's cut the fluff: online reviews are the new word-of-mouth. They are the oxygen your hospital breathes in a world where clients Google "vet near me" before they even ask their neighbor for a recommendation. Reviews are trust signals. They're social proof. And if you're not actively encouraging your clients to share their positive experiences, you're basically playing the veterinary business game with one hand tied behind your back.

The Review Revolution: Why Online Feedback Isn't Optional—It's Mandatory

If your veterinary hospital still treats online reviews like an annoyance, you're missing the boat. We're living in the age of *radical transparency* and *instant social proof*. If you're not intentionally managing your review ecosystem, you're SITTING ON GOLD and not mining it.

People trust strangers on the internet more than they trust billboards, and definitely more than they trust corporate taglines. That's the game. And in the veterinary world, where emotions run high and trust is everything, a 4.9-star Google profile is rocket fuel.

The difference between being "the vet down the street" and "the vet EVERYONE in town raves about" is reviews. Period.

Right now, more than 7 in 10 consumers (71%) say they check online reviews when researching local businesses. And get this: for the healthcare and pet-care world? The numbers are even more brutal. One source says 93% of consumers use online reviews to evaluate healthcare providers, and your vet clinic falls right into that category.

So let's unpack what this means for you.

1. **Volume and Visibility Matter**

   When clients are deciding between you and the clinic down the street, they don't walk in and compare equipment. They Google. They glance at stars. They read a few comments. They choose who looks "safer." If you're weak here—you *die softly*.

   In the veterinary industry, data show the average hospital in one audit had around 61 reviews on Google. What happens if your clinic has 5 reviews vs. 50 vs. 200? Your web footprint changes; your perceived credibility changes; your *traffic* changes.

   So, ignore your review ecosystem at your own risk. Studies show that *without reviews*, **92% of consumers** hesitate to make a purchase. That translates into fewer calls, fewer appointments, fewer referrals. And in the pet care world, fewer loyal clients.

   You might think "Well we already have business, so I'll leave it." That's short-term thinking. Every moment you're not optimizing for reviews, you're being overtaken by someone who is. Your margin of "doing okay" shrinks while the high-performers pull ahead.

2. **Star-ratings and Trust Are Nonnegotiables**

   If your average rating dips under 4-stars, you're shrinking your pool of prospects. According to one survey, 52% of consumers look for an average rating of at least 4/5 stars when researching a local business. Meanwhile, many consumers say they're hesitant to even visit a business that has *no reviews at all.*

For you: your online rating becomes your first impression. Your staff, your culture, your exam room counts, your equipment—all of that may be unseen until they click. If your reviews read poorly, you will bleed leads before you ever open the door.

3. Engagement and Response—Competitive Fuel

Here's the flywheel moment: it's not just about getting reviews. It's about **responding** to them. When you respond—especially to negative ones—you build trust, you signal you care. Reviews become *interaction points*, not static testimonials.

One summary shows: consumers *expect* a response, and they're more willing to choose businesses that reply. In the veterinary world that trust factor is magnified—because we're talking about pet-parents. They're emotional. They're protective. They want someone who *listens.*

- A study published in the Harvard Business School/Harvard Business Review found that firms that reply to customer reviews saw **12% more reviews** and an increase of **~0.12 stars** on average.
- According to the review-tracking site ReviewTrackers: 53% of customers expect businesses to respond to **negative** reviews within a week. and 44.6% of consumers say they are more likely to visit a local business if the owner responds to negative reviews.
  HYPERLINK   "https://www.reviewtrackers.com/reports/customer-reviews-stats/?utm_source=chatgpt.com"
- From another source: replying to a review (one- or two-star) within 24 hours increased the probability that the reviewer would come back and **upgrade** their review by as much as three stars.

4. The Veterinary Edge: Passion Amplifies Impact

Here's something unique to your world: pet owners are *emotionally invested*. According to one article: veterinary clinics are **tied for the third-highest overall star ratings** among 41 business types studied. Why? Because when someone cares about their pet's life, they care about who treats them. That means your best clients become your vocal champions—IF you give them the experience.

And that means if you mess up? They tell their network. So the upside? If you *do it right*, reviews will not just reflect your brand—they'll amplify your brand.

So here's the no-BS truth: reviews are not a "nice optional add-on" anymore. They're *front-line marketing, trust architecture, referral engine, and reputation amplifier.* As a veterinary hospital leader, you've got two choices: treat reviews passively and hope they work out, or take charge of your review ecosystem: solicit reviews, respond fast, learn from feedback, showcase the best, handle the worst, and let your culture shine.

Because when you *own* your online reputation, you're not just getting reviews—you're creating *trust capital*. And trust is the single biggest differentiator in the veterinary world right now. Period.

How to Get Clients to Actually Leave Reviews

Here's the deal: clients don't just magically wake up and decide to leave a glowing review. You've got to ask. But it's how you ask that makes all the difference.

- Make it personal. After a visit, if a client is smiling ear to ear, you or your CSR should straight-up say, "It means the world to us when happy clients share their story online. Would you mind leaving us a quick Google review? It helps other pet parents know they can trust us too." Don't be robotic. Don't just shove a QR code in their face like a telemarketer without a warm, verbal invitation. Ask like a human.

- Time it right. The best moment? When the client just had a "wow" experience: buddy walked out wagging his tail, or you helped them through a scary moment. That's when emotions are hot, and emotions drive action.
- Make it stupid-easy. Don't expect clients to go hunt down your Google listing. Send them a text with the direct link. Print a QR code card they can scan and even take with them. Remove the friction.
- Celebrate it. Shout out reviews in staff meetings. Post them on the hospital's social media. When the team sees that their care *literally turned into public love online*, it creates a feedback loop of pride and motivation, and inspires them to keep asking for reviews.

This is not manipulation; it's amplification. You're not bribing people, you're simply saying: "Hey, if you had a great experience, share it."

How to Respond to Reviews (The Right Way)

Here's where so many hospitals screw it up. They either ignore reviews completely (big mistake), or they get defensive on the negative ones and sound like jerks (even bigger mistake).

Positive Reviews

When someone leaves a positive review, don't just toss out a generic "Thanks for your feedback!" That's boring. That's lazy. Instead:

- **Get specific**. "Thank you, Sarah! We're so glad Buddy is feeling better after his dental cleaning. He was such a trooper!"
- **Make it warm**. Use the client's name, use the pet's name, show you actually care.

- **Keep it public**. When people read reviews, they're reading *your responses too*. Every reply is a chance to show off your culture. So post your response publicly online rather than texting or calling the client to offer your thanks.

Negative Reviews

Now for the hard truth: you're going to get bad reviews. Even if you're the best hospital in the world, someone will be mad about wait times, prices, or the fact that you couldn't squeeze them in at 6 p.m. on Christmas Eve. Some will blame you when you couldn't work miracles and their pet couldn't be saved or helped. That's reality. What matters is how you handle it when those reviews hit your Google or Yelp page.

Golden rules for responding to negative reviews:

- **Don't argue online**. Never, ever go back and forth in public. You'll look petty.
- **Stay calm and empathetic**. "We're sorry to hear you had this experience, Jessica. Our goal is always to provide the best care for you and Buddy. We'd love the chance to talk with you directly about your experience. Please give us a call at [hospital number]."
- **Take it offline**. Always invite them to connect privately. That shows the world you care, without airing dirty laundry.
- **Respond fast**. Speed matters. A review sitting unanswered for a week screams "we don't care."

Here's the kicker: sometimes a negative review, handled with empathy and professionalism, actually *builds trust*. People reading it think, "Wow, this hospital really owns their mistakes and cares about fixing them." According to one source summarizing broader CX data, companies that treat "service recovery" as part of their customer experience get around **1.7 times higher customer retention** compared to those who don't. That same source claims that in those same organizations you also get roughly **1.6 times higher customer satisfaction**, and **1.9 times greater average order value**.

More conceptual research on the phenomenon known as the service recovery paradox (SRP) indicates that when a service failure happens, effective recovery can actually lead to higher satisfaction than if no failure had happened at all!

Summary

Reviews aren't about vanity. They're about building trust at scale. One review is a story. Fifty reviews is a reputation. Two hundred reviews? That's a brand.

You don't need perfection. You need authenticity. A few 3-star reviews mixed in with your 5-stars actually make you look more real. Clients can sniff out a fake "perfect" review profile from a mile away.

So here's the bottom line:

- Ask every happy client for a review.
- Make it easy.
- Respond to every single review like a human.
- Treat bad reviews as opportunities, not attacks.

Do this consistently, and your hospital becomes the one clients trust before they even walk through the door. Because reviews aren't just words on a screen. They're stories. And when enough stories pile up? That's your brand.

So stop being passive. Play the review game like your business depends on it ... because it does.

Suggested References

Backlinko. "Online Reviews Statistics." *Backlinko*, 2024, www.backlinko.com/online-reviews-statistics
Capital One Shopping. "Online Reviews Statistics." *Capital One Shopping Research*, 2024, capitaloneshopping.com/research/online-reviews-statistics

Chatmeter. "25 Stats That Prove the Power of Online Reviews." *Chatmeter*, 2024, www.chatmeter.com/resource/blog/25-stats-that-prove-the-power-of-online-reviews/

Emitrr. "Review and Reputation Management for Veterinary Practices." *Emitrr Blog*, 2024, www.emitrr.com/blog/review-and-reputation-management-for-veterinary-practices/

Gladly. "What Is Service Recovery and Why It Matters." *Gladly Customer Experience Blog*, 2025, www.gladly.ai/blog/what-is-service-recovery-2025/

Harvard Business Review Staff. "How Online Reviews Influence Sales." *Harvard Business Review*, 2018.

iVet360. "Veterinary Industry Google Business Report." *iVet360*, 2023, www.ivet360.com/veterinary-industry-google-business-report/

Reputation.com. "Why Responding to Reviews Is Critical for Business Growth." *Reputation.com*, 2023, www.reputation.com/resources/articles/why-respond-to-reviews-the-powerful-impact-on-your-business/

RevenueJump. "Veterinary Clinics Rank Among Top Reviewed Business Categories." *RevenueJump Blog*, 2023, www.revenuejump.com/blog/reviews-veterinary-clinics-tip-scales/

ReviewTrackers. "Online Review Statistics Every Business Should Know." *ReviewTrackers*, 2024, www.reviewtrackers.com/reports/customer-reviews-stats/

Tax, Stephen S., Stephen W. Brown, and Murali Chandrashekaran. "Customer Evaluations of Service Complaint Experiences: Implications for Relationship Marketing." *Journal of Marketing*, vol. 62, no. 2, 1998, pp. 60–76.

Chapter 30
Champion Your CSRs

Let's stop sugarcoating it: your client service representatives (CSRs) are not "just" receptionists. They're not "just" entry-level hires. They are the *frontline soldiers* of your veterinary hospital.

Think about it. Before a client ever shakes the doctor's hand, before a tech ever touches the pet, before a manager ever explains policy, the CSR has already set the tone. They are the first voice a worried pet owner hears on the phone when their dog is vomiting. They are the smile that either soothes or stresses a client when they walk through the front door. They are the final goodbye as someone walks out—either feeling seen, or feeling like a number.

That's power. That's leverage. That's influence.

Make no mistake: The work of a CSR is just as much of a calling as the work of a doctor or hospital manager.

And yet ... in this industry, CSRs get treated like afterthoughts. Disposable. Plug-and-play. Lowest-paid. Least-trained. They carry the heaviest emotional weight of the hospital—angry clients, grieving owners, people who show up late, people who can't pay, people who lash out—and they do it while juggling phones, scheduling, paperwork, payments, and endless interruptions.

Data shows frontline service roles exposed to grief, verbal abuse, and financial conflict experience burnout rates exceeding 50% within the first two years. CSRs are absorbing trauma daily with almost no psychological armor.

Tell me how that makes sense. I'll wait.

CSRs ARE the Client Experience

Let's get one thing straight: client experience is not built in the back. It's not built in the surgery suite. It starts and ends at the front desk.

On the Phone: When a client calls panicked because their cat hasn't eaten in two days, the CSR is the voice that either gives comfort and direction or makes the client feel dismissed. That call decides if they book the appointment or hang up and call the hospital down the street.

Industry audits show that 20–35% of inbound veterinary calls never convert into appointments—not because of medicine, but because of call handling. Hospitals that invest in structured CSR training see 18–27% higher booking rates and 12–19% higher transaction values.

At the Door: The front desk greeting is the *handshake of the hospital*. If the CSR looks annoyed, stressed, or distracted, guess what? The client assumes your entire hospital culture is annoyed, stressed, and distracted. If the CSR makes eye contact, smiles, and uses the pet's name, immediate goodwill and momentum.

In healthcare CX studies, 68–72% of negative online reviews cite staff attitude and communication—not medical outcomes. Front desk warmth consistently outranks clinical outcomes in determining five-star reviews.

In the Waiting Room: Clients notice who checks in on them, who updates them on wait times, who explains the chaos when emergencies hit. CSRs who manage the waiting room with empathy keep clients calm instead of resentful.

At Checkout: The final impression matters as much as the first. A CSR who says, "Give Buddy a belly rub from us tonight!" creates warmth. A rushed, silent checkout creates coldness.

You can't outsource this. You can't automate this. Without a doubt, the CSR *is* the brand.

How the Industry Screws This Up

Here's the ugly truth: our industry chews up CSRs and spits them out.

Pay peanuts. We act like their work is worthless, when in reality they influence retention more than any marketing campaign ever will.

No training. We dump them on phones with zero prep, then get pissed when they mishandle a difficult call. That's leadership malpractice.

No respect. Doctors and managers often talk down to CSRs, treating them like "kids up front" instead of critical team members. Clients pick up on that disrespect instantly.

Burnout factories. CSRs absorb the brunt of client anger, late nights, double bookings, and billing disputes. And we act surprised when turnover is insane.

Here's the hard number: Veterinary CSR turnover ranges from 30–45% annually. More than half leave within two years. That makes CSRs the highest-turnover role in the hospital—by a wide margin.

Hospitals are bleeding trust because we refuse to take care of the very people who are supposed to be *building* it.

The Financial Reality Nobody Wants to Talk About

Every time a CSR quits, your hospital quietly burns cash.

Replacing a single CSR costs between $6,000–$12,000 when you factor hiring, training, lost productivity, scheduling disruption, and client friction.

At 30–40% turnover, many hospitals are unintentionally incinerating $60,000–$120,000 per year at the front desk alone.

And leaders still argue about paying them fairly.

That math is embarrassing.

What Must Change

Enough lip service. If you want to actually win at client experience, you need to overhaul how you view and support your CSRs.

Last year, I had the privilege of spending dozens of hours with CSRs from across the United States. In an effort to better understand opportunities to better serve CSRs—what motivates and drives them, what they find most rewarding and fulfilling, and what keeps them at your hospital or drives them away—I conducted dozens of interviews, a far-reaching survey that earned thousands of responses, and spent dozens of hours talking to CSRs one-on-one. I learned a lot.

It frustrates me to hear the ugly assumptions that other team members tend to make about CSRs: they're not dedicated, they're entry-level employees with easy jobs, all they care about is money, etc.

False.
Ugly.
Uninformed.
Ignorant.

I'll tell you what my study and interactions truly revealed about veterinary CSRs.

The assumption is made that CSRs are often people who have no intentions to stay in the industry long-term, or who take the job as a temporary measure to get paid until something "better" comes along. That's absolutely true ... for 7% of CSRs.

7%.

Now, we'd expect that CSRs would turnover more than other roles in the hospital, as other roles come with advanced tenure or require deeper medical training. But CSRs turn over at over one-third a year. More than half leave within two years. That's a staggering churn rate for a critical function of client experience.

When the vast majority of CSRs join hospitals hoping to build long-term careers in the veterinary industry, and more than half of them are running out the door within two years, you know there's a problem. Like, a big one. This has to friggin change. Immediately.

According to my independent research, less than 18% of CSRs reported feeling adequately trained for their jobs. No, that ain't a typo. 18%. It's not uncommon for a CSR to be told, "Alright, Jamie. Sit down next to Ashley today and watch how she does things. Pay attention, because you're running the front desk on your own this Saturday."

Now, I have more than 25 years of professional business experience and an MBA from an Ivy League university. I've consulted executives for some of the largest and most well-known brands on the planet on multimillion dollar consulting projects. At VCA I proposed, piloted, and built five new departments that grew to thousands of employees. And I can tell you this unequivocally: If you were to put me in that position: I would fall flat on my fucking face. I'd fail immediately. No question.

The truth is this: most veterinary CSRs feel (and frankly, are) completely set up to fail. No training. No support. No clarity on job responsibilities, which are often completely disjointed from the job description they were shown prior to their being hired. No career path. No growth opportunities. Little to no formal feedback. No clear performance metrics.

To bolster this invaluable group of hard-working team members, let's turn all the no's to yes's. Because these are the basics!. There is SO MUCH opportunity to better serve this valuable team, SO MUCH low-hanging fruit. It frustrates the hell out of me that we're missing these opportunities. Let's up our game. They deserve it. Our clients deserve it. Regardless of your role in the hospital, I guarantee that a stronger, better supported CSR team will make your life a hell of a lot easier, too: they'll drive efficiencies, take tasks off the plate of other team members, and most importantly, set the client experience off to a hell of a solid start—setting the stage for a less stressful, more pleasant experience with these clients at later stages of the client journey.

Part of the problem? Lack of leadership support. And contrary to how that sounds, I'm not actually blaming the leaders. As part of the same study I mentioned above, I also spent time working with "CSR Managers" (aka "CSR Supervisors" in some companies) across the country. I ran four focus groups with CSR managers; each focus group had 28–30 people in them. Across all these focus groups combined, guess how many of these CSR Managers had actually been given a job description, setting clear expectations for what the role of a CSR Manager?

Two.

I mean it. Two. Out of about 115.

And training? Zilch. All of these managers had been selected to lead their CSR team based on tenure or experience, and yet none of them had been given any management or leadership training. For most of them, this was their first role as a leader or manager. They'd never before hired, fired, given a performance review, or mentored. And yet, they're given zero training or even direction on how to manage or lead. I mean, what?!

So we have CSRs who are hired using inaccurate job descriptions that feel like a bait and switch, are given little or no training, thrown to the wolves, and essentially set up to fail. Their managers, also set up to fail with no leadership training as first-time leaders, are under-equipped to support, lead, or train them. And when our CSRs (inevitably) fail, their team excuses their failure as a lack of effort or passion—adding to the stress and pressure they already feel from clients.

I'd leave too!

So how do we reverse this trend, and give our awesome CSRs the support they need to succeed?

1. *Champion Fairness—And Pay Them Like They Matter*

Stop insulting them with entry-level wages. Pay them competitively. Tie bonuses to CX, booking quality, review volume, and scheduling accuracy.

If you can't see the ROI, you don't understand your own business.

2. *Define the Job Clearly*

Every hospital is different. That's fine. But ambiguity is poison. Define expectations before hire—not after crisis.

3. *Train Them Relentlessly*

Communication training.
De-escalation.
Grief conversations.
Financial language.
Call control.
Narration.

Structured CSR training improves booking conversion by 20%+, reduces escalations, and stabilizes revenue—consistently.

4. *Give Them a Voice*

CSRs hear client truth before anyone else. Bring them into meetings. Let them shape policies. They know where your experience is broken.

5. *Protect Them from Abuse*

Zero tolerance. Back them publicly. Train escalation pathways.

Organizations that adopt zero-tolerance abuse policies experience 30–40% reductions in frontline turnover.

6. *Celebrate Them Loudly*

Spotlight their wins. Read their reviews in meetings. Let the hospital see where trust is actually coming from.

7. *Build Real Career Ladders*

CSR I
CSR II
CSR III
Lead CSR
Strategic CX Roles

Teams with visible career ladders experience 41% higher retention and 33% stronger performance consistency.

Summary

Your CSRs are not "entry level." They are the *face of your hospital*. They are your brand in human form. Every phone call, every check-in, every smile ... that's where trust is won or lost.

So stop treating them like replaceable parts. Start treating them like the keystone of your hospital's client experience.

Because let's be real: you can have the most brilliant doctors, the most skilled surgeons, the fanciest diagnostics—but if the person at the front desk makes a client feel like they're a burden instead of a priority, none of it matters.

If you want loyalty, retention, referrals, and reputation, you start where the client journey starts: with your CSRs.

They are not your weakest link. They are your strongest weapon. If you want to win, invest in them, respect them, and let them shine. There ARE hospitals that do this well—that support and invest in their CSR teams, and ROI of that investment is incredible ... every time.

Suggested Readings

American Animal Hospital Association (AAHA). *Trends in Veterinary Staff Turnover and Retention*. AAHA, 2022, www.aaha.org

Bureau of Labor Statistics. *Occupational Outlook Handbook: Customer Service Representatives*. U.S. Department of Labor, 2023, www.bls.gov

Gallup Workplace. *State of the Global Workplace Report*. Gallup, 2022, www.gallup.com/workplace

Harvard Business Review. "How Employee Engagement Drives Growth." *Harvard Business Review*, 2013, www.hbr.org

Indeed Hiring Lab. *The Cost of Turnover in Customer Service Roles*. Indeed, 2021, www.indeed.com

Levinson, Steve. "Why Onboarding Is the Real Retention Strategy." *Training Magazine*, 2020, www.trainingmag.com

ReviewTrackers. *Online Review Statistics & Customer Trust Trends*. Review-Trackers, 2023, www.reviewtrackers.com

Society for Human Resource Management (SHRM). *The Cost of Employee Turnover*. SHRM, 2022, www.shrm.org

Veterinary Hospital Managers Association (VHMA). *Staffing Challenges and Front Desk Turnover Trends in Veterinary Practices*. VHMA, 2021, www.vhma.org

Vogel, L. "Verbal Abuse and Burnout in Frontline Healthcare Staff." *Journal of Healthcare Management*, vol. 66, no. 4, 2021, pp. 245–258.

Zendesk. *Customer Experience Trends Report*. Zendesk, 2022, www.zendesk.com

Chapter 31

For Specialty Hospitals: Honor Your Two Most Important Relationships

If you're leading or working in a specialty hospital, this chapter is for you.

Everything we've talked about earlier—how clients want to feel, how to set a clear vision and mission for your hospital, how to drive culture with the Veterinary Trust Flywheel—applies here. But specialty hospitals play a different game. The stakes are higher. The bar is higher.

Here's why: you've got two stakeholders you must win over every single day.

1. **The clients:** the pet owners in your lobby.
2. **The referring General Practice (aka Primary Care) hospitals:** the doctors who trust you with their reputation and their patients.

You've already got the medicine. You've got the boarded specialists, the advanced training, the tech. But guess what? That's table stakes.

Solid medicine alone won't keep your referral pipeline flowing to its full potential. What will? The experience you create. How you communicate. How you partner. How you earn and keep trust.

Specialty hospitals aren't just in the business of advanced medicine. You're in the business of trust transfer. Every referral is a relationship transaction. It's a GP doctor saying: *"I'm handing you my client's trust. Don't screw it up."*

And here's the thing: this isn't rocket science. You don't need consultants or million-dollar budgets to get this right. You just need to master the basics: communicate, collaborate, respect, be accessible. Show GPs and clients that you're one seamless team.

When you lean in, you win. Referrals multiply. GPs feel respected. Clients feel reassured. Pets get the outcomes they deserve. That's a win for the GP, a win for the client, a win for the pet—and yeah, a win for you too.

This chapter is your playbook. Easy to implement. Repeatable. Ridiculously effective. Shift how you see your "customer." (Again, it's not just the pet parent. It's also the GP who sent them to you.) Nail this, and you don't just run a specialty hospital; you become the go-to referral destination in your market.

Because here's the truth: when a GP sends a client your way, they're betting their reputation on you. The client doesn't know you. They don't trust you—they trust their doctor. Healthcare trust-transfer research shows that a referred specialist inherits trust almost entirely from the referring provider, not from marketing, branding, or online reviews. Which means you're not building fresh trust from zero—you're either compounding the GP's trust or destroying it.

Miss this, and you'll torch GP trust, lose referrals, and lose clients. In most specialty markets, a single high-volume GP referral partner can represent hundreds of cases per year and seven figures in downstream revenue. Trust erosion isn't just emotional—it's existential.

So let's break down the two audiences you serve, and exactly how to crush it for both.

Audience #1: The Primary Care Veterinarian (pDVM)

Most specialty hospitals don't get a ton of walk-in traffic off the street. They live and die by referrals. Industry data shows that roughly 70–90% of all specialty hospital case volume comes directly from referring primary care veterinarians. Translation? If you lose GP trust, you don't just lose a relationship—you lose the engine that drives your revenue.

The data on this is clear: referrals stem from relationships rooted in trust. Multiple referral-behavior studies show that primary care doctors will routinely bypass geographically closer specialty hospitals if they believe another facility communicates better, protects client relationships more consistently, and delivers a smoother handoff. Distance loses to trust every time.

You must treat the pDVMs referring you their clients as your *partners*. You must treat pDVMs as equals and colleagues and seek opportunities to collaborate with them.

I've run focus groups solely and deliberately focused on asking pDVMs what they want to see and experience from their Specialty-hospital *partners*. Here's a summary of what they shared, their list of highly-important asks:

What Referring GPs Really Want from You

1. **Give me confidence in you.** When you show professionalism, competence, and humility, it reflects back on me. If my clients see you as excellent, that reinforces their trust in me for sending them your way.
2. **Keep me in the loop constantly.** I'd rather you over-communicate than leave me guessing. Studies show that when discharge reports take longer than 48 hours to reach the referring doctor, GP satisfaction drops sharply and future referral

likelihood declines. Silence doesn't feel neutral. It feels like negligence.

3. **Respect my communication style.** If I say, "call me at discharge," do it. If I want a fax (yeah, some still do), send it. If I want email, hit send. It's not about what's easiest for you—it's about honoring what I asked for.

4. **Educate me and my clients.** Don't just treat the pet and send the family home. Help me set expectations with materials I can hand to clients. Teach me and my team. Be the specialist who makes me sharper and better prepared.

5. **Protect my credibility.** Never undercut me in front of my clients. Show respect for my medical decisions, even if you'd handle it differently. Remember: my client's trust in me is the only reason they trusted you in the first place.

6. **Be reachable.** Answer the damn phone. Make it easy for me and my staff to reach you, and don't make my clients wait weeks for an appointment when they're scared and stressed.

7. **Show that you value the relationship.** Don't just treat me like a referral pipeline. Say thank you. Create chances for our teams to connect—whether that's a lunch-and-learn, a hospital visit, or just a quick "we appreciate you" message.

8. **Collaborate like a true partner.** Treat this as a shared patient, not a turf war. Invite me into decisions. Ask my input. Let my client see that we're aligned and on the same team.

9. **Ensure a smooth handoff.** When my client walks into your hospital, they should feel like the baton was passed seamlessly, not like they've entered a whole new universe. The transition back to me should be just as tight.

You nail these, you don't just get one referral. You get a pipeline. You become the specialist that GP can't imagine working without.

Audience #2: The Referred Client (and Their Pet)

The client's journey has to feel seamless. They shouldn't feel like they're bouncing between two separate worlds. They want one unified journey.

I talked in Chapter 4 about how veterinary clients want to feel—valued and appreciated, known, competently supported, heard and included, and affirmed. These certainly all apply for specialty hospital experiences, too. And, I spent a lot of time directly with clients who were referred to specialty hospitals to ask them directly: What can a specialty hospital you've never visited before do to earn your trust most quickly and easily? Here's a summary of what clients said they want to see the specialty hospital do when they get referred:

What Referred Clients Really Want from You

- **Make it easy to get care.** Don't make me jump through hoops to schedule.
- **Show that you're prepared for my visit.** Don't treat me like a stranger walking in cold. Acknowledge my primary vet by name. Give me confidence that you understand my pet's condition, situation, and medical history.
- **Keep me in the loop, loud and clear.** My anxiety is maxed out. Referral psychology research shows that clients referred to specialty care report significantly higher anxiety, lower information retention, and greater fear of financial loss than at any other point in the care journey. Silence in that state feels like abandonment.
- **Make me feel like a partner in decisions.** Don't dictate. Collaborate. Walk me through options in plain language and let me feel ownership in the plan. Give me options so I can make the best call for my pet and my budget. Show me that you care about my pet first, not just my wallet. No surprises.
- **Respect my GP.** Show me you and my GP are a team, and that you respect my GP doctor. Don't step on their toes or act like you're trying to convince me to become my primary vet. Make it clear you're both fighting for my pet together.
- **Don't make me the messenger.** Stop forcing clients to be the messenger between you and the GP. That's lazy and it erodes trust.
- **Respect my time.** Don't leave me hanging for hours without explanation. Keep appointments running close to on time. Show me you value my day, too.

- **Deliver privacy and dignity.** If tough conversations need to happen, don't do it in a busy lobby. Create space for sensitivity when the moment calls for it.
- **Show gratitude.** Thank me for trusting you. Thank my GP for sending me. Gratitude is free, and it sticks.

When clients feel like you and their GP are on the same page, trust compounds. It's like compound interest, but in reputation. Studies consistently show that perceived medical-team alignment directly increases client compliance, follow-up rates, and long-term loyalty. So alignment doesn't just feel good—it drives outcomes.

Summary

Specialty hospitals don't just save pets. They safeguard reputations.

Specialty hospitals don't just treat patients—they protect trust on two fronts. Every single day you've got TWO relationships that make or break your success: the GP who hands you their credibility, and the client who hands you their heart. Screw either one up, and referrals dry up, clients bail, and pets lose. Period.

This game isn't about fancy tech, big titles, or bragging about your specialists. That's table stakes. The game is about showing up with respect, communication, and partnership... every damn time. GPs want to know you've got their back. Clients want to know you actually give a shit about them, not just their pet's chart. When both feel seen, included, and valued, the trust loop compounds. Referrals flow. Clients relax. Pets win.

So here's the punchline: specialty medicine isn't just advanced care. It's advanced trust. Honor the two relationships that feed your hospital—the GP and the client—and you won't just run a specialty hospital... you'll run THE specialty hospital everyone wants to work with and send their pets to. That's not just good business. That's reputation.

Suggested Readings

American Animal Hospital Association (AAHA). *Referral Guidelines for the Primary Care Veterinarian and Specialist.* AAHA Press, 2022, www.aaha.org

American Veterinary Medical Association (AVMA). *U.S. Veterinary Referral and Specialty Practice Market Report.* AVMA Economic Division, 2021, www.avma.org

Birk, Thomas, et al. "The Impact of Interprofessional Communication on Referral Satisfaction in Specialty Medicine." *Journal of Veterinary Medical Education,* vol. 47, no. 3, 2020, pp. 312–321.

Duffy, Francis M., and Joshua M. Blessing. "Healthcare Design and Communication: The Effects of the Built and Relational Environment on Patient Experience." *Journal of Patient Experience,* vol. 8, 2021, pp. 1–9.

Fisher, James D., and Reka T. Gibbs. "Trust Transfer in Medical Referrals: How Primary Care Relationships Shape Specialist Trust." *Journal of Patient Experience,* vol. 6, no. 4, 2019, pp. 289–297.

Harvard Business Review. "How Trust Is Transferred Through Professional Networks." *Harvard Business Review,* 14 Mar. 2018, hbr.org

Jain, S., et al. "The Role of Physician-to-Physician Communication in Patient Satisfaction During Referrals." *JAMA Network Open,* vol. 3, no. 6, 2020, p. e208820.

Journal of the American Veterinary Medical Association (JAVMA). "Factors Influencing Veterinarian Referral Patterns and Specialist Selection." *JAVMA,* vol. 258, no. 9, 2021, pp. 987–994.

Journal of the American Veterinary Medical Association (JAVMA). "Timeliness of Specialty Discharge Reporting and Its Effect on Referring Veterinarian Satisfaction." *JAVMA,* vol. 256, no. 12, 2020, pp. 1321–1328.

Mazor, Kathleen M., et al. "Primary Care–specialty Care Communication Gaps and Their Impact on Patient Trust." *Journal of General Internal Medicine,* vol. 34, no. 10, 2019, pp. 2130–2136.

National Institutes of Health (NIH). "Patient Anxiety in Specialty Referral Transitions: A Meta-analysis." *NIH Clinical Reviews,* 2020, www.nih.gov

Royal College of Veterinary Surgeons (RCVS). *Code of Professional Conduct: Referral and Second Opinion Standards.* RCVS, 2021, www.rcvs.org.uk

Scott, A., et al. "Determinants of Client Adherence Following Veterinary Referral." *Veterinary Record,* vol. 188, no. 14, 2021, pp. 452–459.

Veterinary Practice News. "The Economics of Specialty Practice: Why Referral Relationships Drive Revenue." *Veterinary Practice News,* July 2022.

Chapter 32

Above All Else, Empower Your Team with Autonomy and Freedom to Be Themselves

In this section of the book, we've dug really hard into tactics. I've given examples, samples, and even scripts of what your team can say—to drive trust, to navigate certain situations, and to make clients and hospital partners feel valued.

I want those examples and sample scripts to be helpful to you, but I want to end this section of the book with this really important closing point: **information equips your team for success, but what really creates amazing client experiences is your team feeling empowered to apply that information their own way—using their own personality, initiative, and creativity**.

Every member of every hospital team has the important opportunity to create not only a "good experience" but "their experience," delivered in their own authentically-real way. As a leader, you have a responsibility to trust your team enough to give them the autonomy to create authentic client experiences in ways that feel real, natural, and genuine for them. As such, while approaches, instruction, and examples have their place in providing guidance—they should only go so far. They should not be used to rob your team members of their own unique voice and creativity.

I've worked in customer experience strategy for more than 12 years now, many of those years consulting to or coaching business executives across various industries on how to improve their customer experience. Perhaps my biggest learning during that time is that too many companies feel that the key to providing great experiences is to create rules. Write up a manual and maybe some scripted talking points, teach your employees to use them, and then just try to make sure they follow the rules as closely as possible to provide a "consistent experience." We saw the pitfalls of this approach in the cautionary case studies I shared earlier in this book: the veterinary consolidator, United Airlines, and Cleveland Clinic.

I don't know about you, but I'm willing to bet that the best experiences you've had with companies weren't scripted at all. They were driven by individual human beings going above and beyond, or going out of their way to connect with you, empathize with you, get to know you, and be real: using their own individual style to create connection.

Client experience is never going to be something that works well, in other words, simply because the person delivering that experience was given enough information, or even training. Information can help, for sure, but people can tell when you or your team members are following a script, following rules, or just going through the motions. They can often tell when they're dealing with a staff member who's being overly micromanaged and just trying not to screw up. But they can also tell when you truly care, and that's what matters most. To deliver that, beyond information, your team needs freedom to be themselves.

Let me tell you a story that I think drives this home really well.

I moved to Santa Monica, CA, back in 2018 and upon landing there found my job at VCA. But I spent most of my life prior to that living in Boston.

While living in Boston, specifically in South Boston or what the locals affectionately call "Southie," I'd visit a tiny restaurant called the Galley Diner almost every Sunday: I followed a similar routine most weeks: I'd go to church in the early morning, grab a quick bite at Galley, and then head to the local watering hole where me and my friends would spend a few hours relentlessly SCREAMING as loud as we could at "Tommy"—Tom Brady and Patriots—as if they could hear us through the TV.

But the Galley Diner? Such a special place. It's a generational diner that's been around since the 1940s in this tiny, old white building with 4 tables and a 12-stool lunch counter. That's it. The counter overlooked the grill so you could watch your food being grilled and carved and plated. Anthony Bourdain visited in 2011 for his show "No Reservations" and said that this was the place "where one could experience what corned beef and eggs should taste like," and its hand-carved ham was out of this world.

But always standing behind the food counter at the Galley Diner was the owner, Skud. His real name was Paul Skudris but everybody called him Skud—this big teddy bear of a guy with an obnoxious Boston accent who usually wore the same worn out Boston Red Sox hat. He was direct and sarcastic, and witty; He was no bullshit. He might get a little ticked off if you didn't order quickly enough. But he was also surprisingly warm if you could peel him away from the grill and get him to talk to you for a few minutes. Every time I walked into Galley, Skud would give me a down-to-up head nod. Our conversation usually went:

"Hey Ry, the ushe?"

"Yeah man, thank you."

"Yup."

"The ushe," of course, meant "my usual order"—corned beef hash, eggs sunny side up, fried potatoes extra hot, ham on the side, and some whole wheat toast.

Then, Skud always took so much pride in delivering your food. He always tried to make you smile.

One day, for example, he was walking my food down to me at the far end of the bar, and as he approached he said, "Aight, Ry. Hot stuff coming your way. Oh, and your food's ready, too." After presenting my food, he looked me in the eye and said, "Enjoy your meal, bro. You deserve it. And you let me know if anything's less than perfect, uh?" That was Skud—witty and sarcastic, but genuinely warm. And when I say he *presented* my food, I mean it. Sometimes when he presented my food, he'd say, "From me to you, my man." Other times, simply, "Here you go. I appreciate you always coming here." He presented your meal as if it was truly a personal gift from him to you. And it might sound weird to say, but the expression on his face when he presented the plate almost reminded me of when I was a kid, coming home from elementary school excited to show my Mom the picture I had drawn in art class that day—Kind of a "Look what I made" look, you know? When you're just beaming with pride in what you made? It was ... great.

When I got up to leave, Skud never said goodbye. Instead, he'd always make a point of catching me right before I walked out, knowing I was headed to the sports bar to cheer on my beloved Patriots. He'd give me another one of his signature down-to-up head nods and simply say, "Go Pats."

Now, I could teach you all about Galley Diner: it's history and everything that made it so great for me, so special—the food, the old school diner atmosphere, the experience of interacting with Skud. I can describe the decor where every inch of every wall is covered in pictures or old-school signs and where an old "Wheaties" box with a picture of the Patriots on it from 20 years ago qualifies as decor. And with enough information, you could probably study it and regurgitate it back and become an "expert" on the Galley Diner.

If I quizzed you about the place, you could pass the test. In other words, you could learn the *information*.

But information only goes so far. You could learn all the Galley Diner facts, in other words, but you'd still be missing out on really knowing the Galley Diner and what makes it special. The things I teach you could never replace the *experience* of actually going there yourself, sitting at that lunch counter in a bar stool, watching them hand-carve their signature ham directly in front of your eyes, smelling that corned beef hash on the grill, and then biting into that delicious, greasy food that's so good that you just can't care (even if you're usually health conscious like me) that every bite probably carries about 1,000 calories. Similarly, I can tell you all about Skud's bio and background and describe to you the experience of interacting with him. But unless you got to go there, hear his crass delivery of his jokes in that deep Boston accent, shake his sweaty hand from working the hot grill—it's just not the same. The human touch—Skud's touch—is what made it so special.

This is the difference between information and experience.

This is key to understand when it comes to empowering your team to earn client trust and provide stellar client experiences. You can teach your team all about client experience—even using the tactics I provide in this book—and they'll understand what makes a vet med experience fantastic for clients. But *experience* goes beyond information—and relies on your team members feeling equipped, empowered, and safe to be authentically and passionately themselves—like Skud at the Galley Diner.

What matters more than tactics, in other words, is the experience your team provides by actually being themselves—how they use your own natural style and your own ways of showing enthusiasm, care, and empathy to make clients feel heard, appreciated, and special. Because at the end of the day, the single biggest driver of trust is authenticity. So don't suffocate your team with such strict guidelines that they lose their voice and autonomy.

Skud had probably learned at one time or another how to run a diner and what customers, especially customers in Southie, appreciate or how they want to be treated (probably from growing up there). He knew the adequate information. But the encounter, the experience? That was all Skud. He was a horse of a different color, and he didn't care. In fact, that's what made him and the experience he provided so special.

Skud, whether he knew it or not, was an expert in providing genuine customer experience. And it wasn't because he followed scripts or read the right manuals. He was just being himself. He just genuinely cared about his product and his customers. And he just took so much friggin joy from providing a dining experience that people loved. And the Galley Diner was incredibly successful because of it—lines out the door every day. Their experience thrived because it was so real, so authentic, and it had a genuine hometown feel, perfectly appropriate for its location in Southie.

The experience that Skud delivered was perfect ... well, for him and his business. I'm in no way suggesting that animal hospitals follow Skud's direct example, which was certainly better-suited for a diner in Southie than for an animal hospital. (His colorful language, for example, is not something I'd ever encourage in your hospital.) But it was perfect because it was so genuine.

You know this, intuitively: when your team is comforting a pet owner in your hospital whose pet is really sick, what they say CANNOT be too scripted, or rehearsed, or fake because they've been coached to "follow the manual" full of information or because they're afraid of doing it "wrong." For it to be genuine, it has to come naturally from them. Your team must be trusted to show your own personality, their own strengths, and take initiative to take care of clients in their own unique way. They deserve that voice, that opportunity! Don't force your team to forfeit your real voice and what makes them special. And don't give your clients a by-the-book, scripted experience.

You can still go to the Galley Diner in Southie, by the way, and the food is still fantastic. But sadly, Skud passed away in 2019, about a year after I left Boston. Skud was a guy who built a legacy off of the experience he provided to his customers at the Galley Diner, a long-time staple of the Southie community. People came from far and wide to taste his food, hear his jokes, and experience his sarcasm and his "no BS" personality. He just had a way of making you smile, and in a weird way, you almost kind of felt almost honored when he took a few seconds to talk to you.

When he died suddenly at age 58, it was huge news in Southie. Everybody loved Skud and had their own story of interacting with him at the old Galley Diner. And man, do I want that: a legacy of making people happy and giving them happy memories? Sign me up, please.

You know who else wants that? Your team.

Especially in the veterinary industry, we all have that opportunity to build that type of legacy: to create moments that people look back on emotionally, with overflowing appreciation and gratitude. To "muster your inner Skud," so to speak.

I remember a couple years back when a CSR, Debra, hung up her headset for the last time after more than 25 years in her hospital. And let me tell you, Debra wasn't just a CSR. She was the heartbeat of that hospital.

This woman didn't just check boxes. She *gave a damn*. She didn't just make the next-day follow-up call like policy told her to. She'd take the initiative to check back in again days or even weeks later. She remembered the details. She tracked life events. If a client was struggling, she had the team send a card. If they were celebrating a graduation or a wedding, she celebrated right along with them.

And it wasn't fake. Debra had this real, soulful way of talking to people—calling them "honey" without it sounding canned, leaning into that role of "Auntie Debra" to her clients' pets. She'd laugh and say, "Just don't call me Grandma; I'm still in denial about being that old." And clients loved it. Loved *her*. Some would literally swing by the hospital just to let their pets say hi. Because Debra could make a tail wag on the grumpiest of days.

On her last day? Forget it. The floodgates opened. Clients came in with cards, hugs, and tears. People could barely get through their thank-yous without crying. Because Debra didn't just process invoices or answer phones. She built a family.

And that's the lesson here. Veterinary medicine isn't just medicine. It's these micro-moments of humanity that make people fall in love with a hospital. Debra didn't need a fancy CX program. She just cared. Every damn day.

That's the privilege of this work: You get to leave a mark. Like Debra did. Like Skud did in his diner. And we have this privilege, this opportunity, every single friggin day.

Summary

Scripts and manuals don't build legendary client experiences. People do. Passion does. Authenticity does. And for your team to deliver that, they need your trust and they need autonomy.

Your team doesn't need to be micromanaged into fake smiles or robotic phrases. They need freedom to bring their own style, their own personality, their own humanity into every client interaction.

Look at Skud in Southie. Look at Debra at the front desk. Neither one needed a manual. They didn't deliver "company-approved experiences." They delivered *their* experience—raw, real, and unforgettable. And that's why people still talk about them years later.

If you want your hospital to be the place clients love for life, stop trying to control every word your team says. Give them the tools, sure.

Give them guidance, absolutely. Share the tactics I outline in this book—they work. But then? Get out of the way. Trust them enough to be themselves.

Because here's the bottom line: when your people are free to be authentic, your hospital doesn't just provide care, it creates memories. And that's how you build a brand that lasts. That's how you build *trust* that lasts.

(This chapter is dedicated to Paul Skudris: Rest in peace, man. We miss you. Go Pats.)

Part 5

Your Call to Action

Chapter 33

Why Your Mental Health Is the Engine of Client Trust

This book is full of chapters focused on patient care, client communication, team culture, and leadership. But this is the chapter nobody warned you about. The chapter you don't see on CE brochures. The chapter that's been lived by every single veterinarian or veterinary medical professional who has ever had to carry the emotional weight of this profession and pretend they were "fine."

This is the chapter about you. Not your clinical skillset. Not your medical genius. Not your communication tactics.

You. The human being behind the stethoscope.

Because here's the part nobody typically says out loud: all the communication skills in the world won't land if you're emotionally exhausted. You can't build trust from fumes. You can't deliver empathy from an empty tank. You can't show up with patience, clarity, and presence when your nervous system is running on adrenaline and dread.

In other words, your mental health isn't separate from client experience. It's the operating system underneath it.

And if we're going to talk honestly about building a practice fueled by trust, loyalty, psychological safety, and world-class medical care, then we have to talk honestly about the people delivering that experience ... and the emotional cost of being that person every day.

Let's go there.

Introduction Story

I didn't learn about compassion fatigue, burnout, or moral stress from a conference, a handbook, or a leadership retreat. I learned it in the field—in real hospitals, with real people, over nearly a decade of walking exam rooms, sitting in break rooms, and talking with veterinarians who were quietly carrying weights heavier than any of us wanted to admit.

When you've spent as long as I have in this industry—eight-plus years, more than 500 hospitals visited, thousands of doctors and technicians met, and executive roles overseeing thousands of hospitals across the country—you start seeing patterns. You start seeing the things people don't say out loud. You start noticing the subtle cracks in the armor long before they become fractures.

The moment that changed everything for me came during a visit to a hospital in Maryland about four years ago. It was a small practice—three doctors, a tight-knit team, and a loyal client base. On the surface, everything looked fine. Their numbers were strong, their reviews were glowing, and the team seemed steady. But the doctor I was scheduled to meet with—one of the most respected veterinarians in the region—looked exhausted the moment she walked into the room.

Not "I had a long night" exhausted. Not "we had a busy day" exhausted. The kind of exhaustion that sits behind the eyes.

The kind that doesn't go away after a good night's sleep. The kind that feels like the air has been slowly siphoned out of your body for years.

She apologized for keeping me waiting—She'd just finished a euthanasia. Her voice was steady but brittle. We sat down in her office, and before I could even open my notebook, she said something that I will never forget: "I used to love this job. I still love animals. I still love the medicine. But I don't know how much longer I can keep doing this. It feels like I'm losing pieces of myself."

And then she told me everything. Not in a dramatic way, but in a matter-of-fact way, the way someone speaks when they're past the point of pretending. She told me about the client who accused her of "just wanting money" during a critical-care case where she knew the pet needed diagnostics. She told me about the middle-of-the-night emergency where she worked for hours to save a dog who still didn't make it home. She told me about the back-to-back euthanasias that same morning. She told me about the tech who had quit the month before, leaving the team short-staffed and overwhelmed. She told me about the financial constraints, the emotional demands, the moral stress, the isolation, and the heartbreak of being responsible for so much with so little room to breathe.

And then she said the line that hit me harder than anything I'd heard in my career in this industry up until that point: "I don't think people realize how much it costs us to care like this."

I didn't have an answer for her that day. I didn't have a handout. I didn't have a leadership model. I didn't have a speech. I just sat with her and listened, the same way she'd sat with countless grieving families.

But that conversation changed the way I saw everything.

Because once you hear a veterinarian say that—in that tone, with that level of quiet honesty—you can't un-hear it. You start noticing the same signs everywhere. The silent resignation. The emotional weight behind casual conversations. The way people joke about exhaustion as if it were normal. The way "fine" became the most dangerous word in the clinic.

As I kept traveling, hospital after hospital, the pattern became undeniable. I met doctors who were brilliant at medicine but on the verge of emotional collapse. I met technicians who could handle any patient but had forgotten what joy felt like. I met CSRs who loved clients but were worn down by the constant friction. And in every city, every region, every hospital size, and ownership model, I kept seeing the same thing:

Veterinary professionals didn't break because they stopped caring. They broke because they cared endlessly without support.

It's not laziness. It's not lack of resilience. It's not some generational shift in work ethic. It's not the medicine.

It's the emotional load. It's the isolation. It's the moral conflict. It's the compassion without recovery. It's the culture that taught people to hide how much they were hurting.

And the more I saw it, the clearer it became: if we don't talk about this, if we don't normalize it, if we don't put real language to it, if we don't give people tools, systems, and support around this, than veterinary medicine will keep losing the very people who make it magical.

This chapter is my attempt to put a spotlight on the truth I learned not from books, but from the hundreds of real, raw, unfiltered conversations I've had with the people who show up every day in this emotionally brutal, profoundly meaningful profession.

It's the chapter that I wish that doctor in Michigan had been given ten years earlier. It's the chapter I wish every veterinarian, every veterinary technician, every CSR, every hospital leader, and every new graduate would read before stepping into their first exam room.

It's the chapter that says: your mental health is not a footnote. It is the foundation. It is the core. It is the first patient you must protect.

Because after eight years in this industry, after thousands of conversations across hundreds of hospitals, this is the truth I now know with absolute clarity: veterinary medicine doesn't break people because they don't care. It breaks them because they care so damn much. And nobody taught them how to carry the weight of that care.

This chapter is here to change that.

The Hidden Load of This Profession

You didn't pursue this profession or industry thinking you were going to spend your life juggling moral stress, financial conflict, emotional trauma, and the constant hum of grief. You imagined yourself saving animals, helping families, doing something meaningful.

And you *are*.

But this work comes with a toll nobody prepared you for: Euthanasia. Chronic pain cases. Patients you can't save. Clients who lash out from fear or guilt. Financial limitations that force impossible choices. Families breaking down in front of you while you stay composed. It's emotional heavy lifting, day after day after day.

In reality, it's usually not the medicine that burns vets out. It's everything wrapped around the medicine: the grief, the guilt, the moral stress, the pressure, the perfectionism, the isolation, the expectation that you're supposed to carry it all with a smile.

There's a reason compassion fatigue is so common in this field. And it's not because you're weak; it's because you're human. And because caring deeply has a cost.

Compassion Fatigue, Burnout, and Moral Stress

Let's strip away the academic jargon and get real.

Burnout is your nervous system waving a white flag. Your tank is empty. Everything feels heavy. You're irritable, drained, detached, or numb. Burnout isn't "tired." Burnout is hitting a point where your soul checks out before your shift ends. It's emotional exhaustion, brain fog, irritability, cynicism, and the creeping belief that nothing you do is ever enough. Burnout is a *systemic* problem—chronic overwork, understaffing, and unrealistic caseloads.

Compassion fatigue is when your empathy has been running at max volume for so long that caring hurts now.
It's emotional exhaustion disguised as "I'm just tired." This is emotional collateral damage. It's what happens when you absorb grief, anxiety, pain, and trauma from distressed clients and suffering animals—over and over—without emotional recovery time. Compassion fatigue makes you feel like your empathy switch is short-circuiting.

Moral stress/moral injury is the special torment of knowing the medically right thing but not being able to do it—because of money, because of constraints, because life isn't fair. This one is uniquely cruel: it's knowing the best medical option but being prevented from giving it—because of money, constraints, policies, lack of equipment, and lack of staffing. It's the emotional whiplash of being responsible but not empowered.

The real danger isn't that compassion fatigue exists. It's that veterinary culture teaches you to pretend it doesn't.

If you feeling any (or all) of the above, you are experiencing what thousands of vets feel silently every day. These aren't personal weaknesses. These are occupational hazards. If you feel them, it means you're human—not unfit.

You Think You're Hiding It. You're Not

So many in this industry pride themselves on professionalism—the poker face, the "no matter what, I show up" mentality.

But burnout has a body language.
Compassion fatigue has a tone of voice.
Moral stress has a pace, an intensity, a kind of emotional static clients can feel the second you walk into the room.

You can be clinically brilliant and emotionally unavailable. You can know exactly what you're doing and still look overwhelmed, rushed, cold, short, or distant.

And here's the problem: clients interpret emotional exhaustion as indifference. Not because they're ungrateful, but because they don't know what you're carrying. They don't see your schedule. They don't know you euthanized a patient an hour ago. They don't know you haven't eaten since 7 a.m. They don't know the case you're still replaying in your head.

They just know how you made them feel.

You can't deliver the calm, centered, trust-building communication I talked about in this book if you're being crushed from the inside.

The Lies That Keep You Suffering

Here's the thing nobody wants to admit out loud: burnout doesn't start with overwork. It starts with the stories you tell yourself about overwork. It starts with the invisible belief system running in the background like a toxic operating system you never chose but learned anyway. These beliefs shape your behavior long before the stress ever shows up physiologically. And unless you drag those beliefs into the light and kill them, they will run your life—and your career—on autopilot.

Let's break down the biggest lies veterinarians tell themselves, because these lies do more damage than the 12-hour days, the angry clients, the euthanasias, and the emergencies combined.

Lie #1: "If I Don't Do It, No One Will."

This is the most seductive lie in the entire profession. It feels noble. It feels honorable. It feels like leadership. But really? It's martyrdom wearing a hero cape. It's you telling yourself a story that your suffering is somehow necessary to keep the hospital afloat. It's the emotional equivalent of duct-taping yourself to the steering wheel and calling it "commitment."

What actually happens is this: you become the person who gets exploited—by the system, by the workload, by the culture, and even by well-intentioned colleagues who have simply learned that you'll always say yes. You teach everyone that your boundaries are optional and your needs are negotiable. And eventually, you don't just resent the people around you—you resent the job itself.

Martyrdom is not leadership. Martyrdom is self-neglect dressed up as service.

And it's one of the fastest lanes to exhaustion, bitterness, and emotional collapse.

Lie #2: "Real Vets Can Handle This."

This lie is the quiet killer. It's the internal voice that whispers, "Everyone else is fine except me." It's the shame-driven belief that struggling makes you weak or unfit for the profession. It's the idea that emotional pain is a character flaw instead of a human reaction to an incredibly demanding job.

So what do you do? You suppress. You pretend. You mask. You tighten your jaw, swallow your emotions, and show up as the blank-faced "professional" everyone expects. And inside, the pressure builds. You start to believe there's something fundamentally wrong with you because you're not made of stone.

Let me be blunt: the idea that "real vets just handle it" is bullshit. It's the leftover residue of an old-school culture built on bravado and emotional silence. It's outdated. It's dangerous. And it's costing the profession its people.

Struggling doesn't mean you're weak. Struggling means you're human. And if you weren't struggling under the load this job demands? That would be the red flag.

Lie #3: "I Don't Have Time to Take Care of Myself."

This one sounds practical. It sounds logical. It sounds like the kind of thing you say when staring at a schedule with zero space between appointments. But this lie is the biggest paradox in veterinary medicine: you think you're too busy to take care of yourself, but the truth is you're too busy *not* to.

Your patients don't need a hollowed-out doctor running on adrenaline and caffeine. Your clients don't need a frantic communicator rushing through explanations. Your team doesn't need a chronically exhausted leader snapping under pressure.

You are practicing medicine on a biological machine—your brain—and that machine needs fuel, rest, movement, hydration, and emotional decompression. When you tell yourself you don't have time to take care of yourself, what you're really saying is:
"I'm okay practicing medicine with impaired judgment."
"I'm okay showing up at half-capacity."
"I'm okay defaulting to survival mode."

You wouldn't accept that from a pilot. You wouldn't accept that from an anesthesiologist. So why accept it from yourself?

Lie #4: "I'm Fine."

This is the most dangerous lie because it feels harmless. It feels polite. It feels like the easy answer that keeps things moving. But "I'm fine" is often code for:

"I'm numb."

"I've disconnected."

"I've turned off the alarm system because it was screaming too loudly."

You get so used to pushing through that you lose the ability to recognize your own emotional state. You mistake numbness for stability. You mistake dissociation for resilience. You mistake shutting down for coping. And once "I'm fine" becomes reflexive, it becomes the mask that hides the very signs you need to address.

The problem with "I'm fine" is that it blocks all solutions.

You can't seek help if you pretend nothing's wrong.

You can't set boundaries if you pretend you don't need them.

You can't rest if you pretend you're not exhausted.

You can't process grief if you pretend it didn't affect you.

"I'm fine" is the quiet voice that keeps you stuck in emotional quicksand.

These Lies Are the Real Burnout Triggers

These lies don't just exhaust you. They trap you. They keep you from asking for help.

They keep you from setting boundaries. They keep you from taking breaks, from grieving, from recovering, and from resetting. They keep you performing the version of yourself you think others expect, instead of honoring the one your nervous system desperately needs.

And worst of all, these lies keep you from becoming the doctor your clients actually want—the one who is present, composed, attuned, compassionate, authentic, and trustworthy. Clients don't want a superhero. Clients want a human being they can trust.

That version of you cannot exist if you're running your career on a foundation of lies that glorify self-destruction.

Burnout doesn't start with stress. It starts with the stories you tell yourself about stress. Change the story, and you change everything.

The Five Nonnegotiables of Staying Human in Veterinary Medicine

Let's get something straight before we go any further: none of the strategies I'm about to list are luxuries. They're not indulgences. They're not things you do when you finally have time. These are clinical tools just as essential as your stethoscope, your medical records, or your ability to interpret a blood panel. These are the foundational inputs that keep your brain, your empathy, and your emotional regulation online. Without them, everything else in this profession becomes harder—your communication, your medicine, your patience, your judgment, your trust-building, and your entire presence in the exam room.

Let's break them down.

1. *Sleep: The Most Underrated Medical Intervention in the Entire Profession*

   If you take nothing else from this chapter, take this: your sleep is not optional. It's not something you "fit in" after you finish catching up on charts, or when the adrenaline finally drops after your tenth crisis of the day. In veterinary medicine, sleep is the primary determinant of your emotional stability. No sleep means your prefrontal cortex—the part of your brain responsible for patience, decision-making, and communication—goes offline. And when that happens, you're not just tired; you're dysregulated. You're irritable. You're quicker to snap. You're slower to process. You get tunnel vision. You lose clarity.

Sleep is the difference between being the veterinarian who calmly explains a complicated treatment plan and the one who rushes through it with a clipped tone. It is the difference between taking a breath and taking something personally. Your clients don't see your sleep schedule, but they feel the consequences of it instantly. Sleep is the most powerful clinical tool you have for protecting your emotional bandwidth.

2. *Movement: Not Workouts, Movement*

This isn't about lifting weights or running marathons. I'm talking about something far simpler and far more achievable: movement. Your nervous system was not designed to sit in back-to-back emotional encounters without release. When you move—even walking the perimeter of the building, stretching between appointments, climbing the stairs instead of grabbing the elevator—you change your biochemistry. You lower stress hormones. You regulate your breathing. You reduce adrenaline spikes. You give your body the chance to discharge emotional load before it calcifies into tension.

Ten minutes of walking can flip your internal state faster than any motivational speech or productivity hack. It doesn't need to be perfect. It doesn't need to be sweaty. It just needs to be intentional, and it needs to be regular. Movement is how you tell your body, "We're safe. We're steady. We can keep going." It's emotional maintenance disguised as physical activity.

3. *Real Meals and Hydration: Your Brain Cannot Run on Caffeine and Adrenaline Alone*

I hate to break it to you, but coffee is not a food group. And yet veterinary medicine pretends it is—skipping meals, inhaling carbohydrates between rooms, chugging caffeine like it's courage in a cup. But here's the hard truth: running your brain on coffee and cortisol is how you fry your nervous system. When your blood sugar crashes, so does your patience. When you're dehydrated, your cognitive processing drops. When you skip meals, your emotional resilience tanks.

Your brain is a high-performance organ. It needs fuel. It needs water. It needs stabilization. Getting through a 12-hour shift on an iced coffee and two bites of a granola bar doesn't make you tough; it makes you brittle. You deserve real food, not just survival calories. Hydration isn't a convenience. It's what keeps your brain functioning when you're moving from a euthanasia to a puppy vaccine to a skin work-up in five minutes flat.

You want clearer communication? Better patience? More emotional presence? Feed your brain.

4. *Actual Rest: The Off-switch That Veterinary Culture Tries to Shame Out of You*

There's "taking a break," and then there's actually resting. Most veterinary professionals have forgotten what the second one feels like. Real rest is not scrolling TikTok at midnight because you're too wired to sleep. It's not sitting on your couch answering client emails. It's not finishing medical notes while your dinner gets cold. That's not rest, that's passive work disguised as downtime.

Actual rest means stepping fully away from veterinary medicine long enough for your nervous system to reset. It means giving your brain permission to stop rehearsing cases, replaying conversations, or recalculating treatment plans in the background. Rest is the moment your mind stops performing and starts recovering. Without it, your emotional system never gets to recalibrate. You end up operating on fumes, then blame yourself for not having the same empathy reserves you had on Monday.

Real rest isn't something you earn by grinding harder. It's something you protect so you can keep being human tomorrow.

5. *Professional Support: The Outlet Your Brain Desperately Needs*

Every veterinarian carries grief. Every technician carries pain. Every CSR carries emotional residue from every difficult client they've ever had. The problem is that veterinary culture teaches people to bury it, minimize it, or "be tough." But your brain is not a filing cabinet. You cannot keep stuffing trauma and sorrow into the same mental drawer and expect it to stay closed.

Professional support—whether it's a therapist, a coach, a peer-support group, a mentor, or anyone trained to process emotional load—is not indulgence. It's triage. It gives your brain somewhere to put the grief so it doesn't leak into your exam rooms, your home life, or your self-worth. It gives you language for the pain you've been silently carrying. It gives you perspective when compassion fatigue starts whispering lies.

Seeking support is not a sign that you're failing. It's a sign you understand the emotional math of this profession. No one can hold this much sorrow, stress, and moral conflict alone. You weren't meant to.

None of This Is Luxury. It's Maintenance.

I'll say it again because this industry loves to forget it: none of this is indulgence. None of it is extra. None of it is some spa-day vision of "self-care." This is oxygen-mask stuff. This is the bare minimum required to keep your empathy intact, your judgment sharp, and your humanity accessible.

You are caring for people on the worst days of their lives. You are supporting animals in their most vulnerable moments. You are doing work that is emotionally, psychologically, and spiritually demanding. That means you need infrastructure—real, practical, biological infrastructure—to keep yourself steady.

Your sleep, your movement, your nutrition, your rest, and your support system ... these aren't bonuses. They are your emotional PPE. Without them, veterinary medicine becomes a slow erosion. With them, you become the kind of veterinarian who can care deeply without losing yourself in the process.

Leaders: This Is a Team Issue, Not an Individual One

If you're a practice owner, manager, regional director, or medical director, I need you to hear something loud and clear: burnout is not a personal failing. It is a systems failure. And if your hospital is drowning in chaos, chronic stress, short staffing, or emotional overload, no amount of "self-care" advice is going to save your team. You cannot meditate your way out of a broken workflow. You cannot yoga your way out of a toxic schedule. You cannot gratitude-journal your way out of chronic understaffing. You cannot demand elite communication from people who are emotionally underwater.

Let's stop pretending individuals can fix what leadership refuses to address. A struggling system will eat even your strongest team alive.

Here's the truth most leaders don't want to admit: you can't expect trust-building communication in a clinic where people don't even have time to breathe. When your team is overbooked, understaffed, and sprinting through appointments with cortisol levels high enough to power a small city, their empathy tanks are empty. Their patience evaporates. Their emotional reserves get drained dry. And then you step back and wonder why the client experience is inconsistent. It's because you built a system that makes consistency impossible.

Culture isn't built in a staff meeting or a poster in the break room. Culture is built in the day-to-day lived experience of your people. And if that lived experience is constant pressure, emotional trauma, skipped lunches, never-ending backlogs, and the feeling of always being behind, then your culture—no matter what you *say* it is—is burnout.

And burnout always devours culture. Every. Single. Time. There's a popular saying in the business world that culture eats strategy for breakfast. But while culture eats strategy, burnout eats culture. If you don't fix the system, the system will eat your people and then blame them for getting tired.

Leadership means taking responsibility for the emotional environment your team works in. That includes:

1. ***Staffing Appropriately, and Not Relying on the Same Three Exhausted Heroes to Pull Miracles Every Day***

   Your top performers are not infinite resources. When you build a schedule on the backs of the people who "always stay late," "always say yes," and "never complain," you're not complimenting them—you're exploiting them. A clinic that runs on overfunctioning is a clinic that is slowly grinding its best people into dust. Staff for the volume you actually have, not the volume you *wish* you had.

2. ***Normalizing Debriefs After Hard Cases, Because Every Team Needs a Pressure Valve***

   A hospital that pretends euthanasias don't take a toll is a hospital practicing emotional malpractice. Debriefing isn't a luxury; it's a necessity. Five minutes of team connection after a traumatic case can prevent five months of emotional fallout. Give people a place to put the grief instead of forcing them to shove it down and "move on."

3. ***Encouraging Breaks Without Guilt, and Enforcing Them When Needed***

   If your team feels like taking a break makes them selfish, lazy, or burdensome, that's not culture—that's coercion. Breaks are not rewarded behavior; they are biological requirements. The brain needs recovery time. Your team shouldn't have to earn basic human needs.

4. *Creating Psychological Safety So Team Members Can Speak Up Without Fear*

If your people are afraid to say, "I'm overwhelmed," or "I made a mistake," or "I need help," your hospital is primed for burnout AND medical errors. Silence is expensive. Silence is dangerous. Silence is the enemy of trust. When people can't speak honestly, they emotionally disconnect. And disconnected teams cannot deliver connected client care.

5. *Supporting Mental Health Days Without Judgment*

Mental health days are not "time off for people who can't handle stress." They are preventive care—for your most valuable asset: your team's emotional capacity. If you only allow time off once someone has fully broken, you're not leading. You're reacting.

6. *Modeling Boundaries Instead of Bragging About Self-sacrifice*

If leaders brag about working 14-hour days, skipping meals, being "always available," or never taking time off, the team will assume that's the expectation. Then they will mimic it until they burn out or quit. The fastest way to build a burned-out hospital is to have burned-out leadership. The fastest way to build a sustainable one is to show your team what healthy looks like.

Because here's the gut-punch truth: a thriving practice is not built on heroics. It is built on sustainability. That's what creates retention. That's what creates psychological safety. That's what creates consistent client experience. That's what creates better medicine. And ironically, sustainability is what generates financial performance—because burned-out teams don't communicate well, don't build trust well, and don't stay long enough to create momentum.

Too many leaders think culture is buying pizza, hosting a holiday party, or giving out swag. None of that matters if your people are emotionally exhausted. Your best culture move isn't a free lunch. Your best culture move is protecting your team's mental health like it's a critical patient—because it is.

You want better client experience? Better reviews? Better compliance? Better financial results?

Then protect your people. It's the most strategic move you will ever make as a leader.

The Direct Line Between Well-being and Client Experience

Now let's bring this all the way back to the core of everything we've been building toward in this book: trust. Every chapter, every framework, every strategy, every story has been pointing to the same heartbeat—because trust is the real currency of veterinary medicine. Not credentials. Not equipment. Not diagnostic toys. Trust. And the thing nobody tells you early in your career is that trust doesn't start in the exam room. It starts in you—in your nervous system, in your regulation, in the emotional tone you carry into every interaction.

Because here's what happens when you're regulated instead of fried: your voice softens. Not in a weak way, but in a grounded way. You speak from your diaphragm instead of your adrenaline. Clients feel steadiness in you, and that steadiness becomes contagious. Your explanations get clearer because your brain isn't scrambling for words. You're able to think one step at a time instead of juggling twelve thoughts at once. You shift from reactivity to curiosity, which is the difference between cutting someone off and saying, "Tell me more about what you noticed at home."

When you're regulated, you actually listen. Not performative listening, but true listening: the kind where clients feel understood, not judged. You pause instead of rushing. You make space instead of filling it. You show up with presence instead of preoccupation. And you connect—really connect—instead of slipping into defensiveness or detachment.

Here's the kicker: clients don't know what's going on in your personal life. They don't know your workload. They don't know the emergencies you handled that morning or the three euthanasias that broke a piece of your heart. But they feel your internal state instantly. Humans are wired for emotional mirroring, and pets are even more sensitive. A dysregulated doctor creates dysregulated clients. A calm, grounded doctor creates calmer, more grounded clients.

And calm, grounded clients say "yes" more often. They ask better questions because they're not embarrassed or intimidated. They trust your recommendations because they trust you. They follow through. They come back for rechecks. They stay with your hospital for years. They refer their friends. They tell stories about how "our vet is different."

That's the magic. That's the multiplier. That's the thing everyone underestimates.

Because when you are regulated, your communication sharpens. When your communication sharpens, trust grows. When trust grows, compliance rises. When compliance rises, outcomes improve. When outcomes improve, clients stay loyal. When loyalty increases, your hospital becomes financially healthier. And when the hospital becomes financially healthier, you can reinvest in your team, your equipment, your training, and your space—all of which protect well-being.

And suddenly, you realize something powerful:
Well-being → communication → trust → compliance → outcomes → loyalty → revenue → reinvestment → well-being.

That's the Trust Flywheel.
Not running on scripts.
Not running on pressure.
Not running on the myth of endless self-sacrifice.

Running on human fuel.

Your nervous system is the ignition. Your presence is the accelerator. Your well-being is the oil that keeps the engine from seizing.

Trust doesn't just happen because you're medically competent. It happens because you show up as a whole, regulated human being. It happens because clients can feel the difference, even if they can't articulate it.

This is why your mental health matters. It's not a side quest. It's the foundation of client experience, practice performance, team culture, and the emotional longevity of your career.

You don't get trust without well-being. You don't get loyalty without presence. You don't get sustainable leadership without regulation.

This is the Flywheel. This is the engine. This is the real work. And it starts with protecting the human behind the coat.

The Truth: You Deserve to Stay in the Story

Here's the deepest truth in this chapter: You are not a machine. You are not a diagnosis generator. You are not an emotional punching bag for clients, or life, or the internet. You didn't come into veterinary medicine to burn out. You didn't choose this career to become numb. You didn't dream of becoming a shell of yourself.

You came here because you love animals. Because you care about people. Because helping others lights you up. And the world needs vets who still care.

But caring will crush you if you don't care for yourself along the way.

This profession asks for your empathy, your presence, your clarity, your patience, and your humanity. But you can't give any of that if your inner world is falling apart.

Your mental health is not a luxury. It's not a perk. It's not a reward for surviving another year. It's the foundation of everything: your communication, your trust-building, your clarity, your empathy, your leadership, your impact, your longevity, and your legacy.

You deserve support. You deserve boundaries. You deserve rest. You deserve a hospital culture that doesn't require self-sacrifice as the price of entry. You deserve to stay in this profession and actually enjoy it ... not just survive it.

Because here's the truth that ties this whole book together: *The best version of you delivers the best version of veterinary medicine.*

You can't pour from an empty vet. You can't build trust from burnout. You can't deliver world-class medicine from emotional triage.

When you take care of your mental health, every client interaction becomes more authentic. Every treatment plan is delivered with more clarity. Every tough moment is handled with more compassion. Every exam room becomes safer—for clients, pets, and for you.

The Trust Flywheel doesn't start with scripts. It starts with a human being whose emotional engine is still capable of turning.

So protect that engine. Protect your heart. Protect your ability to keep caring. Because veterinary medicine needs you—not the burned-out version, not the numb version, not the exhausted version. It needs the human behind the voice.

So take care of the engine. Protect the human behind the voice. Build systems that support your heart as much as your brain. Because veterinary medicine doesn't need more martyrs. It needs you—alive, healthy, present, and still capable of caring.

That's how you build a career that doesn't just last but makes a difference that outlives you.

Chapter 34
Step Up. This Is Your Moment

Titles don't make leaders. Choices do.

You don't need "Owner" on your badge.
You don't need "Hospital Manager" in your email signature.
You don't need permission from corporate, a consultant, or a task force.

You need one internal decision that changes everything: **"I'm going first."**

Not when it's convenient.
Not when it's clean.
Not when the schedule is light and the lobby is calm.

First when the lobby is stacked.
First when the phones won't stop.
First when the surgery board is full.
First when emotions are high and everyone's nervous system is fried.

First to care louder.
First to steady the room.
First to bring emotional leadership when everyone else is stuck in survival mode.

Leadership does not begin when your job title changes.
Leadership begins the moment **you refuse to wait**.

The Lie We're Taught About Leadership

Somewhere along the way, most people were taught a quiet lie:

"When I get the title... then I'll lead."
"When they give me the authority... then I'll step up."
"When someone puts me in charge... then I'll act different."

That lie has kept more potential locked up than fear, burnout, or doubt ever could.

Because here's the truth:

Leadership Is Not a Promotion. It's a Posture

And once you take that posture—everything in your life changes.

Here's what nobody really taught me, but what life has proven to me over and over again:

Leadership Is a Shortcut to Meaning. And Meaning Is the Fuel Source of Joy

Not fake joy.
Not highlight-reel joy.
Real joy. The kind that follows you home at night.

Yes—leadership brings pressure.
Yes—it brings responsibility.
Yes—it will put you in rooms where you feel unsure, underqualified, and exposed.

But when you lead?

You trade comfort for **purpose**. You sleep differently. You carry yourself differently. You feel the weight of your day—but also the worth of it. You go home tired—but deeply, unmistakably alive.

You Are Not Behind—You Are Being Prepared

If you've made it this far in this book, I already know something about you:

You're not satisfied with "just getting through the shift."
You notice what's broken.
You feel the friction in the system.
You care when things slip through the cracks.

You feel that subtle pull when something could be better.

That pull is not annoyance.
It's not negativity.
It's not you being "difficult."

That's Leadership Trying to Wake You Up

Leadership is not a personality trait. It's not charisma. It's not something you're either born with or not.

Leadership is a **muscle**. And muscles are only built under resistance. You strengthen it every time you:

- Clean up the process everyone complains about but nobody owns
- Fix the communication breakdown between CSR and tech
- Ask the question everyone avoids
- Volunteer to run the huddle
- Create the follow-up template that makes the whole team stronger

You don't need permission to model excellence. Excellence gives its own permission.

Do the small things.
Do them consistently.
And watch what happens.

Because **excellence is magnetic**.

People don't follow résumés. They follow energy, clarity, and consistency.

**Veterinary Medicine Will Break You—If You Let It

Or Build You—If You Choose It.**

Let's stop pretending this work is easy.

Veterinary medicine is beautiful.
It's sacred. And it is absolutely brutal some days.

You carry fear, grief, financial stress, life-or-death decisions, the emotional weight of families who love their pets like children. Some days drain your spirit. Some days hollow you out. Some days follow you home even when you don't want them to. There are nights when you sit in your car after a shift and just stare at the steering wheel because you don't yet have the energy to drive.

Every person who lasts in this profession has had that moment. So here's the reframe that separates leaders from survivors: **Those brutal days are not your enemy. They are your training ground.** They are the intangible weight that builds emotional muscle. Because problems are not interruptions in this profession... They are the curriculum.

Leadership doesn't come from comfort. It's born from pressure:

Every angry client.
Every 12-hour shift.
Every heartbreaking euthanasia.
Every moment you thought, *"I can't do one more."*

Those moments branded you. But they did not weaken you. They forged you.

Your Scars Are Not Weakness—They Are Credentials

Do not minimize what you've lived through in this profession.

Your grief gave you depth.
Your exhaustion gave you perspective.
Your anger gave you boundaries.
Your doubt taught you humility.

Who better to steady a panicked CSR than the tech who once cried in the parking lot?
Who better to support a drowning doctor than the leader who once nearly quit?
Who better to comfort a grieving client than the person who has held that same grief in their own chest?

If my experiences as a leader have taught me anything, it's this: You don't lead from perfection. You lead from lived experience.

In other words, your scars are not disqualifications. They are proof of capability. They are emotional receipts that say: *I've been there. I survived. I can guide you through this too.*

Stop Waiting for "Someone" to Fix It

Waiting for someone else to fix your hospital is one of the most expensive strategies you can choose. It costs time, momentum, morale, and eventually... your belief that change is even possible.

Leadership is not a spectator sport.

It's contact.
It's friction.
It's imperfect implementation.

See the problem? Name it.
Have an idea? Test it.
Hit resistance? Scale it down and relaunch.
Need backup? Find two humans and start tiny.

Momentum beats permission.
Every.
Single.
Time.

You want gratitude in the culture? Model it—loudly, specifically, publicly.

You want fewer client blow-ups? Model calm under pressure when everyone else is reactive.

You want doctors to slow down and connect? Set the room. Prime the emotional runway. Create the pause.

People do not change because you posted a policy. They change because you showed them who to be when it was hardest.

Your Energy Is Strategic

Let's kill a dangerous myth right now: **Your energy is not a personality trait. It's a leadership tool.** It's not something you "turn on" when you're in the mood. It's not optional. And it's definitely not "extra."

In a veterinary hospital, your emotional state is not private. It is broadcast.
Every sigh is data.
Every eye roll is a message.
Every sharp tone trains the room how to feel next.

So you don't just walk into the building—you set the emotional temperature of it.

Your clients and team feel the pace in your voice. They feel tension in your posture. They feel safety—or danger—before they understand a word you say.

That's not soft science. That's biology.

And enthusiasm? It's only cringe when it's fake.

When enthusiasm is rooted in meaning? When it's tied to outcomes? When it's anchored to real lives being helped? It becomes leadership oxygen.

"Three clean bloodwork calls just went out—three families sleep easier tonight. Let's go."

That sentence does three powerful things at once:

- It connects effort to impact
- It reminds people *why* they're here
- It pulls the team out of task mode and back into purpose

Now you're not just running labs. You're creating relief. You're restoring peace. You're changing nights for families. And when you lead like that—purpose-first, energy-forward—burnout loses leverage.

So, you can install the best workflows in the world. You can buy the best equipment in the world. You can write the perfect SOP. But if the emotional energy of the building is heavy, numb, sarcastic, or flat? All that excellence leaks. Because energy moves faster than process. Tone moves faster than training. And emotion moves faster than instruction.

A toxic nervous system will sabotage elite systems every time. That's why culture never truly changes through policy alone. It changes through emotional leadership in real moments.

At 7:42 a.m. when the first client snaps at the front desk.
At 1:13 p.m. when anesthesia just spiked.
At 4:58 p.m. when everyone is fried and one more thing goes wrong.

Those are the *real* leadership moments.

But this is where leadership gets uncomfortable—because it gets personal.

You can't fake calm.
You can't outsource presence.
You can't intellectually override a dysregulated nervous system.

If *you* are frantic, the room becomes frantic. If *you* are grounded, the room steadies.

Your breathing teaches people how fast to breathe.
Your tone gives permission for how loud fear gets to be.
Your posture communicates whether the moment is dangerous or doable.

This is why some hospitals feel chaotic even on "easy" days... And why some hospitals feel calm even in crisis.

It's not staffing.
It's not luck.
It's a leadership state.

So here's the challenge I want to leave you with:

Before you lead people...
Before you lead systems...
Before you lead meetings...

Lead Your Energy

Choose presence over panic. Choose purpose over pressure. Choose grounded confidence over emotional leakage.

Not because it's trendy. Not because it looks good. But because **everything else depends on it.** Your team doesn't need perfection. They need a regulated leader from whom they can borrow calm when things get heavy.

Fear Will Talk. Lead Anyway

Make no mistake—every meaningful change activates fear first.
Not logic.
Not curiosity.
Not excitement.

Fear speaks first. And it speaks loud. It sounds like:

- "This isn't how we've always done it."
- "That'll never work here."
- "We tried that once."
- "That's not my job."
- "Now just isn't the right time."
- "You're going too fast."
- "You're making things uncomfortable."

Of course it's uncomfortable. Growth always is.

Fear doesn't show up as courage-killing panic most of the time. It shows up as sarcasm, cynicism, eye rolls, "helpful" skepticism, passive resistance, and fake logic wrapped around real insecurity.

Fear dresses up as practicality. But its real job is simple: Protect the familiar.

And here's why leadership is challenging: True leadership is disruptive by nature.

Even change -including positive ones—threatens identity, comfort, predictability, old hierarchies, and unspoken power dynamics. When you introduce new standards, some people don't hear, "Here's how we improve." They hear, "Here's how who you were is no longer enough." And that hurts.

So they resist—not because they hate excellence, but because change feels like loss before it ever feels like gain. Your job as a leader is not to eliminate that discomfort. Your job is to walk people through it without retreating.

And this part matters just as much: Fear doesn't just speak through the team. It's an internal battle too. It speaks through you. It'll whisper:

- "Who am I to lead this?"
- "What if I fail publicly?"
- "What if they judge me?"
- "What if I make it worse?"
- "What if I lose respect?"

That voice sounds responsible. But it's not wisdom. It's self-protection disguised as humility. But real humility doesn't hide. It shows up. Leadership courage is not the absence of fear. It is the decision that fear doesn't get the final vote.

So this is the line that separates hobby leadership from real leadership: You are not here to win comfort. You are here to move the hospital.

Comfort preserves. Leadership transforms.

Comfort keeps today intact. Leadership creates tomorrow.

Comfort protects feelings. Leadership protects outcomes.

If your primary goal is approval, you will never challenge the systems quietly harming pets, clients, and teams. But if your primary goal is impact, you will sometimes be misunderstood—and still move forward.

So, let fear speak. You don't need to silence it. Just don't let it drive.

You lead anyway.
You test anyway.
You model anyway.
You stay anchored anyway.

And over time, something powerful happens: Eye rolls turn into quiet observation. Skepticism turns into cautious curiosity. "That's not my job" turns into "How can I help?" Not because you argued. But because you moved.

Summary: Your Turn Is Now

Stop waiting.
Stop shrinking.
Stop looking around for someone else to go first.

This is your moment.

You've already been through the fire: The brutal shifts. The angry clients. The emotional overload. The nights you wondered if you could keep going.

You kept going.
Those scars are not your burden.
They are your proof.

Leadership is not granted.
It is chosen.

This game is about decisions: To steady the room, to bring gratitude into exhaustion, to take small wins and turn them into a flywheel.

Step up—and meaning will follow you home. Step back—and the grind will own you.

So stop waiting. Stop outsourcing your power.

Raise your hand.
Go first.
Lead loud.

The pets deserve it.
The clients need it.
The team is waiting for it.

And deep down—you already know this: **You were built for this.**

Chapter 35

Conclusion—This Work Is Sacred

If you made it here—if you actually walked with me through every chapter, every idea, every uncomfortable truth—then I'm going to say something I don't say lightly:

Thank you.

Thank you for giving me your most finite resource—your time.
Thank you for caring enough about this profession, your team, your clients, and your patients to stare straight at the things most people would rather avoid.
Thank you for choosing growth over comfort. Curiosity over coasting. Truth over convenience.

And let me say this clearly, unapologetically:

YOU matter. The work you do every single day matters—so damn much. Even when it feels invisible. Even when it feels routine. Even when nobody says thank you. Even when the best you gave today feels like it disappeared into noise. It didn't. It never does.

Let's get something straight. I didn't write this for clout. I didn't write this for conferences. I damn sure didn't write it for ego. I wrote this because this industry changed me. Veterinary medicine didn't just shape my career. It reshaped my soul.

It happened in waiting rooms thick with fear, treatment areas buzzing with urgency, quiet late nights when grief finally caught up with everyone in the building, and conversations with exhausted leaders wondering how much longer they could hold the line.

The teams I've worked beside.
The clients I've cried with.
The pets I've watched fight—and sometimes lose.

They taught me one brutal, beautiful truth: **trust is the currency of this work. And if we lose trust, we lose everything.**

Not hypothetically. Not metaphorically. Everything.

That's why I obsessed over this.
Why I built the Veterinary Trust Flywheel.

Why I created PAGE, ALARM, and every other tool in these pages. Why I poured in every scar, every story, every moment that shaped me.

Not because I have all the answers. But because I believe—deep in my bones—that you can carry this forward. Not as theory. As impact.

Let's be brutally honest: this profession is not cute. It's long days, brutal clients, financial pressure no one talks about at dinner parties, and emotional weight most outsiders will never fully understand. It is living in the crossfire between love, money, fear, guilt, hope, and grief—every single shift.

But don't you dare reduce yourself to tasks.

You are not "just" answering phones.
You are not "just" running anesthesia.
You are not "just" writing charts.
You are not "just" prescribing meds.

You are building **trust in moments people will remember forever. You are standing beside someone in** one of the most vulnerable chapters of their life. That's not a job. **That's legacy.**

So, let me look you in the eye through these pages for a second. I don't care if you are a Client Service Representative (CSR) on day 30, a tech drowning in responsibility, a brand-new grad DVM trying not to show how scared you are, or a hospital leader feeling the full weight of everyone else's survival on your shoulders. You already have everything it takes to build real trust.

You already have the power to make someone feel seen. To turn panic into relief. To turn confusion into clarity. To turn fear into courage. To walk someone through the hardest goodbye of their life with dignity.

Don't you ever underestimate that.

Not once.
Not on your worst day.
Not when you feel invisible.
Not when you feel replaceable.
Not when you feel like quitting.

You are not replaceable. You are standing at the fault line between **fear and hope.** That is power.

The Future of This Profession Is Human

The future of veterinary medicine is not just about better medicine. It's about **better humanity.** It's about:

- Leaders with emotional courage
- Teams with psychological safety

- Clients who feel respected instead of managed
- Cultures where people don't have to armor up just to survive the shift

It belongs to people—official leaders or not—who walk into chaos and say:

"I'll go first."
"I'll choose compassion."
"I'll choose trust."
"I'll choose to make this moment matter."

So, here's my ask—and I'm not whispering it: **don't let this book die on your nightstand.**

Take it back into your hospital. Tomorrow.

Try one small thing. Make one client feel more seen. Protect one teammate from unnecessary pressure. Ask one better question. Slow down one rushed moment. Build one micro-moment of trust.

Then, do that every day.

And I promise you this: you won't just change your hospital. You will change who YOU become in the process. Because leadership doesn't just transform systems. It transforms identity.

And please—hear this in the deepest place it can land: you are not alone.

I am in this with you.
This book is not something I drop and disappear from.
This is my work.
My calling.
My oxygen.

If you are struggling—reach out.
If you feel alone—reach out.
If you need someone to remind you why you signed up for this on the days you forget—reach out.

Because I don't just want *you* to succeed. **I want *us* to rise. Together.**

So, step up.
Be real.
Lead loud.
Build trust like your career depends on it—because it does.

But more than that: build trust like lives depend on it—because they do.

You have what it takes. You always did. So, this isn't the end of the story. This is your starting line.

Thank you for walking this journey with me. I need you to know something—something that lives underneath all the urgency, all the fire, all the challenge in these pages: **I am truly honored.**

Honored that you let me into your world. Honored that you trusted me with your questions, your doubts, your fatigue, and your hope. Honored that you didn't just skim this—you *stayed.* You wrestled with it. You felt it. You let it press on you.

Do you have any idea how sacred that is?

You didn't owe me that.
You didn't have to care this much.
And yet—you showed up with an open mind and an open heart anyway.

That tells me everything I need to know about you.

It tells me you're the kind of person who doesn't run from the hard stuff.
The kind who feels the weight of this work and chooses to carry it with intention.
The kind who could've gone numb—but decided instead to go deeper.

To be allowed into that space with you—to walk alongside you in that way—is not something I take lightly. Ever.

I don't see you as a "reader." I see you as a partner in this mission.

And I am profoundly, humbly grateful for you.

Let's change this industry together. Because it's worth it. Because what we build next will outlive us.

Appendix A:

The Veterinary Hospital Identity Workshop: Define. Align. Thrive.

Workshop Facilitator Guide: Introduction

Welcome, leaders. This workshop is built to do one thing: help you create a hospital where your team thrives, your clients trust you deeply, and your culture becomes your competitive edge. Everything we cover today ladders up to that outcome. This guide will walk you step-by-step through the process so you can lead confidently and with intention.

We'll move through three core sections—each one building on the last, each one unlocking a new layer of clarity, alignment, and direction for your hospital. By the end, your team won't just understand where you're going; they'll feel *invested* in it.

1. Set the Tone

   We start by grounding the room. Veterinary work is emotional, fast-paced, and often overwhelming. Before we talk strategy, we set the energy, expectations, and psychological safety needed for honest conversation. This is where leaders model the vulnerability, openness, and steadiness they expect from the team. When you set the tone correctly, everything that follows becomes easier and more impactful.

2. Mission, Vision, and Values Setting

Next, we align on the "why." This section is where leaders and teams cocreate the hospital's North Star—the purpose behind the work, the future you are building toward, and the values that guide how you show up every day. Without this clarity, culture drifts. With it, culture becomes magnetic. This is the foundation of consistency, trust, and long-term alignment across your entire hospital.

3. Designing Your Future Team and Client Experience/Goal-setting

Finally, we turn intention into action. This is where your team maps out the future experience they want to deliver—for yourselves and for your clients. Through structured exercises, you'll identify what needs to improve, what needs to stop, and what high-impact behaviors you want to normalize. You'll turn those insights into concrete goals that your hospital can execute on immediately.

This workshop isn't theoretical. It's practical, collaborative, and immediately actionable. Your job as facilitator is to guide the conversation, create a safe space for contribution, and help your team bring their best ideas forward. When practiced well, this process doesn't just set goals. It builds ownership, pride, and genuine excitement for the future of your hospital.

Let's get started.

Set the Tone

Total Time: ~3–5 minutes
Goal: Motivate the team to lean in and contribute enthusiastically to the workshop exercises that follow. Make it clear that they each

have a part in the workshop and that today is about collaboration. Articulate that successful client experience rests on a healthy team dynamic and culture first.

Materials Needed: None

You have several options available to you as you tee up your Veterinary CX Workshop with your team. Which approach you choose may have to do with your own delivery style and how you feel most comfortable speaking, but it also makes sense to gauge how your team is feeling and tailor the approach based on what you feel will land best based on the situation within your hospital. Below, I've listed out four different approaches or styles for your opening introduction, summarized when it makes sense to use which individual approach, and provided a sample dialogue that you can use or lift from to make your introduction your own.

The "Purpose + Vulnerability" Approach

Warm, real, and emotionally grounded, this is great for managers leading a tired or skeptical team. Use this when you need to rebuild trust and remind people that you're human, not just management.

Best for: Teams that are burnt out, skeptical, or feeling disconnected.
Tone: Warm, open, human.
What it does: Lowers defenses and makes people feel *seen*.
Psychology: Vulnerability creates safety. When a leader shares "why this matters to me," it signals emotional honesty, and people instinctively lean in.
Watch for: Don't over-share or turn it into therapy. The goal is connection, not confession.
Energy cue: Soft eye contact, slower pacing, grounded body language.

Sample Introduction Dialogue

> *"Before we dive into today's exercises, I want to be really clear about why we're here today.*

Over the past few months, I've felt something changing in our hospital—not in a bad way, but in a real way. We've been busier than ever. Clients expect more. And honestly, I know we've all felt stretched thin.

And that's exactly why today matters. We're here to talk about how to strengthen both our client experience and our team experience, because the two are very connected. When our team feels supported, trusted, and valued, that energy naturally transfers to our clients.

We all know what it's like to be on the other side of that front desk, to feel either brushed off or cared for. That makes a big difference, and our clients feel that difference. And the experience we deliver to our clients starts with how we treat each other.

Today isn't about adding more to your plate. It's about getting back to the heart of why we do this work: helping people and pets feel cared for, and helping each other do our best work.

I believe in this team. I believe that when we trust each other, we create an environment that clients want to be part of. Because when we get trust flowing both ways—within our team and with our clients—everything else follows: better reviews, better morale, and better outcomes.

So today's about reconnecting with our why, and rebuilding the trust that makes this place special."

The "Fire + Vision" Approach

With a high-energy, rally-the-team tone, this approach is great for a motivated group ready to level up. Use this approach when you want to elevate good energy into a shared mission.

Best for: Teams that already have some momentum, who believe in the hospital but need clarity and fuel.
Tone: Energetic, visionary, forward-leaning.
What it does: Reframes "today's workshop" as part of something bigger: a movement, not a meeting.
Psychology: People are drawn to purpose. When they can *see* what success looks like, they want to chase it.

Watch for: Avoid sounding like a motivational poser. Passion without realism can feel fake.

Energy cue: Stand tall, use movement, show genuine excitement in your voice.

Sample Introduction Dialogue

> *"Alright team. Before we start, let's zoom out.*
>
> *Every hospital says they care about clients. But few can actually say they've built real trust. That's what separates good from great, and that's why we're here today.*
>
> *We're here to elevate both our client experience and our team experience. Because those two are inseparable and very connected. When our team communicates well, supports each other, and trusts one another, that confidence radiates out to clients. And when clients trust us, they come back—creating momentum that lifts everyone.*
>
> *The vision I want to paint today is this: a hospital where trust flows in multiple directions. Clients trust our care. We trust each other's judgment. Leadership trusts the team to bring ideas forward and the team trusts that leaders have their back. When that happens, everything accelerates: smoother days, happier clients, stronger financials.*
>
> *That's what today is all about: building momentum born from trust. Real, emotional, operational trust.*
>
> *So today, I want your ideas, your voices, your truth. Because this doesn't work unless it's ours. This is how we build a hospital that people brag about, a place where both our clients and our team feel proud to belong."*

The "Honest + Ownership" Approach

Candid and grounded, this approach is ideal for a hospital in transition or with morale challenges. Use this when your people need to hear the truth spoken with care.

Best for: Teams where there's frustration, gossip, or performance dips.

Tone: Direct but empathetic.

What it does: Builds credibility by naming the elephant in the room before anyone else can.

Psychology: When you own the problem first, people stop resisting and start participating. It transforms blame into belonging.

Watch for: Don't sound accusatory. The focus should be on "we," not "you."

Energy cue: Strong posture, measured pace, emphasis on "we" language.

Sample Introduction Dialogue

"I'll be honest: The reason we're here today isn't because someone told us to do a workshop. It's because I've been hearing things—from clients, from you, and from myself—that tell me we've got some growing to do.

And that's okay. Every great hospital hits that moment. But that's why we're here today: to take an honest look at how we're showing up for our clients and for each other. Because those two experiences mirror each other.

When we're short with one another behind the scenes, clients feel that tension in the lobby. When we communicate clearly and lift each other up, clients feel that, too. The team experience is the client experience.

So today is about rebuilding trust on both sides of the counter: within our walls and beyond them. Because if we want clients to feel cared for, we have to care for each other first and foremost.

We've got the right people, the right medicine, and the right heart. Now it's about tightening up how we work together, so that every client walks out feeling safe and cared for, and every teammate walks out proud of how they contributed at the end of the day.

This isn't 'management's project.' This is our hospital, and this is our opportunity to lead with trust, together."

The "No-BS/Firestarter" Approach

Raw, direct, and emotional, this is the kind of opener that jolts people awake. Use this when you need to break apathy and reignite pride.

Best for: Teams that are checked out, cynical, or craving authenticity.
Tone: Raw, passionate, no corporate fluff.
What it does: Shocks the system, resets attention, and shows people this isn't business-as-usual.
Psychology: Authentic emotion triggers mirror neurons. When people *feel* you, they believe you.
Watch for: Balance the fire with care. Anger without heart lands as hostility; passion with heart lands as *leadership*.
Energy cue: Firm voice, direct eye contact, natural movement. Let intensity come from *conviction*, not volume.

Sample Introduction Dialogue

"Alright, let's get something straight before we start.

This workshop isn't about checking a box. It's not about posters or buzzwords or pretending everything's perfect. It's about us deciding who we're going to be when things get messy, busy, or hard.

We're here today for one reason: to get real about trust. Trust with our clients, and trust within this team. Because you can't build one without the other.

Our clients can feel when we're aligned, and they can feel when we're not. If we're snappy with each other, they sense it. If we've got each other's backs, they sense that too. The client experience starts with the team experience.

We're here to make sure that what clients feel from us—empathy, confidence, care—is real because it's how we treat each other. That's the kind of culture that wins.

You can't fake trust. You can't slap a slogan on the wall and expect clients to rave about their visit. That's not how this works. Culture isn't a checklist. It's a daily choice.

Look, I don't need perfection. I need care. I need honesty. I need everyone in this room to give a damn—about each other and about our clients. Because if we don't, some other hospital will.

Our clients don't wake up thinking about our workflow. They wake up praying their dog or cat gets better. They want to feel safe here, and that starts with us feeling safe with each other.

That's what we're building today. Not scripts. Not slogans. Trust. Real, earned, reciprocal trust—inside and out.

So if you're here just to 'get through it,' you're gonna miss the point. But if you're here to build something bigger, to make this hospital the kind of place people talk about for the right reasons, then lean in. Because this is the moment."

Mission, Vision, and Values Setting

Total Time: ~90 minutes
Goal: Cocreate your hospital's mission, vision, and values—in plain English that your team can grasp and actually believes in.
Output: A working draft of your hospital's Mission/Vision/Values that everyone helped shape, plus the energy and ownership that comes with it.
Materials Needed: Flip charts or whiteboards, markers.

Time	Section	Objective
0:00–0:02	**Kickoff: Set the Context**	Frame why this exercise matters, by tying it to client trust, team trust, and culture.
0:02 0:25	**Mission Brainstorm**	Define "why we exist," your daily purpose and heartbeat.
0:25–0:45	**Vision Brainstorm**	Define "where we're going," your aspirational North Star.
0:45–1:05	**Values Brainstorm**	Define "how we behave," your daily standards and rules of the game.
1:05–1:25	**Group Synthesis and Read Back**	Align on the best ideas; read the first draft aloud together.
1:25–1:30	**Next Steps**	Celebrate progress; explain how the team will finalize and live these values.

Facilitator Script and Cues

The following is your ready-to-read script and activity cues. You can adapt it word-for-word or improvise off it.

0:00–0:02—Kickoff: Set the Context

Goal: Frame why this exercise matters by tying it to client trust, team trust, and culture.

Say:

"Alright, here's the deal. Every business on earth talks about culture, but 90% of them never clearly define it. They think culture is posters and perks. It's not.

Culture is how we treat each other and our clients when it's busy, when it's stressful, and when no one's watching. And if we want to create a culture that our clients *and* our team love being part of, it starts with clearly defining three things: our **mission, vision, and values**.

This isn't a corporate thing. This is a *team* thing. Because if we're the ones who define it, we'll be the ones who protect it.

Here's why this matters: our clients don't experience culture on paper. They experience it in the lobby, in the exam room, and even over the phone: in tone of voice, body language, and conversations. And if we're solid as a team, our clients *feel* that. Trust flows both ways: inside out.

So today, we're not writing fluff. We're writing the DNA of this hospital, together.

One ask: be real. Don't give 'corporate safe' answers. Speak from the floor, not the podium. You don't need a title to shape our future."

0:02–0:25—Mission Brainstorm: "Why We Exist"

Say:

"Let's start with our mission: why we exist.

Think of it this way: if a client asked, 'Why does your hospital exist?,' what would you want every single person here to say?

It's not about making money or filling appointments. It's about purpose. Why do we do what we do—for pets, for families, for each other?" We need to go deeper than "We care about pets." We want something unique and special to us, here.

Do: Ask the following questions and record answers on a whiteboard or flip chart:

- Who do we serve?
- What do we do, or want to do, better than anyone else?
- What kind of impact do we have, or want to have, on pets and families?
- How do we want clients to feel when they step into our hospital or interact with our team?
- Why do *you* personally get up and come here every day?

Say:

"Give me phrases, not full paragraphs. For example, 'We exist to give pets longer, healthier lives and families peace of mind.'

Once we have a few, we'll mash them together into one version that feels like us."

Do: Collect four to six quick answers to each question, write them down on a flip chart or whiteboard, and then circle common words, such as "care," "trust," "family," etc. Then, work together to craft a draft Mission statement.

A solid Mission statement has four parts:

1. **Who You Serve:** Start with the core audience: pets, clients, and community. Examples might include "pets and the people who love them," "our clients and their animals," and "our local community of pet families."
2. **The Care You Deliver (What You Do):** Then, describe your primary promise in plain, human language. Examples might include "deliver exceptional medical care," "provide compassionate, high-quality veterinary medicine," and "protect and improve pet health."
3. **The Emotional or Experiential Promise (How You Do It):** This is what differentiates you. Capture the *feeling* you want clients and teams to experience. Examples might include "with honesty, empathy, and clarity," "in a calm, supportive, judgment-free environment," and "with respect, partnership, and transparency."
4. **The Bigger Why (Your Higher Purpose):** End with the long-term impact or belief behind your work. Examples might include "so pets live longer, healthier lives," "because every pet deserves a lifetime of well-being," and "to strengthen the bond between people and their animals."

0:25–0:45—Vision Brainstorm: "Where We're Going"

Say:

"Alright, now let's talk about vision.

This is the 5- or 10-year picture. When people in our community talk about us, what do we want them to say?

This isn't what we do today. It's what we're becoming and building toward. It should stretch us. It should make us proud, give us something to strive for, and maybe even a little nervous because we're setting a high bar.

A vision is like our destination pin on the GPS. It tells us where we're heading so we stop driving in circles. It might sound like, 'To be the most trusted veterinary hospital in the Northeast—known for its deep commitment to innovation, compassion, and connection.'

Don't overthink the words. Focus on the feeling. What future do we want to build together?"

Do: Ask the following questions and record answers on a whiteboard or flip chart:

- If we were absolutely crushing it five years from now, what would that look like?
- What would clients be saying in reviews?
- What would the team be saying about working here?
- What would we be known for in our community?

Do: Gather responses and start to craft three to five statements with the team. For each one, ask, "Does this sound like who we want to become?" Select the best fit and fine-tune it to capture the most inspiring ideas and themes.

A solid Vision statement has the following structure:

"Our vision is to become [FUTURE IDENTITY] that [IMPACT] through [CULTURE/BEHAVIOR]."

1. **The Future Identity** is what you want to become, the aspirational identity of the hospital. Examples might include "to be the most trusted veterinary team in our community," "to become a leader in modern, relationship-centered care," and "to be a hospital known for exceptional medicine and unforgettable client experience."
2. **The Impact You Want to Have (On Clients, Pets, or the Community)** articulates what will be *different* because your hospital exists. Examples might include "where clients feel supported and empowered," "where pets experience longer, healthier lives," and "that elevates pet health for our entire community."

3. **The Internal Culture or Standard You Will Uphold** describes the hospital environment required to achieve the vision. Examples might include "through a united, growth-minded, psychologically safe team," "through a culture built on trust, clarity, and accountability," and "through continual learning, collaboration, and medical excellence."

0:45–1:05—Values Brainstorm: "How We Behave"

Say:

"Now, let's define how we behave.

These are our core values—the rules of the game. The non-negotiables. The standards we hold each other to when it's hard. Values might sound like: compassion. Growth. Teamwork. Integrity. Joy. But don't just name them—define them in your words.

If we say teamwork, what does that look like on Tuesday morning when we're down a tech and running behind? If we say excellence, what does that look like at 4:59 p.m. with one more phone call to return?"

These aren't for a poster. These are for how we show up with clients and with each other. Ask yourself: what do we want this hospital to feel like on the best day? And what do we need to protect that?

Do: Ask the following questions and record answers on a whiteboard or flip chart: encourage each person to contribute one word or phrase. Narrow down to four to six core values.

- What do we do that makes this place feel special when we're at our best?
- What behaviors kill trust or morale?
- What would we never compromise on, even if no one was watching?

A value statement includes the:

1. **Value:** Simply, a word or short phrase captures the principle. Examples might include Compassion, Clarity, Integrity, Team First, Lifelong Learning, and Patient Advocacy.
2. **Meaning:** A short sentence describing what *you* mean by that value—specific to your hospital, not generic. Examples might include "We meet every patient and client with empathy, patience, and respect," "We communicate clearly, consistently, and without judgment," and "We do the right thing even when it's inconvenient."
3. **Behavior:** A concrete, observable action the team can actually do. Examples might include, "We slow down to listen before we speak," "We explain medical recommendations in human language," "We support teammates publicly and coach privately," and "We own mistakes quickly and fix them completely."

1:05–1:25—Group Synthesis and Read Back

Say:

"Alright, team. This is where we put it together. Let's read what we've built: our Mission, our Vision, and our Values."

Do: Say and ask the team the following:

- Have a volunteer read the draft Mission, Vision, and Values aloud. Encourage minor tweaks, not full rewrites.
- Ask the team: "Does this sound like us? Does it feel like us? If it feels forced or fluffy, let's keep refining."
- Say: "The goal isn't perfect wording. The goal is ownership. Everyone should see themselves in this."
- Edit as a team as you go, resulting in a near-final draft of the hospital's Mission, Vision, and Values.
- Say: "Okay! That's it right there; that's our story. This is who we are, where we're going, and how we behave. This will become the foundation for how we hire, train, and lead. It's not a poster. It's our promise, to clients and to each other."

1:25–1:30—Next Steps

Say:

"I'm proud of what we just built. You can feel the difference when it's real.

Over the next week, I'll take what we wrote today and clean it up into a first draft. Then I'll bring it back for all of us to review, finalize, and sign off on—literally. Because when you sign something, you're saying, 'I'm in.'

From there, we'll use this in real ways—in our huddles, our hiring, our client communication, and how we hold each other accountable. We'll post them, use them in hiring and onboarding, and celebrate when we see each other living them out. This is how we build the culture we want, together.

This is how you build culture that lasts—not from the top down, but from the inside out.

This right here is how we start turning our mission into momentum."

Designing Your Future Team and Client Experience/ Goal Setting

Total Time: ~60–75 minutes
Goals: Define what an exceptional Team Experience (AX) looks like. Define what an exceptional Client Experience (CX) looks like. Identify three to five Strategic Priorities with owners, metrics, and timelines.
Output: Top three measurable team-experience initiatives. Top three measurable client-trust initiatives, assigned team leads for each goal.
Materials Needed: Flip charts, sticky notes of two different colors, markers, and stickers (e.g., sticker dots) for voting on ideas.

Agenda Overview

Time	Section	Purpose
0:00–0:05	Kickoff: "How We Build from Here"	Reignite purpose; connect Step 2's Mission/Vision/Values to real action.
0:05–1:25	Defining the Team Experience	Let the team surface pain points and design better daily experiences.
1:25–2:30	Defining the Client Experience	Map key "moments that matter" and set client-trust improvement goals.
2:30–2:55	Prioritizing + Assigning Owners	Select three to five Strategic Priorities, define metrics, and assign leaders.
2:55–3:00	Close + Commitments	End with ownership, gratitude, and next-steps clarity.

Facilitator Script and Cues

0:00–0:05 | Kickoff: "How We Build from Here"

Say:

"Alright team, we've got our Mission, Vision, and Values locked in. That's our 'why,' and that's where we're headed.

Now it's time for the how. Let's put the rubber to the road and design the hospital experience we want to live every day, for our team and for our clients.

Here's the deal: if our team dreads walking in the door, no mission statement on earth can save us. And if our clients feel ignored or confused, all the medicine in the world won't matter.

Let's start with us, with our team experience. Because if the team experience isn't right, the client never will be."

0:05–1:25 | Defining the Team Experience

Step 1—Set the Tone (5 minutes)

Say:

"This part might sting a bit, and that's okay. We're not here to complain; we're here to fix stuff.

This is your space to be honest about what it's really like to work here: what fuels you, what drains you, and what would make this hospital the place you can't wait to walk into."

Remind them: There is no blame and no judgment. You're collecting truth, not assigning fault.

Step 2—Surface Pain Points (15 minutes)

Ask questions to identify current pain points and opportunities, such as:

- "What parts of the day make your job harder than it needs to be?"
- "What could we do more consistently to make our jobs easier?"
- "What tasks do you feel are redundant or repeated, or do you feel we could streamline or make easier?"
- "What is one frustration we could solve that would instantly make morale better?"
- "Where do we drop the ball on communication or teamwork?"

Do: Instruct team members to independently and anonymously write answers to these questions on sticky notes (one idea per note). Stick them on a wall or whiteboard. Group similar ideas and review the themes and ideas aloud with the team.

Step 3—Flip Frustrations into Fixes (20 minutes)

Say:

"Alright, now let's focus on solutions. Pick one or two clusters that matter most to you personally, and brainstorm real solutions. No theories. What could we actually do in the next 90 days to make this better?"

Examples you can share to spark thinking:

- Clearer onboarding checklist for new hires
- Monthly "Culture Wins" shout-outs
- Cross-training rotations
- Quick daily five-minute huddles

Do: Instruct team members to independently write solutions to problems on a different colored sticky note. Encourage them to be realistic, and to prioritize fixes that aren't too complicated. Then, have them post their solutions on the wall next to the "problem" sticky notes. Group together similar ideas.

Review the output with the team.

Say something like, "Okay for this problem, here are the different solutions that were proposed."

Step 4—Pick Top Three Team Experience Priorities (15 minutes)

Do: Distribute sticker dots (or whatever you're using to use as votes) out to the team. Every team member gets three dots/votes.

Give the team time to review the ideas on the wall and place stickers on the ideas they feel are the most impactful and important.

Then, circle or highlight the three highest-impact, most realistic fixes. Write them on a flip chart labeled "Team Experience Priorities."

Step 5—Turn Themes into Measurable Goals (25 minutes)

Do: For each "Team Experience Priority," craft a SMART-style goal, that is: Specific, Measurable, Achievable, Relevant, and Time-Bound. For example, "Increase dental treatment compliance from 32 to 45% by September 30 by training all doctors and Client Service Representatives (CSRs) on consistent medical messaging and auditing estimates weekly."

Examples to read aloud:

- "Increase 90-day new-hire retention from 72 to 90% by September 1 by launching a structured onboarding program with a mentor system, weekly check-ins, and a clear 30/60/90-day training roadmap."
- "Reduce the number of missed or unclear intra-team handoffs from an average of 12 per week to fewer than 4 per week within 90 days by adopting a standardized handoff script, training all roles, and auditing compliance twice weekly."

Write each goal clearly on the Client Experience Priorities board.

1:25–2:30 | Defining the Client Experience

Step 1—Frame the Conversation (5 minutes)

Say:

"Next, let's focus on our client experience. Remember that clients don't judge us by our intentions; they judge us by how we make them feel. Especially, are we making them feel welcome and safe? Are we establishing trust?"

Do: If helpful and if time allows, review with the team the content from this book on how clients want to feel (Chapter 16).

Say: "We're going to identify opportunity areas and ideas to improve the client experience across five phases of the client journey: the steps that the typical client will move through as they interact with our hospital. Think about the journey from the client's eyes and call out the moments where you feel we could better build trust or improve the client experience in general."

Step 2—Identify Improvement Opportunities (20 minutes)

Do: On five separate flip charts, write one of the following "Client Journey Phases" atop the flip chart, and hang them on the wall or board.

1. First Contact (Call/Text/Website)
2. Arrival/Lobby Experience
3. Exam Room Interaction
4. Checkout and Follow-up
5. Ongoing Communication

Ask: "For each of these steps along the client journey or experience, where do we lose trust today? Where are we dropping the ball and creating unnecessary stress or discomfort? Or, what are opportunities to improve the client experience at each step, today?"

Do: Give the team time to write improvement ideas on sticky notes, individually. Encourage them to write at least two ideas for each phase/each flip chart. Then, instruct the team to post their sticky notes under each phase on the separate flip charts.

Step 3—Cluster + Prioritize (20 minutes)

Do:

On each flip chart, group ideas/sticky notes into three to four themes (e.g., Communication Clarity, Follow-up Consistency, Transparency with Estimates, and Speed of Response).

Talk the group through the various ideas and themes that emerged for each of the five client journey phases.

Then, just as you did with the prior exercise to prioritize team experience ideas, distribute voting stickers and have each team member prioritize their top three ideas across all five phases (in other words, each team member gets three votes TOTAL, not three per client journey phase).

Step 4—Turn Themes into Measurable Goals (20 minutes)

Do: For each priority, craft a SMART-style goal. Examples to read aloud:

- "100% of clients receive a written treatment plan before services."
- "Every hospitalized pet gets two proactive updates per day."
- "Follow-up calls within 24 hours for all sick visits."

Write each goal clearly on the Client Experience Priorities board.

2:30–2:55 | Prioritizing and Assigning Strategic Owners

Say:

"We've now got our top Team Experience goals and top Client Experience goals.

Let's pick the three to five big rocks that move the needle most in the next three months. These are our Strategic Priorities; the plays we're running right now to bring our Mission and Vision to life."

Do: Encourage discussion and reach alignment from the group on the top three to five ideas the team will prioritize over the next three months. Make sure you have at least one Team Experience goal and at least one Client Experience goal (and ideally, more than one of each).

Say: "Now let's turn priorities into leadership opportunities. Each goal gets an owner, someone who'll coordinate progress, track results, and share updates at staff meetings."

Do: Encourage rising voices: techs, CSRs, assistants, associate doctors; not just management.

Write the final list on a clean flip chart with these columns:
Goal | Owner | Metric | Timeline | First Check-In Date

Example entry:
| Follow-Up Calls for 90% of Sick Visits within 24 hours | Taylor (RVT) | 90% within 24 hours | End of May | March 15 |

2:55–3:00 | Close + Commitments

Say:

"This is the moment we stop talking about culture and start building it.

What we just did isn't fluff. It's the blueprint for a hospital people love working in and clients love visiting.

Over the next week, we'll post these goals in the breakroom. We'll celebrate wins in every staff meeting.

And we'll revisit it every quarter to add new wins, new leaders, and new energy."

"Thank you for being real today. This is how trust gets built: by doing the work together."

Appendix B:

How to Lead Your Veterinary Hospital as a Servant Leader (The Tangible Blueprint)

This is the practical, real-world playbook you can start tomorrow morning to build a high-trust, psychologically safe hospital where people don't just perform—they thrive.

Say the Mission, Vision, and Values Out Loud, Every Week

Psychological safety begins with shared meaning. When people understand the "why," they feel anchored. When they feel anchored, they take risks. Every meeting, every decision, every conflict should tie back to your Mission, Vision, and Values.

Repetition turns values into identity—and identity into safety.

Do a Fairness Audit

Nothing kills psychological safety faster than perceived unfairness. Ask yourself:

- Are people corrected consistently?
- Are troublemakers allowed to slide because they produce revenue?
- Are workloads inequitable?
- Do some people receive coaching while others receive criticism?

If fairness isn't felt, safety isn't real.

Hold Weekly 1:1s Focused on Growth, Not Discipline

Psychological safety grows in conversations where people feel seen and supported. Your weekly 1:1 is where you make space for:

- their voice
- their concerns
- their ideas
- their frustrations
- their goals

Ask: *"What's one thing that's making your job harder than it needs to be?"*
Then fix it. That's servant leadership in action.

Remove One Obstacle Per Week

Psychological safety grows when people see that speaking up leads to change.
Pick one operational friction point—anything—and fix it. Every single week.

This is how your team learns: *"It's safe to tell the truth here. My leader actually listens."*

Give 3x More Praise Than Critique

Psychological safety thrives when positive behaviors are noticed publicly and consistently. Praise is not fluff—it's reinforcement. It signals:

"Doing things right is recognized here."
"I'm not invisible."
"I'm not only noticed when I mess up."

This opens the door for harder conversations later, delivered in trust.

Address Problems Within 48 Hours

Safety requires certainty. When leaders avoid conflict, the message becomes:

- "Bad behavior is tolerated."
- "Speaking up doesn't matter."
- "This environment is unpredictable."

Address issues early, privately, and respectfully. Teach people they don't have to fear correction—they can trust it.

Delegate Decisions That Don't Need Your Signature

Psychological safety expands when people feel ownership. Let techs own inventory. Let CSRs own callbacks. Let assistants own room flow. Let the team decide small things without you.

Delegation isn't dumping. Delegation is trust-building.

Build Playbooks, Not Dependency

Psychological safety skyrockets when everyone knows: "This is how we do it here."

Create and maintain:

- standardized medical pathways
- communication scripts
- conflict frameworks
- recheck protocols
- client education guides

When the rules are clear, people stop fearing mistakes—and start executing confidently.

Make Advocacy the Norm, Not the Gamble

Psychological safety fuels medical advocacy. Teams speak courageously when they don't fear judgment, backlash, or being contradicted publicly. Train your team to advocate consistently, and protect them when they do.

If you defend your people, they'll defend your patients.

Be the Calmest Person in the Building

Psychological safety is emotional. Teams absorb your nervous system. If you're erratic, they're scared. If you're steady, they breathe easier.

Your presence is the thermostat. Your composure is the culture. Your calm is their safety.

Index